MONT ☑ **W9-COW-231**
ROCKVILLE CAMPUS LIBRARY
ROCKVILLE, MARYLAND

MULTICULTURAL BIOMEDICAL ETHICS AND GLOBAL BIOSOPHICAL MORAL LOGIC

Suzan S. Parhizgar, Ph.D.

and

Kamal Dean Parhizgar, Ph.D.

University Press of America,® Inc.
Lanham · Boulder · New York · Toronto · Plymouth, UK

9 o 8 44 9

AUG 0 5 2009.

Copyright © 2008 by
University Press of America®, Inc.
4501 Forbes Boulevard
Suite 200
Lanham, Maryland 20706
UPA Acquisitions Department (301) 459-3366

Estover Road
Plymouth PL6 7PY
United Kingdom

All rights reserved
Printed in the United States of America
British Library Cataloging in Publication Information Available

Library of Congress Control Number: 2007942935
ISBN-13: 978-0-7618-3998-9 (paperback : alk. paper)
ISBN-10: 0-7618-3998-4 (paperback : alk. paper)

™ The paper used in this publication meets the minimum requirements of American National Standard for Information Sciences—Permanence of Paper for Printed Library Materials, ANSI Z39.48—1984

To Parhizgar Family Members: Ozra Mitra Esfandiari,
Robert R. Parhizgar, and Fuzhan F. Parhizgar
with whom we have a very happy life.

We have written the book of
Multicultural Biomedical Ethics and Global Biosophical Moral Logic;
So we care about humanity and humaneness in the book above.

You can forget our names or remember them as you wish;
So we will be remembered by the book of
Multicultural Biomedical Ethics and Global Biosophical Moral Logic.

Suzan S. Parhizgar and Kamal Dean Parhizgar

TABLE OF CONTENTS

CHAPTER 8:   MELIORISTIC GLOBAL BIOETHICS OF HUMAN SUBJECT IN BIORESEARCH.................277

CCHAPTER 9: BIOETHICAL DIMENSIONS OF ORGAN AND BODY MATERIAL TRANSPLANTATION...309

INTRODUCTION

This book stems from the confluence of two subjects that have been integrated into a unified one: multicultural biomedical ethics as a foundation for institutionalizing scientific valuable systems and the cause and effect of rational reasoning as an application of biosophical moral logic. Bioemedical ethics has been fortunate in being able to integrate intellectual thoughts in the areas of phenomenology, hermeneutics, and the philosophies of casuistry, as well as ethical and moral based approaches in universal rights, natural rights, human rights, and civil rights. The ability of biomedical ethics to absorb such powerfully integrated divergent fields of inquiry is based upon its indicative of the breadth of this topic and the increasing sensitivity to its sophistication.

Historically, there are critical questions such as: How much attention or vigilance should we devote to our bioscientific deliberations in the effort to maximize observation of universal rights, natural rights, human rights, and civil rights in bioresearch? How much control should we allow biotechno scientists to have over our DNA, genes, and other body materials? To what extent should we supervise our efforts to improve our life longevity? To what extending limit should we promote sick care, well care, and total quality care and remove causes and effects of suffering and pain among human beings? Yet if these and other similar questions are virtually included in the mainstream of biomedical ethics, we should strive to avoid abusing and exploiting our thoughts and actions. If our biosophical analogies are so strong then why shouldn't our contemporary biotechno scientists and bioresearchers be promoted? Therefore, we should not deceive ourselves in our progressive scientific technological obsession and ignore the fact of natural imperfect living conditions on earth.

Philosophers such as Plato, Francis Bacon, Rene Descartes, Jean Lamarck, and Charles Darwin looked at the pragmatic biosophy of life actualization. Nevertheless, since relief from suffering and pain and the expansion of satisfactory choices are laudable objectives of having a happy life, there should be a trend in determining what kind of happiness should be promoted and what types of choices are best to be pursued. There is a dual argument that calls for enhancing human genes and eliminating harmful ones. Within such a complex domain of argument, it strikes us that bioethics is not only an academic pursuit but it is also a pragmatic social movement in which theosophists, biosophists, philosophers, and ethicists are, in a literal sense, searching to answer to the validity of the principles of bioethical and biomedical solutions.

What is more? It is the comparative analysis of biosophy and biophilia in our arguments concerning socio-cultural and politico-economic considerations. This book explores the historical multicultural roots and socio-economic ramifications of bioethics as a pivotal phenomenon of lifetime human integrity. If you turn on major global broadcasts like CNN, CBS, NBC, and Fox, and if you have satellite and/or Internet connections, and if you read newspapers, magazines, and professional journal articles or analyze your daily social life, you will find events, crises, or problems related to biomedical activities. Through your personal moral and global ethical convictions, you quickly question: Who is at fault? Who is fair or unfair? Who is just or unjust? Who is liable and should pay damages? Who acted responsibly? Who did not? Then you wonder: Are these issues and problems inherent in the nature of human beings, or are they holistic by-products of socio-cultural and politico-economical beliefs and desires of interest groups among nations?

Multicultural biomedical ethics is an invisible aspect of biosciences and biotechnologies. It intersects between an individual's desire and group interests and raises a special curiosity in the minds of scientists, technologists, professional medical clinicians, and the biopharmaceutical industry around the world. The magnitude of competitive academic enterprise makes it imperative that bioscientists and biotechnologists have developed multicultural codes of ethics, codes of moral behavior, and codes of legal conduct in order to deal with today's global cultural diversity.

The diverse cultural and religious needs among nations and the universal integrity of academia must be viewed as a reality in bioresearch. Multicultural biomedical ethics is a positive phenomenon, associated with accelerated novelty and the creation of global integrity and honesty. It stands alone in its concern with contentious problems such as political ideologies, ethnicity, race, gender, color, and religious faiths. In our ecological environments, the most problematic issue is the friction generated by nations and their industrial operational functions along with the consideration and integration of different cultural values and perceptions.

In the Twentieth century, we witnessed how ignorance, fanaticism, prejudice, inhumanness, and atrocity mingled with religious cultural egoism and political racism, and how they ignored the spiritual dimension of humanity and the integrity of the human species. Understanding *Multicultural Biomedical Ethics and Global Biosophical Moral Logic* is crucial to every scientist who belongs to and leads within an academic center. In recognition of the development and rapidly growing importance of international relations and the need to educate future professional experts, bioethics mandates colleges and universities to examine various approaches and arguments concerning bioethical and biomoral conclusions.

Multicultural Biomedical Ethics and Global Biosophical Moral Logic is a sort of imaginative coverage of multi-moral, ethical, and legal cultural differences and similarities for future use by students in the fields of biology, medicine, pharmacology, health care, and the biopharmaceutical industry. The similarities and differences in the various approaches to bioethics among nations lead us to an unavoidable conclusion: The moral dimensions of human existence cannot be captured by a single culture. The multiethical approaches and views to biosciences that we explore in this book are different paths to a common ground of the interpretation of humanity. Each cultural view in its own term and trend suggests that, although principlism is valuable, it also has conclusive means and ends in each sociocultural and politico-economic endeavor. Topics in this text are presented in a smooth and logical fashion.

The authors' intention was to establish, as powerfully as possible, a frame of reference that expressed this judgment and method of study, which was appropriate to multicultural biomedical ethics. Several bioethics texts are available to the community of scholars. This book was written not only to be useful for practicing international bioethics, but also to be used for understanding and appreciating similar and different ethical and moral values among nations.

Suzan S. Parhiagar, Ph.D.
Texas Tech University

Kamal Dean Parhizgar, Ph.D.
Texas A&M International University

ACKNOWLEDGMENTS

We sincerely thank, first and foremost, Dr. Peter J. Syapin and Dr. Kathryn K. McMahon, Professors of the Department of Pharmacology and Neuroscience at Texas Tech University Health Sciences Center who professionally advised and mentored our academic mission. We want to express our appreciation to the above professors for creating environments in which ideas are encouraged and supported.

We are pleased to express our sincere appreciation to those people who deserve to be valued as professors and advisors that professionally and sincerely contributed their knowledge and shared their experiences with students. Each in their own unique way has taught students something that was new and several made useful academic contributions that have improved intellectual abilities of the community of scholars. We want to identify some individuals who have been especially helpful in the long and arduous process of our academic journey. Particularly, we want to thank the following professors at Texas Tech University Health Sciences Center: Dr. Reid N. Norman, Professor and Chair, Department of Pharmacology and Neuroscience; Dr. Michael P. Blanton; Dr. Barry Lombardini; Dr. Thomas E. Tenner, Jr.; Dr. Arthur S. Freeman; Dr. Ali Roghani; Dr. Lisa Popp; Dr. Richard L. Dickerson; Dr. Lynn T. Frame, and Dr. Barbara C. Pence.

Several colleagues have substantially supported the final product of this text. We want to thank the following scholars at Texas A&M International University: Dr. Ray M. Keck, President; Dr. Dan Jones, Provost and Vice-President for Academic Affairs at Texas A&M International University.

Special thanks to Dr. Bernell K. Dalley, Associate Dean of the Texas Tech University School of Medicine; Professor Kitten S. Linton, M.D., Professor of Clinical Family Medicine, Texas Tech University School of Medicine; Dr. Manoucher Mohseni Parsa, Professor of Industrial Sociology, University of Teheran, Iran and Ms. Kathleen Flacy, Ph.D. student at Texas A&M University, College Station for their supports.

Particularly, we thank Ms. Patti Belcher, Acquisition Editor, University Press of America Inc., and Mr. Brian DeRocco, Editorial Administration, University Press of America Inc. We must also appreciate the staff at the University Press of America, Inc.

Finally, without help of our family members this textbook could never have been completed. Thanks to our family members Mrs. Ozra M. Esfandiari Parhizgar, Fuzhan F. Parhizgar, and Robert R. Parhizgar who encouraged and supported us to complete such an important textbook.

Suzan S. Parhizgar, Ph.D. Post-Doctoral
Associate Researcher, Texas Tech Medical School

Kamal Dean Parhizgar, Ph.D.
Professor of Management and Business Ethics

CHAPTER 1

AN OVERVIEW: MULTICULTURAL BIOMEDICAL ETHICS AND GLOBAL BIOSOPHICAL LOGIC

When a business is lost, something is lost;

When liberty is lost, democracy is lost;

When the judiciary system is lost, justice is lost;

When a personality is lost, reputation is lost;

When morality is lost, dignity is lost;

When ethics is lost, integrity is lost;

When honesty is lost, faith is lost;

When decency is lost, humanity is lost;

When honor is lost, all is lost.

Kamal Dean Parhizgar and Robert R. Parhizgar (2006)

CHAPTER OBJECTIVES

When you have read this chapter you should be able to do the following:

- Develop conceptual skills to integrate human dynamic innovations.
- Indicate why bioethics in diverse cultures is an essential phenomenon.
- Understand the increased role of the level of biotechnology through bioscientific synergy and prodigy.
- Develop a framework of analysis to enable a student to discuss how bioscientific advances and biotechnological breakthroughs will change human nature.
- Develop an understanding of the scope of biotechnological innovation and how it differs from the natural somatic structures.
- Develop an ability to analyze and evaluate qualitative bioethical value systems for the future of human race.

PLAN OF THIS CHAPTER

Our objectives in this chapter are to present an account of morality and ethicality that is systematic, accessible, and usable in bioscientific and biotechnological endeavors. One of the objectives of this chapter is to introduce the ethical and moral perspectives of biosciences and biotechnologies. These common core concepts will be explicated and grounded for the common benefit of the human race. Making scientific and technological progress is still the only way a branch of academic discipline can survive. However, the well being of the human race, the integrating of the natural environment, and the purity of psychosomatic factors of humanity should be the major concerns of the strategic objective

Another objective of this chapter is to provide the theoretical and pragmatic knowledge needed in today's research and development in the fields of biosciences and biotechnology within the ethical and moral context of humanity. In addition, in this opening chapter, we will introduce many issues that from the standpoint of our bioethical considerations are vital for the present and future of the human species. We start with an opening discussion on the legitimacy of the changing bioethical perspectives of the biosciences, biomedicine, and biotechnology.

THE BASIS OF BIOMEDICAL ETHICS

From ancient times, biologists, biophysicists, biochemists, and biotechnologists believed that the wellbeing of humanity depended upon the moral right of having pragmatic freedom in bioresearch in order to discover the truth, to uphold the truth, to complete the truth, and to pursue the application of the truth. Scientific research issues, and more specifically experimental research activities in the fields of biosciences, biotechnology, and biomedical practices have become the controversial socio-political debate that exerts an impact on bioethical analysis. Not everyone is happy with the current state of bioethics, and much of the discontent is focused on the questions of methodology. Meilaender (1995: 2) echoed this concern:

> From where should bioethics take its direction? From within the practice of medicine itself, or from more general moral norms applied to medicine? Do we need a moral theory to guide our bioethical reflection, or can we make our way from case to case, gradually mapping the territory? Are the most common bioethical approaches focused too much on the language of rights, able to offer only a thin and minimal ethics that gives little real wisdom about how to ought to live and die?

In reality, responding to these and other similar questions we need to pay special attention to a general territory of bioethics. We should indicate that bioethics is not only to be concerned about pragmatic ethics in the field of medicine; but also that it covers bio-techno-scientific research and biosocial concerns.

Bioethical debates on human, animal, and plant genetics have been the subject areas in research and development in the past centuries. Historically, each generation of bioscientists, biotechnologists, and biomedical practitioners including physicians have been confronted by critical issues in positioning from cautious approval, to wait-and-see attitudes, and/or complete rejection and condemnation of the progressive paths of bio-techno-scientific efforts.

There are several critical issues and debates concerning genetic testing, predictive gene diagnosis, treatment, and prognosis, somatic cell gene therapy, germ-line gene intervention, organ transplantation, genetic innovation and engineering, genetic information, embryonic research, cloning humans and animals, and diverting the natural evolutionary path of human species into a new global biohierarchy of the human species. Also, the completions of sequencing of the genomic DNA, genomic manipulation, genomic alteration, genomic development and innovation of the eugenics of hierarchical society have attracted the attention of bioethicists.

In viewing the present and future holistic lifestyle of human beings, bio-techno-scientific research will no longer be able to stand apart as an independent form of discipline in inquiring and discovering novel possibilities for a better understanding of the mystery of life. In the past, politicians, biotechnologists, and biopharmaceutical ventures tried to separate bio-techno-scientific research from cultural values, ethical beliefs, moral philosophies, and religious faiths. They tried to limit bio-techno-scientific research within a closed system of inquiry in laboratories. Most sociologists, anthropologists, psychologists, ethicists, and theologians have been left out the picture of bioresearch. Yet never, before now, has bio-techno-scientific experimentation been such an important part of our daily life. Today, as never before, bio-techno-scientific experimental efforts have become the object of morality, ethicality, and legality. We will thus, from the viewpoint of bioethicists, analyze the debates over the tension between freedom of research, on one hand and protection of human rights, on the other. Such a cross-firing line of debate will eventually lead us to ethical, moral, and legal mandates to establish a doctrine to guide bio-techno-scientists to holistically focus and pursue their research activities.

Bio-techno-scientific research will no longer be separated from socio-political and commercial activities. There will be a time for future generations to formulate strategic public policy and regulate bio-techno-scientific options to be made by democratic choices. There will be a time in which humanity will integrate the bio-techno-scientific objectives within the conceptual scope of the general public demand, religious fervor, and bioethical views.

THE HOLARCHY OF GLOBAL BIOETHICS

Biosophy (a biosystem of thought) and/or biophilia (a thoughtful tendency towards life) are the holarchic bedrocks of bioethics. They are the holistic global innate sympathetic affinity for the sanctity of life and the beauty of the synergistic natural and artificial world in which we live. Such globally incorporated visionary thoughts encompass global bioethics to integrate human life and the nonhuman realms of life. Bioethicists and biosophers bridge various spheres of concern and contemporary environmental issues into a cohesive whole picture of global legitimate reasoning. Global bioethics brings together ethical principles back to life. Our brand new thoughts of biosophy and biophilia appreciate and promote a sacred unity, integrity, and interdependence of natural life. Thus, with such a metaphysical aspiration, global bioethics bridges the spiritual and the material, the religious and the secular, and the academia and the public into meaningful perceptual lives. A holarchic integration of biosophical and biospiritual bases for the enlightened sustainable life can create harmony and respect for all creatures and creation.

The holarchic biosophical and biophilia of bio-techno-scientific thoughts and practices integrate respect for autonomy, beneficence, non-malfeasance, and justice in bioresearch. People apply this holarchic integrated value system to avoid inhumane treatment of human subjects. The holarchic integrated biosophy and biophilia articulate ethical theories such as causalism, consequentialism, institutionalism, and contractualism to evade the chaos of conflicting bioethical judgments. We need to take into consideration how bionic life can maintain the sanctity of humans, animals, plants, and ecosystems in a harmonious endeavor. In practical terms it means providing appropriate natural rights for humans, rabbits, plants, butterflies, ants, and bees for the natural fullness of their being.

Bioethical principles and biomoral convictions require human beings to avoid harming themselves and our ecosystem. Our bio-techno-scientific power must be tempered by the higher power of humanity and compassion, not by atrocity and thoughtlessness. These powers are expressed in the biosophical principles of life ethics. *Ahimsa* in Indian culture is the doctrine of avoiding harm to other sentient beings. It is cardinal to sacred living in accord with life ethics. It is tasteless and shameful for violence (*hisma*) to intrude in human affairs, as whenever there is a conflict of opinions and ideas to use biological weapons and biochemical warfare, including radioactive poisoning, tear gas, and pepper spray, to suppress free ideas and free speech. Furthermore, global bioethics is inclined neither to political ideologies nor to religious faiths. It is inclined to life for the present and future generations. It is a holistic philosophy to integrate all ages and generations in the realm of nature. Biosophy and biophilia can be defined as the clarification of bioconcepts, analysis and structural arguments concerning enriched life, the weighing of alternative life values, and advising of a preferable course of bio-techno-scientific action towards excellence.

The central contribution of bioethics is based upon its independent valuable systems of thoughts. By valuable systems of thoughts we mean that bioethics provides the biosophical topography of arguments, objectives, options, and justifications to value and enhance human life. The fundamental ethos of holarchic biosophy and biophilia in bio-techno-scientific research and bionic innovativeness lie in analyzing intellectual strategic frameworks, prodigical techno-scientific methodologies, bioinformational data, languages, programs, and knowledge to institutionalize the validation of human life. The holarchy of bioethics argues the validity of problematic situations in which some causes-effects of bioresearch trial and error will condone the situation, and others will condemn it.

By religious faith all elements in the kingdom of God and/or in nature (in an existential belief) have specific purposes and missions. Nature is not anarchy. Nature includes different elements with different missions to achieve a specific objective. Those objectives are *life, life processes, life cycles* and continuity or discontinuity of *species*. All elements support holistic symbiotic relationships in coexistence. All material objects and spiritual elements in living things observe the inherent rule of symbiosis. Humanity and nature are highly interdependent and interconnected. When one is harmed, so is the other. The famous Persian poet Moslehed Dean Saadi, (1184-1291 A.D.) who is a philosopher, writer, poet, and biosophist with his biophilia idea said:

> *The Children of Adam are limbs of one another,*
> *Created from one essence, each from the order,*
> *When life's calamities to one cause pain,*
> *The other limbs cannot in rest remain*
> (From Flower Garden, *Gulestan*).

Within the biosophy of bioethics there is no hierarchy for all material elements, because the existence and functions of each is highly related to the others. Violating the holarchy or circle of life interrupts continuity of human survival. In the absence of global bioethics, the deterioration of environmental elements and abuses of human rights adversely affect sanctity and purity of human integrity, which deteriorates the level of morality in present and future generations (see Figure 1.1).

Global bioethics is not only concerned with the present and future human generations, but it is also concerned with other biological elements including animals, plants, and ecosystem. We need to find appropriate, innovative ways to fulfill our sincere causes and avoid coetaneous evil and harm to ourselves and to this planet. Multicultural bioethics and global moral reasoning will help human beings to integrate the human mind with nature and prevents us being inhumane. In the state of biosophy, bioethics plays an important role as bridge between humans, animals, and nature. To be an intellectually oriented creature, observation of the epitome of honesty, humaneness, humus (soil), humility, and harmony (5Hs) is a must.

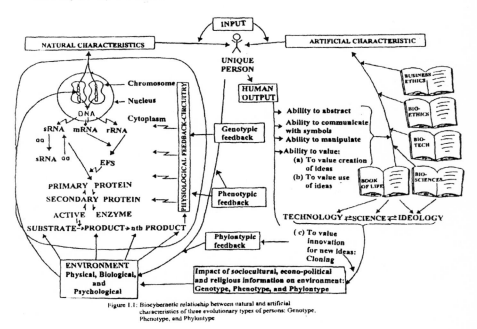

Figure 1.1: Biocybernetic relatioship between natural and artificial characteristics of three evolutionary types of persons: Genotype, Phenotype, and Phylontype

Poter and Poter (1995: 185) stated:

> Enlightened anthropocentrism calls for control of human fertility and sees the human species in the context of the total biosphere... We need a global bioethics that will guide good intentions and harness the will to power. Global bioethics calls for good intentions and harness the will to power. Global bioethics calls for good intentions that are covered by five realistic virtues: humility, responsibility, interdisciplinary competence, intercultural competence, and compassion.

The revival of humaneness and the survival of the human species are not only related to the pursuit of economic well being, but it is also related to the biosophy of global bioethics.

BIO-TECHNO-SCIENTIFIC RESEARCH AND BIOETHICS

Discussions on bio-techno-scientific research and bioethics frequently have emphasized refractory and unclear situations, perhaps to show drama and novelty. Denying the rights of an individual or a group of experts to freely pursue research has been considered unethical and illegal in most, though not all, parts of the world. This general misunderstanding stems from the Mosaic Law, the Code of Hammurabi, Roman law, and other sources, and is part of a general ethics favoring truth going back at least 3,000 years (Steiner and Steiner, 2003: 199).

Overall, ethical and moral traditions that apply to bioethics support the protection of human life, respect for rights, concentrate on the goodness of mankind, and respect the sanctity of religious faiths. In bio-techno-scientific endeavor, lying, deception, and negligence are condemned. According to Bailar III (1993: 104) some scientific practices may distort scientific inferences (see Table 1.1).

Table 1.1: Some Bio-Scientific Practices That Distort Scientific Inferences

<ul><li>Failure to deal honestly with readers about non-random error (bias).</li><li>*Post hoc* hypothesis.</li><li>Multiple comparisons and data dredging.</li><li>Inappropriate statistical tests and other statistical procedures.</li><li>Fragmentation of reports.</li><li>Low statistical power.</li><li>Suppressing, trimming, or adjusting data; or undisclosed repetition of unsatisfactory results.</li><li>Selective reporting of findings.</li></ul>
Source: Baillar III, J. C. (1993). "Science, Statistics, and Deception." In R. E. Bulger, E. Heitman, and S. J. Reiser, (Eds.). *The Ethical Dimensions of the Biological Sciences.* Cambridge: Cambridge University Press, 104.

Deliberate ignorance, carelessness, and greed end up with catastrophes. Honesty is the main characteristic of scientists because they claim that they are enlightened intellectuals. Bio-techno-scientists are dealing with the life and death of people through application of scientific methods to diagnose sicknesses and illnesses. For example, a deceptive research finding is the statistical testing of *post hoc* hypotheses. It is widely recognized that *t*-test, chi-square tests, and other statistical tests provide a basis for probability statements only when the hypothesis is fully developed before the data are examined in any way. Statistical tests are also sometimes used in non-probability cases as rough measures of the size of an effect, rather than to test hypotheses. Bio-techno-scientists apply experimental data to draw conclusions or make deductions from imperfect data to formulate their scientific hypotheses to cure patients. The effectiveness and/or side effects of any drug depend on the viability and reliability of bio-techno-scientists' and bioresearchers' truthful statements of their experiments. Biopharmaceutical companies rely on bioresearhers' scientific experimental statements. Nevertheless, if bio-techno-scientists and bioresearchers neglect their academic professional integrity, they jeopardize human lives.

Different nations have expressed their reactions to bioscientific and biotechnological research differently. In the Central America, Jehovah's Witnesses are against blood transfusions, as they are considered morally obscene. In the country of geographical areas between Burma and Laos, Jains banned the killing of mosquitoes on moral grounds; despite the fact that the region suffers from one of the highest rates of malaria in the world.

From another point of view, bioscientists have long been fascinated by the ability of other species to regrow damaged body parts. Worms can repair themselves almost entirely; lizards can reproduce a tail, and even opossums; if enough can replace a limb. Why can't humans? If bioresearchers can unravel this mystery, they may discover a biological foundation of youth. If they succeed, medicine will enter a new era. Brain-damaged by Alzheimer's or Parkinson's disease could be regenerated to normal. Embryos have this ability because they are essentially clusters of stem cells. A developed cell produces, on average, about 50 copies of itself before dying (Griffith, 2001: 11). Most European countries and the United States are ethically and morally opposed the usage of embryos for stem cell research and have banned it. Of course there are three major types of stem cells: embryonic, fetal, and adult stem cells. In Spain, the government ordered Bernat Soria, head of the Bioengineering Institute at Miguel Hernandez University in Alicante, to halt his work, after it was discovered he had obtained embryonic stem cells from Israel. For the first time in 2001 bioscientists from the biotechnology company, Advanced Cell Technology reported their first, crude attempts to clone human cells. Essentially they took DNA from human skin, placed it inside human eggs from which the chromosomes had been removed, and coaxed the resulting cells to divide a couple of times. The U.S. House of Representatives has passed a bill outlawing the cloning of human cells for medical purposes. Consequently, the U.S. Senate ratified the same bill and legislated a penalty for violators to earn a person ten years in jail and a $1 million fine. Switzerland has held a national referendum on the possibility of banning all transgenetic research. Most of the above nations banned biotechnologies for questionable moral reasoning (Barlow, 2001: 11).

From a utilitarian standpoint, the decision to test drugs voluntarily on a human being might be an acceptable ethical decision for a medical viewpoint, because presumably a majority of a population would benefit from that experimentation. In recent years, a growing concern has emerged over abusive practices in applied biosciences at all levels of expertise including individual bioscientists, bioindustries, and bioresearch institutions. Such animosity is the result of an axiomatic system that works by reduction of human rights and which consequently cannot be sensitive to different cultures and practices. We may agree with much of the criticism, but we may not agree with doing nothing for the welfare of human race. For an adequate account of morality and ethics we need to know how to appreciate and be inspired by goodness and avoid badness. We must recognize a close collaboration between governments and academicians in order to sufficiently observe our moral and ethical obligations in such a complex and implicated subject matter.

Any civilized society possesses a highly systematic system of checks and balances. Some biochemical, biophysics, biotechnological, and pharmaceutical products and services are not produced under free market conditions, and governments act to supply them. In this category there are clean air, clean water, toxic waste disposal, eugenic technologies and biochemical and biogerm weapons. Other goods and services might be exploited in free market conditions, and if they are important, the government regulates their research and development (R&D) and their use. This concern has always been a cause for federal regulation. Unethical and immoral actions of some bioscientists, bioindustries, and on some occasion's covert governmental biochemical and biogerm weapons programs are, of course, reasons for acute concern about global regulations.

Over 200 years ago, the Founding Fathers of the United States of America established a constitutional system of government that had two major purposes. First, it established a government with powers to act in order to safeguard citizens' rights and national independence. Second, it attempted to prevent the tyranny of a minority of elite power-holders over a majority or *vice versa*. Within the contextual boundaries of the American constitution, the Founding Fathers created a system that morally and ethically dispersed political power and decision-making authority among the various branches of government. The underlying principle behind such a system was that it would lead to a system of checks and balances. Such a system is based upon the assumption that other branches of government and/or classes of people would check an attempt to prevent too much power or abuse its powers. James Madison (1962: 320), one of the most influential delegates at the Constitutional Convention, brilliantly argued in *The Federalist Papers* (No. 51), "Ambition must be made to counteract ambition."

EMERGENCE OF BIOSCIENTIFIC DISCOVERIES

The Nineteenth century biology of Darwin's formulation of the theory of organic evolution and Mendel's statement of the laws of transmission genetics, and the Twentieth century's outstanding accomplishments of understanding molecular structures and processes and genetic inheritance are the three great achievements that have given rise to the considerable complexity of moral and ethical issues. Biotechnology is sometimes used to refer to technologies with long histories, such as brewing and animal breeding, which do not involve direct manipulation of genetic materials. In the late Nineteenth and early Twentieth centuries, bioscientists and medical researchers began to integrate basic and pure sciences such as chemistry, physics, mathematics, and statistics into their research projects. In the 1860s, George Mendel, abbot of the Augustinian monastery of Brno in Austria, mathematically calculated the inherited characteristics of pea plants that he bred in his monastery garden (Olby, 1966). A century later, in 1953 James Watson and Francis H. Crick in 1953 discovered the molecular structure of nucleic acids. They described the deoxyribonucleic acid molecule (DNA), a fragment of matter hidden in the nucleus of almost all animal cells, as "two helical chains each coiled around the same axis," (Watson and Crick, 1953: 737). There is no entity in the known universe that stores and processes information more efficiently than the DNA molecule. Furthermore, the cellular basis of physiology and pathology and the germ theory of disease required scientists to use technological instruments such as the stethoscope and thermometer.

Among other scientific discoveries, penicillin was discovered in 1928 and first applied clinically during Word War I. Penicillin was produced synthetically, making this rare drug available to treat patients with pneumonia and other serious infections. In 1946, streptomycin began to be given on a wide scale to patients with tuberculosis, closing hundreds of sanatoriums. In 1947, the drug methotrexate was first used to treat acute leukemia, initiating the era of cancer chemotherapy. In 1949, poliovirus was cultivated in human tissue, making possible the development of the polio vaccines that were introduced in the mid 1950s, and lithium was administered to patients with manic disease. In 1952, antihypertensive drugs were discovered. Also, in 1952 chlorpromazine became available for agitated schizophrenia and the first open heart surgery was performed (Jonsen, 1998:12). These are but some of the other numerous medical discoveries, including treatments and surgical procedures, developed within the past century.

These and other issues can cause ethical and moral resentments among people, culture to culture. People are aware of the late "messiness of the everyday world" in political-legal, socio-cultural, economical, and ethical issues related to gene and cloning technologies. Unlike Dolly, the first cloned ewe, and Gene, the first cloned calf; increasingly animals cloned are transgenic; programmed with another species' gene, making them valuable economic machinery. Animal cloning is developing as a commercial means of bringing products, such as drugs, to the market (Bowe, 1999: 6). However, the alarming trend manifests unknown and unpredictable consequential results over generations. If we review the historical progressive trends of biosciences and biotechnologies, we can discover a mixture of ethical feelings concerning all innovations. For example, in their genetic engineering project for many years, bioscientists and biotechnologists at the University of Illinois gave two genes, a cow gene and a synthetic one, to cows in hopes of increasing the mother's milk production and her piglets' ability to digest milk so they would grow faster. In 2001, researchers at the University of Illinois reported to the FDA authorities those pigs that multiple tests showed were not transgenic. However, in 2003, the FDA discovered that the University of Illinois had sent 386 of the animals to a livestock dealer who in turn may have sent them to be slaughtered rather than to be destroyed. Such an unethical decision may cause contamination of the food industry and cause side-effects on human beings, when as in the Twentieth century British bioscientists experimented with the "meat and bone meal (MBM)" for livestock and caused the emergence of Mad Cow disease among livestock and the Creutzfeldt-Jacob Disease (nvCJD) among human beings (*CNN*, 2003).

Parallel to all the above bioscientific discoveries, other ethical and unethical incidents happened during the Twentieth century. In the 1960s, Dr. Christian Barnard, a South African surgeon, conducted the first heart implant surgery. In such a revolutionary scientific era, scientific medicine was transformed into medical technology. In 1952, the external cardiac pacemaker was applied for cardiac arrhythmia and its implantable transistorized form appeared eight years later. Later on, a human valve was replaced for the first time. External cardiac stimulation reversed acute myocardial infarction. In 1958, the electrical defibrillator was introduced and Fulkl cardiopulmonary resuscitation was introduced. Cardiac catheterization allowed visualization of heart disease. In 1962, hemodialysis was initiated and secrets of metabolism were discovered. Later on, in the endocrine system, the mechanisms of immunity and wound healing were discovered, and in the biology of reproduction, the secrets of the genetic code were revealed (Jonsen, 1998: 12).

Back in 1970, Robert White and his colleagues of the Case Western Reserve University School of Medicine in Cleveland did with rhesus monkeys. The creatures lived for as long as eight days; fully conscious and with complete cranial nerve function as measured by wakefulness, aggressiveness, and ability to eat and to follow movements in the room with their eyes. White indicates: "I'm a brain surgeon. I believe almost all our organs will be mechanical; or we'll be able to replace them using genetic techniques. It seems to me that what is implied here is that the physical repository of the sole is really the brain." He concluded that there are no qualms about the prospect of attaching a living human head to a living, but brain-dead, donor body. It is much easier for the foreseeable future to transfer the wet ware still connected to its original input devices and snug in its handy carrying case. White also believes:

> If you and I are willing to agree that when brain death occurs you're no
> longer alive, or I like the other side of the coin: if everything else has been
> replaced   and   the   brain   is   still   there,   you're   alive,   then   brain
> transplantation, or body transplantation, depending on your perspective,
> should be no problem (Weber 2000: 16).

Research   indicates   that   hearts,   lungs,   livers,   kidneys,   and   pancreas   are
regularly transplanted, but there is a paucity of donor organs and rejection rates
are high. After a transplant, almost one in three livers, one in three lungs, one in
four pancreas, one in five hearts, and one in six kidneys will fail before a year is
out. But mechanical or bioprosthetic limbs substitute that will not trigger the
immune response are well along in the research pipeline. In one mode, cells
derived from either a human or pig organs are enclosed in a tube or a membrane
through which the patient's blood is circulated. More promising still are the neo-
organs researchers are growing in laboratories or in patients from human stem
cells (Weber, 2000: 19).

From another point of view, Darwin's natural selection binds life to the
conditions of existence. It binds humanity to the conditions of life, and binds the
mind's affinity to the conversion of the individual's mind into the kinesthetic life.
It   is   asserted   that   Darwin's   use   of   analogy   between   natural   and   artificial
selections   makes   sense   when   comparing   the   human   mind   with   artificial
intelligence, because both forms are the differentiated and synthesized results of
compounded elements of kinesthetic intelligence. Natural intelligence is the
human mind's virtual beauty, artificial intelligence is the mind's virtual reality,
and kinesthetic intelligence is the prodigy of the mind's creativity. All are the
products of bioscientific and biotechnological innovative prodigies.

In October 1838, Darwin stated:

> Being   well   prepared   to   appreciate   the   struggle   for   existence   which
> everywhere goes on from long-continued observation of habits of animals
> and plants, it at once struck me that under these circumstances favorable
> variations   would   tend   to   be   preserved,   and   unfavorable   ones   to   be
> destroyed. The result of this would be the formation of a new species
> (Darwin, 1958: 120).

If Darwin's evolutionary theory is about elective affinity as a chemist uses
such a term, then Darwin plunges us into the bioscientific innovativeness.

Berman (1993: 404) on behalf of the computer scientist, Hans Moravec
stated:

> Future Human isn't a human at all. Future Human is a machine... The rate
> at which computers are gaining in power is about thousand fold every
> twenty years. In ten years we should be seeing the first generation of
> universal robots... Machines eventually outdistance their human creators
> in all aspects. If Darwin's evolutionary theory is true and Moravec's
> theory of artificial intelligence revolutionary theory is right also,
> biotechnological evolutionary theory makes a link between natural

intelligence (the human's mind) and artificial intelligence is searching for
the one best way to perceive the reality of life.

They will be intelligent beyond our comprehension; they will be curious and
creative; they will be immortal. And what will happen to people?
From another dimension, cognitive mapping of the informational system,
within the brain of an individual person, can be easily manipulated towards preplanned objectives. Cognitive science is the hegemony of the mind. The cognitive
mapping of kinesthetic intelligence is conceived as the result of the pragmatic
application of molar cognitive techniques to process the contextual paradigm of
the human's mind by providing a second-by-second (or even a nanosecond by
nanosecond) nano-genetic picture of the learning, processing, and recognizing of
facts. In fact, kinesthetic intelligence's ultimate objective is to scrupulously
provide the holistic pictorial conceptions of the mind through implantation of
nano-machines in the human body, to manifest the virtual beauty of the human's
mind in a continuity of its mental life. Scientists have learned to build tiny
machines just a few atoms wide. Nano-machines are built by specific structural
design components that make the machines from tiny strands of carbon. The
nano-microscopic machines can inspect individual atoms of materials. The nano-
machines can manipulate atoms and molecules one by one in order to form new
shapes and structures of genes. These nano-machines are invisible to the eye
(Harvey, 2001:16).

EMERGENCE AND FUTURE OF BIOTECHNOLOGY

There are many terms that are used interchangeably by some scientists and
ethicists such as biotechnology, genetic engineering, gene technology,
transgenetics cloning technology, and eugenic technology. There is increasing
evidence that biotechnology has accelerated the pace of bioscientific
innovativeness. Among such technological developments is the transplantation of
organ from one human being to another, despite the body's immunological
defense against such intrusion. There is also increasing evidence of the ability to
construct artificial organs either through stem cell cloning in labs or artificial
hearts and artificial kidneys.
Transplantation of bio-cloned parts and artificial robotics machines raises
bioethical issues for the recipients. There are some ethical issues, such as cost and
benefit analysis, use of scarce resources, and religious mandates that are
conscientiously important for performing such operations. They may prevent the
patient's natural organs to function normally (Sidel, 1971: 147). Clark (1997: 17)
has suggested that advocacy groups help people consider the social and ethical
implications of genetic testing. Still others (Rubenstein, Anderson, and Hall,
1996: 103) have suggested a specific DNA technology, such as DNA analysis in

forensic science, as a mechanism for considering the legal implications of biotechnology.

There are debated pros and cons of the human genome research. Genetic engineering manipulations can accidentally and/or deliberately cause the disruption of normal heredity patterns and create abnormalities. The genome project can be used to screen people and provide specific information to employers concerning those people who are suspected of having cancerous genes and so be denied employment and/or health and life insurance. The bio-techno scientific capabilities could also lead to a new era of gene enhancement where desired traits such as intelligence, immunity, disease resistance, and longevity might be realized through the insertion of new genes into developing human embryos.

One of the dangerous spin-off from the human genome project could lead to ethnic bombs such as biological germs, engineered bacteria, or viruses that will be harmful to one particular ethnic group of people. Mahnaimi and Colvin (1998) stated that in the international community of scholars, experts called for controlling the proliferation of such ethnic bombs. The moral and ethical commitments of bio-techno-scientists are profound and crucial for the survival peace and security among nations.

It is important to understand how rapidly the field of biotechnology has passed through developmental phases and how the current phases will evolve in the future. Also, it is crucial to search for more opportunities to influence the commercialization of the market-based process of biotechnological and biopharmaceutical growth to cure human diseases.

The biotechnologies, hand-in-hand with biopharmaceutical research and development grew up dramatically over the 1990s. Such tremendous volumes of bioinformation caused the establishment of a bureaucratic infrastructure among nations, mainly due to their unique cost structures. As result, bioscientists, bioresearchers, biotechnologists, and biomedical practitioners including specialized physicians left their employers and formed joint venture startup firms. Such joint venture partnerships caused a mixed phenomenon of amoral feelings among bioscientists and physicians to create new techniques of recombinant DNA to find therapies to cure major diseases and/or to conduct gene canceling to prevent fatal diseases among family members. There is a basic ethical question concerning all these efforts: How well are bioscientists, biotechnologists, and biomedical researchers (physicians) conducting their new drug testing with possibilities of long range side-effects on present and future generations? For example Schoen, Hogan, and Falchek (2000: 141) indicated diethylstilbestrol (DES) was a synthetic form of drug used as a substitute for natural estrogen, a female sex hormone crucial to sexual development and fertility. This synthetic hormone was used by thousands of women from the late 1940s through the late 1960s, until it became evident that women who used DES while pregnant had complications with their offspring, especially the females. In 1971, the FDA banned the use of DES during pregnancy (36 Fed. Reg. 21, 537 -1971). Through their research, biomedical scientists found that the offspring of those females who consumed DES were born with physical deformities and abnormalities in their reproductive systems.

Clearly, biopharmaceutical producers in consultation with specialized physicians should have tested the drug for complications not only in the generations that were taking the drug but also on the impact that drug could have had on the next generations. Both biotechnologists and biopharmacists have come under an enormous amount of criticism for their irresponsible behavior by providing unnecessary medication that is really not needed.

Flowers (1998: 1740) categorized four phases for contemporary biotechnological development as follows:

> 1985-1990: The First Period: Developing Tools. Pharmaceutical companies found that they had to develop the tools of biotechnological research in order to do the biotechnological research. This doubled the time necessary to develop a marketable drug.
>
> 1991-2020: The Second Period: Curing Diseases. The tools of biotechnology are used to produce the first period of major medical/biotechnological disease cures, the successfully marketed cures offer new promise; to cure disease when antibiotics have become ineffective; to fight the coming plagues.
>
> 2020-2075: The Third Period: Genetic Modifications. Medical modifications of the body begin to include modifications not needed to cure diseases or inherited mistakes in the genome. Special purposeful modifications of the body are brought about by somatic therapy and other treatments for uses of such as enhancing life in outer space, space exploration, and adapting colonists for life on other planets. By cloning human beings, biotechnological modifications may create new classes of people and new unions based on enhanced physical attributes. Consequently, the social morphology begins to change because of genetic modifications. In addition, theories of genetic engineering, genetic modifications, and genetic evolution will be tested to discover how to enhance human intelligence.
>
> 2075-2200: The Fourth Period: Redesigning the Human Genome. Billingham, (1982) believed that humanity makes long-term strategic decisions and actions on how to use biotechnologies to improve the odds of human survival in a hostile universe. For such reasons, biotechnologies, biopharmaceutical drugs, and cloning can create new human-made diseases for both natural and cloned human species. Naturally, humanity will be exposed to a messy and hostile new world order. Should humanity have the power to redesign their human successors; super intelligent men and women? If the answer is yes, then all of the above phases of biotechnologies and biopharmaceutical processes and conclusions will be subject to bioethics.

Once biotechnologies and biopharmaceutical products cure diseases, or repair hereditary genetic defects, there is an additional issue as to whether it is ethical to effect the cure in such a way that the cure is passed on to the offspring of natural and cloned human species. Should biotechnological and biopharmaceutical companies be ethically, morally, and legally responsible to compensate the offspring of humans for side-effects, and/or to charge them with a fee for a cure that was given to their parents because of a therapeutic procedure given or a drug taken by their parents?

In conclusion, both biotech and biopharmaceutical institutions have undergone an enormous amount of ethical criticism for their apparent greedy behavior in various areas.

THE REBIRTH OF BIOETHICS

A human being is like the egg which might develop into a chicken, but which also, among other things, could become an egg sandwich. Rationality is no more natural to human beings than eating, singing, or possessing material things. Humans are not unique among other animals merely because they could be rational. They are also the only animals that commit suicide, crime, fraud, and that laugh and enjoy killing each other. If it were argued that rationality is the important essence of humans, this overlooks humans' egoism and selfishness. What should be developed in human beings depends upon some ideals of rational appropriateness in the present and future, because humans are dual entities. Feelings, emotions, rationality, and the like are good or bad depending on historical social contexts and outcomes. To be sure, humans have intellect and morals as well as emotions in their nature; sometimes they are constructive and other times they are destructive. Among these things they are moving on two directional of highways (depending in which direction they are pursuing) good or bad. Sometimes they are faced with crossroads that creates the possibility of getting lost. What do they need not to be lost? They need to have a thoughtful roadmap, morality and ethics, in order to provide them appropriate guidance to pursue the right direction in order to get to the right destination. We shall regard bioethics as a good guidance merely because it provides bio-techno-scientists and bioresearchers with the knowledge of what is good and what they should pursue to achieve goodness.

The bioethical voyage started before the industrial revolution where philosophers, scientists, physicians, and practitioners recognized the value of life. Bioethicists recognized its birth from ancient scholars who relentlessly pursued their curiosity to enhance human life. Generally, there are five phases of development from its birth to its rebirth: in the first phase which is extended from human curiosity to 1945, bioscientists pursued it through their individual humanitarian fervor, in the second phase which was between 1945-1966, bioscientists pursued it through professional commitments to humanity, in the third phase, which was between 1966-1974, bioscientists were confronted with social responsibilities and ethical questions concerning their activities; the fourth phase which was between 1975-1989, was a challenging time to create bioknowledge through bio-techno-scientific discoveries, and in the fifth phase which started in 1990, bioscientists started to institutionalize bioethical discourse.

Bioethics is a new pragmatic ethics. It is new because it bears different meanings at different times. Albert Jonsen (1993) dates "the rebirth of bioethics" from the *Hastings Center Report # 23*, when Shana Alexander's article entitled: They Decide Who Lives, Who Dies, which appeared in *Life* magazine in 1962 and described the Seattle dialysis selection committee. Beecher (1966: 1354) exposed scientific abuses in human experimentations by scientists for the first time. Rothman (1991: 3) described 1965-75 as the formative decade for bioethics in the Twentieth century. In addition, simultaneously, a new generation of ethicists appeared not only in the field of medicine, but also appeared in the field of bioscientific and biopharmaceutical activities. They established their academic role as authorities in bioresearch centers and medical laboratories.

Porter (1971) perceived the term bioethics as the science of survival in the ecological sense, an interdisciplinary approach to ensuring the preservation of the biosphere through *earthcare, peoplecare, animalcare*, and *healthcare*. According to such a biosophical perception, bioethics is termed simply ethics for the sanctity of life and for living. Bioethics entails the global assessment of how multicultural values, political-legal ideologies, and religious faiths affect humanity, animals, and environment.

Fox (2001: 29) extended the description, adding that: "Bioethics also incorporates *biosophy*, the wisdom derived from a scientific (especially biological and ecological) and empathic understanding of life." What Wilson reinforces as biosophy, Keller (1993) called *biophilia,* our innate sympathetic affinity for the life and beauty of the natural world, which is the spiritual ethos of the deep ecology and animal rights movements (Fox, 1990).

Medical and biological technologies have forced societies to reexamine the absolute roles of bioscientific systems. Gradually, the development of bioethics has emerged as a reaction to notable and unethical events in the history of biosciences. It is an accumulation of reactions to the ambiguity of the practices of medical research that brought forth a new concern, namely bioethics. The emergence of bioethics is the result of the efforts of medical scientists and researchers challenging traditional medical ethics. Traditional medical ethics had an absolute respect for the sanctity of life and this imperative supported the ethics of medicine. It seems, that the work of healing and convictions about right and wrong behavior have always been tightly linked. Historically, medical ethics was incarnated in a doctor's behavior and character and in the social arrangements that sustained the solidarity, respectability, and educated competence of the profession.

Bioethics traces the views of Dr. Chauncey Leake (1896-1987), a pharmacologist by training, who criticized the traditional writings of the English physician, Thomas Percival. Percival wrote the first book of *Medical Ethics* in 1803. The major theme of Percival's book is based on the combination of the traditional virtues of medical decorum with novel injunctions about the behavior of physicians among themselves. Percival insisted that the duties of office had been granted to doctors by society as public trusts, by encouraging urbanity and rectitude among physicians. Leake criticizes Percival saying that he misconceived medical ethics from the beginning. He accused Percival of ignoring the philosophical literature of ethics and thus of elaborating an etiquette rather than an ethic. Leake's (1927: 18) perception concerning medical ethical philosophy is not only attesting that physicians should have ethical behavior among themselves, but also, they should be concerned about their ethical behavior toward their patients and society at large. Leake indicated:

> The term *medical ethics*, introduced by Percival is really a misnomer. Based on Greek traditions of good taste and on Thomas Percival's Code, [1803] it refers chiefly to the rules of etiquette developed in the profession to regulate the professional contacts of its members with each other... Medical ethics should be concerned with the ultimate consequences of the conduct of physicians toward their individual patients and toward society as a whole (Jones: 1924).

In addition, Leake (1928: 343) wrote:

> Changing conditions in medical practice are making the matter acute. It is becoming apparent that group practice, health insurances, and periodic health examinations, as well as various aspects of public health measures, are profoundly altering the view of the physician.

Later on, on the basis of Leake's advocacy views, the ideal bioethics appeared in academia. Dr. Richard Cabot (1869-1939) (1919), professor of clinical medicine at Harvard Medical School and Social Ethics in Harvard College, insisted that doctors, on the basis of their clinical competence and ethical duties, should reinforce the confidence in scientific research in order to convert medicine into an effective healing art. Medical scientific knowledge should be the primacy of doctors' moral repertoire.

Medical historian Chester Burns (1977: 368) appraised Cabot's contribution in the medical ethics as he stated:

> As much as other physician of his day Richard Cabot demonstrated the validity of the new bases for professional goodness... What counted was whether a practitioner understood the specific diseases, their causes, signs, symptoms, courses, prognoses, treatments, and whether each practitioner applied this understanding in the assessment and management of each individual patient.

Cabot (1919) believed that physicians should attain scientific somatic knowledge and skills. There are new ways to measure medical knowledge and skills through advances in scientific absorbency in physiology, pathology, and bacteriology, and learn to use "quantitative methods to evaluate results of treatment, knowledge, and skill become more measurable."

The new prominence of bioethics can be traced to further deliberations of ethicists in relationship with biotechnology. Most biologists and biotechnologists studied life sciences by taking cells apart and examining their effects on the whole organ. They assumed that the whole is equal to the sum of its parts and can be explained in terms of its parts. Nevertheless, life is viewed as an integrative whole containing synergy. Higgins, (1994: 61) defined: "Synergy means that combined and coordinated actions of the parts (subsystems) of a system achieve more than all of the parts acting independently could achieve." Synergy possesses two different directions: (1) positive, and (2) negative. The negative effects of the meat and bone meal (MBM) on cattle and human beings are beyond imaginable consequential results.

It is quite correct that in the early part of the Twentieth century British biologists discovered a new method to change the natural vegetarian feeding system chain of livestock to cannibalism the meat and bone meal (MBM) in order to provide cattle extra protein. Such a method, scientifically, was very successful to such an extent that the British government made it obligatory for all livestock feed to contain MBM. This innovative scientific method allowed most European farmers and ranchers to save money and make extra profit. However, because of long-term incubation of new diseases; bovine spongiform encephalopathy (BSE) for cattle, and variant Creutzfeldt-Jakob disease (nvCJD), or BSE for humans, the mad cow disease (BSE) caused the death of thousands of cattle and about a hundred humans. The experiment of the BSE and the MBM resulted in the infectious diseases that are forms of the prion protein (PrPSc) that derived from cellular PrP (PrPC) in a conversion reaction involving a dramatic reorganization of the secondary and tertiary structure in the spinal cord and brain and the emergence of variant Creutzfeldt-Jacob Disease (nvCJD). Bioethisists, in contrast, study life sciences by putting things together and assuming that the whole is greater than the sum of its parts (synergy).

In the modern history of European bioethics, the rebirth of bioethics stems from medical and social ethics of post-World War II. It started in 1947 as the result of the Nuremberg Tribunal conviction of twenty-three physicians for war crimes committed under the guise of medical experiments, and it promulgated the Nuremberg Code. The Nuremberg trial initiated a reexamination of traditional medical ethics. Its principles prevailed in science and law through modern interdisciplinary scholarly efforts to discover new methods of diagnosis and treatment of patients through scientific experimental research in the fields of genetic engineering, reproductive technology, organ transplantation, and plastic surgery. Specifically, many German authorities that fled from Germany and sheltered in Latin American countries needed to go through facial and surface-finger print surgeries in order to get away from the Nuremberg Tribunal Crime Trial.

BIOETHICS AND BIO-TEST EXPERIMENTS

It is important to understand how the rapidly developing fields of biosciences, biotechnologies, and biopharmaceutical activities have passed through historical phases and have offered unique opportunities for bioscientists, biotechnologists, and biopharmacists to conduct research in these areas in order to cure human diseases and extend life. Because of such humanitarian intellectual objectives, medical practitioners, including physicians, work hand-in-hand with these researchers to perform the work that results in marketable drugs and biotechnological procedures to cure diseases. Although physicians are deeply involved in the application of biosciences and biomedical technology they are particularly susceptible to ethical and moral persuasion because of the human focus of their profession and because of their specific altruistic ethical and moral commitments. Nevertheless, physicians have had a continuing interest in the ethical and moral issues of biosciences and biotechnologies because the ethics of the biopharmaceutical industry is one control factor that keeps doctors at the center of medical and health delivery power structure as biosciences and biotechnologies continue to chip away at their professional domains (Flowers, 1998: 1737).

From an ethical point of view, the Twentieth century's growing concern about bioscientific and biotechnological research on human beings has created controversial debates. The use of human subjects in research has become alarming due to the violation of human rights. The July 26, 1972 edition of *The New York Times* disclosed a shocking story:

> For forty years, the United States Public Health Service had conducted a study in which human beings with syphilis, who were induced to serve as guinea pigs, had gone without treatment for the disease... the study was conducted to determine from autopsies what the disease does to human body. The human subject of that experimental research was about 600 men, mostly poor and uneducated, from Tuskegee, Alabama (Heller, 1972: A1, A8).

In another scientific mistake in the Twentieth century, the man-made catastrophic incidents of the emergence of bovine spongiform encephalopathy (BSE) among European cattle and the appearance of variant Creutzfeldt-Jakob disease (nvCJD) among human beings are simplified as the mad cow disease. The BSE has cost most European countries billions of dollars because of the need to slaughter and destroy million of tons of contaminated beef (Coockson, 2000: 11). In the late twentieth century a biologist, Stanley Prusiner (1997:13363), discovered a slow virus known as prion. Through their research, Prusiner and his associates discovered that prions are composed largely of a modified form of the prion protein (PrP) designated PrPSc. Prions do not have a nucleic acid genome to direct the synthesis of their progeny. A post-translational, conformational change features in the conversion of the cellular PrP (PrPC) into PrPSc, during which alpha helices are transformed into beta-sheets. Prion diseases can be both inherited and infectious. Investigation of prion strains has led to the conclusion that variations in disease phenotypes are determined by conformation of PrPSc (Prusiner, 1997; Viles *et al.*, 1999; Supattapone *et al.*, 1999; Liu *et al.*, 1999). Furthermore, contaminated ashes of incinerated cows can contaminate the environment and cause ecological effects on plants, animals, and humans. Scientists have found that prion protein selectively binds copper (II) ions (Stockel *et al.*, 2001: 799). The cellular prion protein binds copper in vivo (Brown *et. al.*, 1997: 684). Copper stimulates endocytosis of the prion protein. Prion diseases result from a confrontational alteration of PrPC, a cell surface glycoprotein expressed in brain, spinal cord, and several peripheral tissues, into PrPSc, a protease-resistant isoform that is the principal component of infectious prion principles. The possibility of PrPC may play a role in the metabolism of copper and the effect of this metal ion on the endocytic trafficking of PrPC in cultured neuroblastoma cells. This effect may be physiologically relevant in that PrPC could serve as a recycling receptor for uptake of copper ions from the extra cellular milieu (Pauly and Harris, 1998: 33107). However, Swedish people were among the European farmers who quickly banned the use of such a scientifically mistaken technique. Soon after, in 1987, Swedish farmers themselves introduced a voluntary ban on the use of all meat and fish products in nearly all-animal fodder, with a total ban becoming law in 1991. The Swedish Farmers Association (SFA) declared that: "For ethical reasons we stopped" (George, 2000: 2).

The Willowbrook State School in Staten Island, New York, is an institution devoted to housing and caring for mentally retarded children. In 1956 a research group led by Saul Krugman and Joan P. Giles of the New York University School of Medicine conducted a long-range research experiment of viral hepatitis. The children confined there were made experimental subjects of the study. Krugman and Giles were interested in determining the natural history of viral hepatitis, the mode of infection and the course of disease over time. They also wanted to test the effectiveness of gamma globulin as an agent for inoculating against hepatitis. (Gamma globulin is a protein complex extracted from the blood serum that contains antigens, substances that trigger the production of specific antibodies to counter infectious agents). Krugman and Giles decided to deliberately infect some of the incoming children with the strain of the hepatitis virus prevalent at Willowbrook. They obtained what they considered to adequate consent from the parents of the children during a preliminary interview. Serious moral doubts had been raised about the nature and conduct of the experiments, especially the use of retarded children as experimental subjects, and the ways in which these researchers obtained the consent from the parents of the children (Munson, 1983: 239-241). Fluehr-Lobban (2000: B24) reported:

> Journalist Patrick Tierney's investigation relates that in 1968, thousands of samples of Yanomami blood and other biological data were collected for research. At the same time, a measles vaccine known to be virulent in genetically isolated populations was injected into the Yanomami as part of

a project designed by James V. Neel, of the University of Michigan,
allegedly inspired by eugenic theories.

The story Tierney tells grows more sinister, as an epidemic rapidly ensued
and the research team allegedly was advised not to provide any medical
assistance to the sick and dying Yanomami.

In biological experimental research projects documentation of informed
consents of human subjects needs to be recorded in writing, using the language of
the people studied as well as of the researchers. There is a legal argument that
needs to be analyzed in the field of bioethics. Some international bioethicists
believe that cross-cultural research needs to consider human rights. Some
scientists might argue that informed consent is a specialized Western ethical and
cultural principle from which research outside a country is exempt. Politicians
might say that some underdeveloped countries are primitive people incapable of
giving consent because they are isolated people who do not have highly
sophisticated citizens' rights and cannot understand the scientific purpose of
genetic or social research or its ramifications. These are major concerns in the
field of international bioethics.

The unfolding power of the microchip and the unlocking of human's genetic
code pushed on in the late Twentieth century. Life sciences celebrated a historic
achievement, with the announcement by researchers from academia and biotech
industry that they had assembled a first draft of the human genome; the *Book of
Life* that provides biochemical blueprint in 3billions genetic letters. What is next
after genetic decoding? J. Craig Venter and Francis Collins stated: 'With
mapping of the human genome, man will be able to lengthen his life-span by
eradicating many of the existing causes of diseases and death."

The evolution of science and technology has brought many changes upon all
aspects of society. Technology has allowed mankind to accomplish many
remarkable things and directed the standard of living in a prosperous path. In a
system of "donating" gametes, in which banking is the dominant metaphor, sperm
and eggs are naturally sorted by "worth." We do not like to speak of eugenic
anymore, but it is hard not to think of eugenics when people are actively seeking
the very best genes money can buy (Rothman, 1999: A52). From another point of
view, the mapping of the human genome by J. Craig Venter and Francis Collin
will allow people to lengthen their life spans by eradicating many of the existing
causes of disease and death. With genetic decoding we will be able to control our
feelings and desires. As the Human Genome Project has reminded us, the genetic
chemical DNA has an awesome capacity for information storage; the microscopic
nucleus of every cell in our body contains enough DNA to make a complete
person (Malik, 2000: 15). The *Book of Life* provides our biochemical blueprint in
3 billion genetic letters. Critics say that knowing the full genome is unnecessary
for most biomedical applications, because only a small fraction of human DNA
really represents genes; the working units of heredity and molecular biology
(Financial Times, 2000: 16).

THE NATURE OF BIOETHICAL
PROBLEMS AND ISSUES

Considering the above scientific adventures and other biotechnological breakthroughs all raise many questions concerning the moral, ethical, and legal dimensions of human life. This text investigates the relationship between biosciences biotechnology, and bioethics. This study will analyze whether bioscientific and biotechnological tests or whether the use of sampling data affects the perceptions of people concerning their lives. Since this text is a heuristic study, no specific framework that measures the impact of people's perceptions on biosciences and biotechnology has been suggested. Thus, it is important to develop a comprehensive framework. Within the general boundary of this text, there are some general concerns about bioethics and biotechnology. These concerns are:

- Are eugenic and biotechnological breakthroughs providing humanity with a continuity of promising excellence in our ecological lives?
- Do eugenics and biotechnology serve humanity with moral, ethical, and legal ordinations?
- Do organ transplants and kinesthetic intelligence elevate human dignity and integrity?

If so, what are the main causes, processes, and effects of such important endeavors on mammals, including human beings? These and other similar eugenic and biotechnological breakthroughs raise controversial moral, ethical, and legal questions of how we should or should not reengineer the future generations. Notwithstanding that in today's pragmatic and instrumental times of crisis, it is urgent to construct all our rational conduct in technological terms. Since eugenic and biotechnology construe the basic logical form of human action toward excellence, they are viewed as exhibitions of the idea of taking good means towards good ends. What would make such a judgment very complex, what is a moral wisdom concerning reasoning from ethical values and reasoning from legal values? These issues are the main subject areas that will be analyzed in this text.

The problem of eugenic and biotechnological research is widely acknowledged by ethicists, and is also attested by numerous philosophers and scientists. That is the distinguished practical deliberation from theoretical deliberation as primarily is concerned with pursuit of the good more than pursuit of the truth. Eugenic and biotechnological research has the greatest magnitude of fascinated interest among scientists, technologists, sophists, and ethicists. Each group has expressed their point of views. In this text, a literature review will be done to catalog the major research dimensions of these activities such as: the eugenic path of the future of mammals including pocket-sized smart cloning human beings; organ transplants, gene-therapy; chemotherapy; genetic engineering; chimerical mutation (the combination of human and mammal cells); kinesthetic intelligence (the combination of the natural mind with implanted magnetic nano-computer chips in the human brain); bio-artificial tissues; forensic DNA testing; genomic life; mammalian genetics; genetic modified foods; genetic quantum super computers; anti-ageism organic transformation; biological warfare, anti-bio-terrorist warfare; toxin weapons; and pharmaceutical engineering. Each of the above scientific activities will be reviewed through application of moral, ethical, and legal views.

THE TRIADIC SYLLOGISM OF BIOETHICS

Bioscientific, biotechnologial, and biomedical research have long subscribed to a body of moral and ethical knowledge developed primarily for the preservation and protection of mankind. Members of these professions both researchers and practitioners must recognize their ethical and moral responsibilities not only to their academic professions, but also to humanity. An important emphasis in our introductory work is the hope for readers to understand the individualistic moral convictions and the pluralistic ethical commitments of bioscientists, biotechnologists, and biomedical practitioners. The ultimate objective of these professionals should be based upon doing well and avoiding doing evil. Gert, Culver, and Clouser (1997: 2) stated:

> Bioethics has often been derisively referred to as quandary ethics or dilemma ethics, implying thereby that it consists of puzzles which, though they may fascinate or entertain, are not amenable to systematic analysis and resolution, and hence almost any answer to any one does, suffice. This implies a lack of system, in that the answer to any one puzzle is unrelated to the answer to any other, and this in turn implies that there is no way to show whether the answers to two distinct dilemmas are consistent with each other.

Thereby, a mass of ethical principles, moral values, and legal standards concerned with what conduct *ought* to be existed to guide these professionals is confused.

One of the major problems in the field of bioethics is related to anthological theories of ethics. Typically, several different ethical theories are presented with no attempt to reconcile them. For example, John Rawls (1971) analyzed the virtue of social institutions termed with justice. In an ethical term, Rawls supplied the distinction between justness and fairness, *distributive justice.* John Stuart Mill (1806-1873) stated that the ethical efficacy of a social institution is based upon the greatest happiness for the greatest majority of people; *utilitarianism.* Mill (1957: 62) stated:

> Whether justice consists in depriving a person of a possession, or in breaking faith with him, or in treating him worse than he deserves, or

worse than other people who have no greater claims in each case the supposition implies two things: [1] a wrong done, and [2] some assignable person who is wronged... It seems to me that this feature to the moral obligation constitutes the specific difference between justice and generosity or benevolence. Justice implies something which is not only right to do, and wrong not to do, but which some individual person can claim from us as his moral right.

Also, Mill believed that ethical evaluation is directed to actions and to the manner in which they affect the general happiness; *hedonism* (Albert, Denise, and Peterfreund, 1984: 233).

Immanuel Kant (1724-1804) analyzed the ethical effectiveness of a social institution as based upon not the intention or the mission to produce happiness, but to produce a good will. He did not deny that happiness is a desirable moral obligation, but he also believed that it should be based upon a good will. He asserted that institutions of good products and/or services with good will deserve happiness (Albert, Denise, and Peterfreund, 1984: 203). By analyzing the above views concerning bioinstitutions, the readers naturally conclude that moral and ethical theories are confused, irrelevant, or completely relative.

Within such a wide magnitude of reality in bioethics, we need to follow the syllogism of judgmental moral and ethical reasoning rules in terms of anthological methodology to be valid. What is a valid syllogistic anthology? It is a basic triadic structure that requires that there should be three propositions to question the answers, not to answer the questions. To much better understand such a triadic reasoning structure within the domain of syllogistic correctness and soundness, there are six rules that govern the validity of syllogistic anthology in terms of: (1) major reasoning, (2) middle reasoning, and (3) minor reasoning, according to Corbett (1991: 32). First, each rule will be listed, and then they will be explained as follows:

- There must be three terms and only three terms in assessing a syllogistic validity: major terms, middle terms, and minor terms. The major reasoning in biosciences is to discover the pragmatic somatic truth. The middle term is to apply the truth to help people to avoid suffering. The minor term is related to the expansion of biosciences and biotechnology.

- The middle term must be distributed at least once. This means any scientific effort needs to be effective for enhancing human life. In the syllogism we just looked at, the middle term *human beings/human being* is distributed by the *all* in front of it in the first proposition. Bioscientists need to be concerned about dignity and integrity of the human race. They should not violate their natural rights.

- No term may be distributed in the conclusion if it was not distributed in the premises. What this term is trying to guard against is the use of a term in a wider extension in the conclusion that was used in one of the premises. The conclusion is therefore, human beings are moral and ethical.

- No conclusion may be drawn from two particular premises. This means that bioethical predicates need to draw from all three domains. We should not ignore one or two dimensions of bioscientific, biotechnological, and biomedical endeavors. It is a holistic judgment concerning doing right things and avoiding doing wrong things.

- No conclusion may be drawn from two negative premises. If we understand in the field of biosciences what a particular positive premise is and what a negative premise is, then rationally our syllogistic reasoning is self-explanatory. But we need to apply these three terms to our sample syllogism to see whether they have been observed.

- If one of the premises is negative, the conclusion must be negative. Since bioscientific, biotechnological, and biomedical research is based upon trial and error, we need to assess negative effects in our experiments and then to conclude the validity of our experimental data. If we find one negative premise among experiments, we need to conclude that such an experiment is not valid; it may have side effects. From an ethical and moral view, bioscientific discoveries need to have positive impacts on human life.

If you have read this far, you have been told more about the syllogism than you care to know. But even if you have not understood how to construct a valid syllogism or to test the validity of your syllogistic experiments, you may have understood something valuable about the mechanism of the deductive processes. Thus, syllogism is a schematization of how the scientific mind deductively presents it's reasoning   for discovering truth.

TRIANGULATION IN BIOETHICS

Qualitative and quantitative bioethical considerations are distinct in both experiential and experimental research. Yet almost in all bioscientific research findings, quantitative orientations are given more respect, this may reflect the tendency of the expertise to regard life sciences as related to numbers and implying precision by logical reasoning to solve bioproblems. It is not the objective of this text to argue against quantitative research procedures. Nevertheless, any type of quantitative research represents both deductive and inductive qualitative interpretations concerning fact-findings. Thus, the orientation of this text does not entirely either embrace or reject Kaplan's (1964: 206) claim: "If you can measure it, that ain't it!"

Triangulation is a term in fact finding through three major steps: (1) biomap making via formation of scientific hypothetical assumptions, (2) bionavigation through conducting experimental research projects to examine viability and reliability of the research hypothetical assumptions, and (3) generalization of bioscientific formulas for future problem solving. Most bioresearchers have at least one methodological technique they feel most comfortable using, which often becomes their favorite or only approach to conduct a research project. Many bioresearchers perceive their research methods as empirical. The ethical and moral problems surface when they are considering dignity and integrity of human subjects. Furthermore, many bioresearchers perceive their research methods as conclusive end results to summarize their fact-findings. The major flaw in such domains of inquiry concerning a theoretical assumption has already been made; specially, that reality is fairly constant and stable. Within these domains of inquiry the direct observations of all particularities are assumed reality and are deeply affected by actions and reactions of all subjects including themselves. Nevertheless, each researcher and each research project with specific methodology reveals slightly different facets of reality. Every research methodology is a different line of sight directed to the same point of discovery. By combining several lines of sights with different attached dimensions researchers can conclude more substantive picture of reality. The use of multiple lines of sight is frequently called *triangulation* (Berg, 1995: 5). It should be indicated that bioresearch projects and bioresearchers are not immune to *triangle of error*. They may conclude their experiential research projects to present a new drug to treat patients, but also they may ignore the long-term side effects of their products (e.g., Viox, DES, Estrogen, etc.).

Within the domain of bioethical triangulation, there are three major components with three major lines of objectives: (1) individual(s) as researchers, (2) industries as major beneficence; biopharmaceutical and biotechnological, and (3) institutions as major regulatory agencies; Food and Drug Administration (FDA). Nevertheless the best estimate of the true location of bioethical point of objectives is the center of the triangle, assuming that the three lines of objectives could be equal in error. Although, validity of sightings could be done with two sightings line objective intersecting (researchers and industries) at one point, the third line objective (FDA) validates the scientific effective applicability of a more accurate estimate of the proven points or formulas for problem solving.

By looking at the Figure 1.2 we can analyze the triangulation domains of bioethics in three major societal constituencies:

- Individual bioscientists, biotechnologists, biochemists, biophysicists, bioinformationalists, and biomedical practitioners.
- Bioindustries including biochemistry, biophysics, bioinformation, biotechnology, biopharmaceutical, and biomedical laboratories.

- Bioinstitutions including private bioresearch centers, governmental bioregulatory agencies, universities, health research centers, hospitals, and military bioresearch centers.

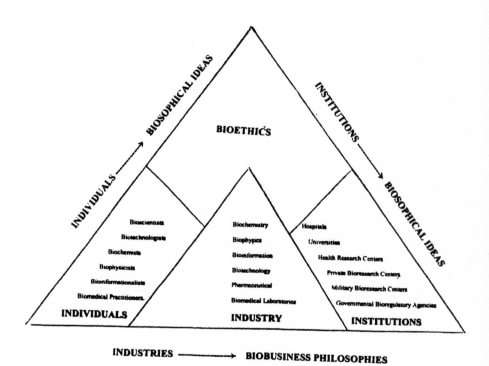

Figure 1-2: The Triangulation Syllogistic Biosophical, Biophilia, and Philosophical Integration in Bioethics

ON DEMARCATING THE SYLLOGISM OF BIOETHICAL AND BIOMORAL REASONING

Recognition of the importance of scientific advancements and technological breakthroughs is closely related to the need for the maintenance of human dignity. Human dignity refers to the realization and deliberation of wisdom in accordance with virtue. If the nature and the purpose of wisdom is assumed as the bed-rock of science and technology towards excellence, then the functions of bioscientific and biotechnological efforts must be oriented toward goodness. Ethical excellence is a type of virtue in which scientific thoughts come into relationship with practical goodness. The nature of bioethics is first and foremost a state of somatic well being, even for those who pursue it as finality in spiritual happiness.

In our modern world many of the newest and most controversial bioscientific advancements and biotechnological breakthroughs begin with being thrust upon researchers involved in cloning, stem cell therapies, and genetic engineering activities that provoke moral and ethical debates. Often, bioscientists and biotechnologists argue that the means of bioscientific and biotechnological advancement is the enhancement of human life, while on the other side there are those ethicists and moralists who question the beneficial ends that we expect from the same work. The major ethical and moral issue between these opposing groups is related as being between those who opposite the means and those who laud the ends. In order to get to a middle ground of fairness, we need to examine a means of assurance that a particular line of bioresearch is worthy to justify the worthwhile ends. In order to analyze such a debatable issue, we need to examine the natures of the biosciences from triadic dimensions: (1) biosciences and biotechnologies are pure, (2) biosciences and biotechnologies are impure, and (3) biosciences and biotechnologies are neutral.

Clearly, biosciences and biotechnologies have changed societies and their values. They often do so in ways that confront naturalists' beliefs head on, bringing about significant ethical anxiety and legal restraints. The result of such a complexity is the ending spasms of an old moral and ethical order in the process of being supplanted by a new notion of scientific advancement (Edwards, 1999:24). Nevertheless, the knowledge and attitudes of bioscientists and biotechnologies toward many biotechnological changes are unlikely to be mediated by predictable hypotheses about bioethical determinants and changes in biogenetic engineering. These hypotheses can be based on either ethical or legal assumptions that are mutually affected by events and norms or values. Michael, Grimyer, and Turner (1997:13) concluded that there are two major discourses among people: (1) science and technology are impure, and (2) science and technology are pure in the professional laboratory where their uncertainties and contingencies were considered less in evidence. These hypothetical assumptions could be summarized as the following:

H-1: Biosciences and Biotechnologies Are Pure and They Can Generate Goodness for Human Race

Consider for a moment what would you do if you were exposed to an acute illness:

- Where would you like to go?

- To whom you trust to submit your life?
- What type of professionals would you believe possess an appropriate knowledge to diagnose, treat, and prognoses your illness?
- How would you know what types of medical procedures and medications can be effective for your recovery?

Answering these and other similar questions would lead you to the persons that you trust and he/she is a physician. The point is that one must already know that a physician possesses sufficient scientific medical knowledge. This .work of demarcation is an important step for humanity.

We believe that beyond the messy world of politics and economics, biosciences and biotechnologies are idealized realms in which useful scientific knowledge can be initiated and practiced. We believe that the words ought, should, and must are the rational language to be used in bioethics. We believe that the surest methods to solve our somatic problems are biosciences and their applications through biotechnologies. We believe that knowledge is based upon application of pragmatic rational rules, ideals, and procedures that constitute the clearest indication for building trust and confidence among people. Thus, we believe that scientific values direct the path of new biotechnological innovativeness and promote the more frequent application of new bioscientific results for the goodness of humanity. In addition, we believe that it is the responsibility of bioscientists and biotechnologists to explicate, clarify, and organize bioethical and biomoral rules. Now we turn to the opposite side of bioscientific and biotechnological goodness.

H-2: Biosciences and Biotechnologies Are Impure, and They May Cause Harm to Human Race and Environment

The opposite point is the corollary of the first: that just because bioscientific and biotechnological research are useful, there is no reason to assume that the means of bioresearch is good. For example, during World War II, new treatments for malaria and vaccines for typhus were developed in concentration camp experiments (Barlow, 2001: 11); doing well in the nature of bad or doing badly in the nature of good. Most people today agree that it was wrong to murder someone in the interests of bioresearch, no matter what good may have come from it for either bioscience in general or for humanity at large.

From the global practical view, we are living in a challenging environment that sometimes mandates us to follow social Darwinism ideology: "The survival of the fittest and the demise of the weakest and/or the sickest." What are global scientific efforts for, and whose values, beliefs, and interests may be at risk? Are they binding upon bioscientists, biotechnologists, bioinformationalists, and biomedical practitioners in an independent political and economic environment; namely as a nation? If the answer is related to the national interest, then it creates a mixture of opinion; should bioscientific advancements and biotechnological breakthroughs be helpful or harmful to whom? This can create unethical and immoral conditions to ignore or violate human natural and civil rights.

In reality biosciences and biotechnologies are part and parcel of the messy world of politics and economics. Therefore, they need to safeguard their innovative efforts for the benefit of interest groups. Patents of eugenic innovations change and formalize the new bioscientific and biotechnological directions and will increase the frequency of application of progressive directed trends of bioscientific and biotechnological testing methods towards more aggressive intended ends.

From another view, within the human's brain, biotechnological systems as knowledge-based processes are known as systems of perceiving and learning. Manipulated holistic functioning and processing systems of biotechnologies are based upon the existence of natural intelligence that is aided through cognitive and cybernetic systems. Bioinformation systems are not only modern interdisciplinary forms of knowledge but are also examples of the usage of cognitive mapping of human beings; cloning. Bioinformation systems such as Robotic Bacteria Endotoxin Test (RBET), Robotic Assay Development (RAD), Medical Computer Aided Manufacturing Systems (MCAMS), Biocomputer Numerically Controlled Systems (BNCS), Surgical Navigated Computer Controlled Robotics Systems (SNCCRS), Computer Aided Gene Engineering Design Systems (CAGDS), and Biotech Integrated Manufacturing Systems (BIMS) make possible not only the acceleration of modern biosciences and biotech abilities of scientists, but they also play an active medium role between bioscientists and biotechnologists, to establish a set of systemized multi-linkages to the sources of research discoveries. For example, recently, IBM scientists have built a transistor array out of carbon nanotubes, "cylindrical structures of carbon atoms" that are 10,000 times thinner than the diameter of a human hair. It is an invisible machine with components only a few atoms thick. The carbon nanotubes are vital to the future of the semiconductor industry, specifically in the field of biomedical research (Spooner, 2001).

Consider for a moment what would make a difference between bioscientific endeavors, namely: (1) biochemical and biological germs and biotechnological weapons, and (2) biopharmaceutical sedative products. These pragmatic bioscientific procedures are based upon subjective and manipulated derivative goals. Within the contextual boundaries of such visions, bioscientists and biotechnologists observe their tasks to respond to their specific elite interest groups. They identify different sets of objectives to meet their own personal and clientele demands.

By viewing impure biosciences and biotechnologies, researchers and practitioners postulate three bases for their professional objectives: the self, their employers, and other people within the biospherical environments. In other words, researchers avoid their commitments to their professional codes of ethics, and only observe their professional codes of conduct. Do you find differences between these two codes? We will discuss the differences of the two views in future chapters.

H-3: Biosciences and Biotechnologies Are Neutral and They May or May Not Cause Harm to the Human Race and Environment

Bioscientific and biotechnological neutrality is a more complex concept than is generally recognized. Neutrality means not being in favor of one more than another, and it is viewed as equivalent to fairness to all parties. Bioscientific and biotechnological neutrality does not, by itself, guarantee moral intentions and/or ethical actions. They are amoral. Amorality means telling a portion of truth not the whole. Since bioscientific and biotechnological research is a continuous process of unlimited discoveries of truth, it is not possible to predict all possible innovative side effects. They are multiple objectively oriented endeavors with multiple trials and errors.

The vision of bio-techno-scientific research would appear to oscillate between two opposed radical conceptions. The first is that of reductionalist positivistic epistemology, that is to state a position of the neutrality of biosciences, invariably considered as certain through its concealment of margins of uncertainty. The second is that of extreme epistemological pessimism, in which biosciences are viewed as totally undecidable, and in which biotechnologists and bioscientists take arbitrary decisions on the rationality of their scientific applied methodologies. The first conception has two variants: the first is taking for granted scientific certainty and the second is to hide scientific uncertainty.

Since bioscientific advancements and biotechnological developments are not complete products of individual scientists and/or researchers, therefore their ends are related impartiality to all individuals and groups. So an adequate account of the impartiality requires by morality, not amorality to be related to all individuals and groups. Bioethics should serve all human beings who can feel pleasure and pain. Therefore, impartial bioethicality and biomorality today are often more complicated and more in the public eye that they were a hundred years ago. This situation stems from validity of recent advancements in cybernetic scientific medicine. When you get to the cybermedicine, there is no privacy. Scientifically, you can have access to all types of information and specimens. Such a vague and open-ended discussion creates new problems.

The advent of the genetic testing and genetic engineering may have a radical impact on the natural and civil rights and life styles of all people including future generations. Some health, business, occupational, and governmental agencies claim that they should be entitled to ask for the results of the genetic testing or genetic engineering of their clients. For example, genetic testing can identify the risk of all individuals of developing particular diseases. The results can provide a breakthrough for employers and insurance companies not to hire or to make these individuals uninsurable. Also, genetic testing puts individuals and families in health at risk, because people lose their trust in physicians, hospitals, clinics, and governmental agencies disclosing their genetic characteristics. People will avoid being exposed to any kind of separation of disease symptoms to be tested in the labs. It is a fact that the natural environment is not a safe place for a perfect human being. Genetically, some people have a predisposition to develop specific diseases, some environmental factors develop illnesses, and some medical diagnoses, treatments, and prognoses develop side effects. If we do not maintain impartiality in biosciences and biotechnologies, the ends may create social catastrophe.

ISSUES, PROBLEMS, AND AREAS OF CONCERN IN BIOSCIENCES AND BIOTECHNOLOGIES

People today appreciate scientific advancements and technological breakthroughs because of effective innovative interventions into their lives. While biosciences have provided us with an astonishing amount of know-why, know-how, and know-what knowledge about living creatures, they have promised us little about the humanities. Nevertheless, phrases such as the "failure of nerve," (Murray, 1925), "future shock," (Tofler, 1970), and "civilization malaise," (Heilbroner, 1974) have been coined to convey the feeling that a void seems to have been created and sustained when experiences no longer make sense to individuals (Trosko, 1984: 70). As Gregory (1984: 11) stated: "Why do the natural sciences and the humanities need each other? The presupposition was these two great divisions of knowledge are capable of existing separately, which of course has been the case at least three generations." In sum, we feel that there is a void between bioscientific and biotechnological developments and humanities. People unconsciously live in that void. Some people would say that there is no such thing as bioethics, because they believe that biosciences and biotechnologies are changing the pure nature of humanity. Therefore, they advocate that biosciences and biotechnologies do not go together with bioethics. This kind of perception could be meant to imply that bioscientific and biotechnological functions by their natures are amoral.

People are more comfortable when discussing human suffering and ailments. They believe that physicians and bioscientists should do everything in order to cure patients, more in terms of their bottom-line impact than in terms of their ethical impact. The cardinal modes of human control over the use of biosciences and biotechnologies may be categorized according to two axes: societal concerns (legal or ethical) and personal concern (vocational or professional).

In many countries, societal concerns, including legal and ethical issues, are subject to the formalization of the political controlling systems, while in others they are subjected to their cultural and religious value systems. Legal controls are formalized as a result of perceiving unmet needs in ethical control mechanisms. This means that in as much as people in a society are more unethical, that society moves more toward legal controlling systems. Similarly, failures in a vocational control system can call forth professional controls. What does it mean? The theory argues that in so far as vocational individuals are not tuned to their social career responsibilities, society is moving more toward professional controlling systems in order to impose a more professional code of ethics (see Figure 1.3). There is a difference between ethical and legal rights. One may have a legal right to do something unethical, or an ethical right without any corresponding legal guarantee.

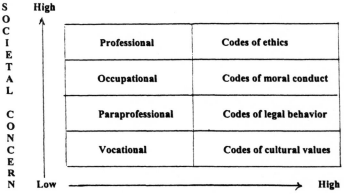

PERSONAL CONCERN

Figure 1. 3: Peoples' Perceptional Concern in Bioethics

Ethical rights are derived from a basis of criticizing legal rights. Legal rights exist independently from religious faith and humanitarian beliefs. Legal rights are derived from political ideologies. This means that political ideologies convert all socio-cultural and econo-political beliefs of nations into constitutions, judiciary systems, legislative enactments, case law, and executive orders of the highest bureaucratic officials in a nation. Beauchamp and Childress (1994) indicated that legal rights can be eliminated by lawful amendments or by a *coup d'etat*, but moral rights cannot be eroded or banished by political votes, powers, or amendments. For example, one of the major issues concerning human values is patenting bioscientific and biotechnological discoveries. To most people, the idea of body ownership by an individual may sound obvious without further explanation. People assume that their brains, hearts, lungs, kidneys, arms, legs, eyes, or all other somatic organs belong to them as long as they are alive. Nevertheless, people often complain that their genes, cells, tissues, eggs, ovaries, and stem cells which are isolated from their bodies by physicians, researchers, bioscientists, hospitals, biotech corporations, and governmental agencies are viewed as commodities to be bought or sold. In such a course of business transactions, the business of biosciences and bioetechnologies is to make a profit out of their discoveries. Therefore, bioscientific and biotechnological innovativeness becomes concerned with discovering and producing bio-products or services to be sold in order to make a profit. Biotech corporations, pharmaceutical companies, medical laboratories, hospitals, clinics, and medical groups' primary objectives are buying and selling materials and products, developing new products or services, increasing their market shares, extending longer product life cycles (PLCs), product positions, and other business activities, rather than with their moral and ethical duties to humanity. These types of business transactions convert biosciences and biotechnologies into biobusinesses.

Biotech corporations, pharmaceutical companies, and medical groups (e.g., HMOs, clinics, and universities) are trying to ask government to grant them patents for body parts or life; namely cloned human beings such as Eve. Through such a legal processing system, government can grant biotech and pharmaceutical companies and bioresearch centers patents that would enable them to store, cut, slice, and paste the human cells, genes, tissues, eggs, ovaries, limbs and other human and animal somatic organs and transplant them to other people's organs for profit.

The patent of human organs and life creates, no doubt, a very controversial ethical and moral dilemma. It goes beyond the limits of economical, political, and cultural value systems. It casts doubts concerning the ownership of human body parts and life controlled by governmental agencies, corporations, and individuals. Hildyard and Sexton (2000: 73) stated: "The push for patents on genes (or human organs) is not altruism... It is about privatizing the very basis of life. Biotech patenting has little to do with the public good and much to do with private greed."

FOUNDATIONS OF MULTIBIOETHICS

Bioethicalism means a healthy environment where everyone, regardless of his or her religious faith, cultural beliefs, political ideologies, ethnicity, color, or gender, has an appropriate, safe place in their particular society. In a humanistic society, people respect each other regardless of their differences and/or group affiliation. Therefore, multibioethicalism is the means of bioscientific and biotechnological collaborative participation among multicultures in humanity. It shares their mutual understanding for navigating the whole human life system towards a state of excellence.

The concepts and perceptions of multibioethicalism are lively and practical. These features are:

- Multibioethicalism can create a universal scientific sense of interdependence, interrelatedness, and above all correlated· human synergies. Multibioethical synergies seek an effort with combined performances that create greater efforts than the total of the sum of their parts.
- Multiethicalism is building a peaceful place for all cultural beliefs and human values. It is driving international relations towards civilized synergy, no valuable human thoughts, scientific efforts, and technological innovativeness to be given up or lost. There are four

foundational principals that should be considered in studying multibioethicalism: (1) religious faiths, (2) cultural beliefs, (3) political ideologies, and (4) universal human values.

Religious Faith

Religious faith is an emotional enforcement in believing reality. It is a meaningful reliance on a strong belief that psychologically can be used as reinforcement for a faith. Faith is for eradicating anxieties, to ceasing the self-doubt, and strengthening the belief in truthfulness, worthiness, and righteousness. Religious faith is the presumable factual reinforcement of the attitudes that peace and revelation (the reduction of fear, misery, and inferiority feelings) are the only ends for a human being. Finally, religious faith is an emotional and sensational fidelity and loyalty to a phenomenon, person, promise, and/or an oath. Failure to fulfill the obligation would be breaking the faith. For example, in somewhat the same way that the pantheist (the doctrine that God is the transcendent reality of the material universe and human beings are the only creatures who can perceive God everywhere) sees God in the trees and the birds and the very air, religious and/or political beliefs are also ubiquitous, albeit in more concrete forms.

Cultural Beliefs

Beliefs are inferences made by and observed about underlying states of expectancy. Beliefs seem to form the core conceptual ideas and opinions concerning the acceptability of something or to be denominated by some faiths. Sproul (1981: 204) defines: "A belief is understanding that represents credible relationships between objects, properties, and ideas." Beliefs are imbued with powerful emotional feelings. The fervor with which people hold their religious or dogmatic ideologies is good examples. Beliefs are viewed as confidence in the truth or existence of something not immediately susceptible to rigorous proof. In religious terms, beliefs are tenets to the acceptance of the truthful existence of God.

Political Ideologies

As a factual belief, human beings are living within two integrated environments:

- The natural (we can identify it as ecological)
- The artificial (we can identify it as a culture).

From the standpoint of a materialistic view, the ecological environment provides all organic elements, including human beings, animals, and plants, with the appropriate conditions to survive. However, the artificial environment provides specific human-made conditions to survive. Those conditions, which are authoritatively approved sets of political ideas, are called ideologies. Thus, the specificity of conditions of human ideas could be called ideologies. Political ideology is a set of diplomatic ideas, a formalized belief system that explains and justifies a preferred political order for society. Ideologies offer a socio-political and cultural strategy (processes, institutional arrangements, programs, and hierarchical power) for their attainment (Mullins, 1972: 498-511). For example, Lane (1962: 3-15), in his *Book of Political Ideology*, undertook to discover the latent political ideology of the American urban common man through in-depth interviews with fifteen American males. He described ideologies as "group beliefs that individuals borrow."

As Marger (1985: 16) indicated: "Ideologies comprise beliefs that, through constant articulation, become accepted as descriptions of the true state of affairs." Ideologies are worldviews, which are built upon and reinforced a set of powerful dominant class of beliefs and values in societal interactions. For example, the idea of progress, which has been a defining ideology in the traditional Western civilization, was built on a set of beliefs of capitalism. Capitalist ideology included economic efficiency, self-interest as a major motivator, and exploitation of resources through impersonal market mechanism. Capitalistic ideology has created enormous inequalities of wealth and opportunities among people and nations. On the other hand in the modern American democracy, the beliefs and practices of the ideology of democracy are a combination of popular sovereignty, political equality, and majority rule. American culture continuously seeks to reconcile these competing beliefs and values. However, Barrett (1991: 194) has found six notions in defining ideology, explained as:

- The opposite of material reality (illusory)
- A sublimate of material life-processes serving class interests (Class-bound)
- An expression of the dominant material relationships (Superstructure)
- A terrain of struggle resulting from material transformations (Revolution)
- Mediation between classes as a postponement of class rule (Bonapartism)
- Reification or mystification (Fetishism of Commodities)

In a multicultural analysis, in all of the above approaches, an ideology implies a thoughtful reality that concludes the subjectivity of the world in which we live.

Humane Values

Values are preferred and standardized expected modes of apperception and behavior in human civilization. Terpstra and David (1991: 106) defined:

> Values are priorities for sorting out the options and, when one has the will and the resources to do so, for implementing one code of behavior rather than others... Values direct society's people to selectively attend to some goals and to subordinate others.

They are the ways an individual expects all people to think and behave, when individuals are faced with a given situation. For example, in the field of bioethical value systems, in the Moslem faith, the human corpse is viewed as sacred. All organs of a dead body should be buried together in one grave. Even before burial ceremonies, the dead body needs to be cleaned and washed and all nails need to be taken off. The corpse needs to be wrapped in a clean white cloth. No part of the Moslem's dead body should be transplanted into another human being. Interestingly, in the Moslem medical schools, students are not allowed to use a Moslem's cadaver for their pathological experimental analysis. Moslem medical schools import their cadavers from those cultures that do not believe in sacredness of the human corpse; like Hinduism and Buddhism. Hindus and Buddhists cremate their dead bodies.

Values are rationally charged priorities for the sociability of an individual to be accepted in a society. An individual without values is assumed to be a savage. Values usually manifest the underlying assumptions of the surface behavior of people about faith, beliefs, trust, and confidence in self and others. Norms are expectations of ways people should ideally act, not anticipations of the ways people really will act. Values are expectations of proper behavior, not requirements for that behavior. There is a difference between cultural values and legal values. Cultural values are not published, may not even be obeyed, and cannot be enforced; but they are expected. Legal values are published and should be enforced (Hosmer, 1987: 82).

DOMAIN OF BIOETHICS

The evolution of integrated biological sciences and biotechnologies has brought many changes upon all aspects of our lives. Technology has allowed mankind to accomplish many remarkable things and put the standard of living in a progressive path of unknown destination. This is not a subjective guess in modern civilization. It is an objective one. It is a fact, in a scientific hypothetical assumption, to not only know when an objective's mean is true, but we also may deduct why the subjective end is true too. This is the reality of the unknown path of biopharmaceutical advancements and biotechnological developments.

The human species can no longer be subordinated to natural selection. It can be in a position to intervene in the natural selection. We no longer have to consider ourselves subject to the blind processes of natural selection. Biologist Dobzhansky (1967: 409) expressed his opinion this way: "Evolution needs no longer be a destiny imposed from without; it may conceivably be controlled by man, in accordance with his wisdom and technology." Those who are in favor of the advocacy of the biopharmaceutical excellent philosophy, favor diffusion of scientific advancements with socio-cultural practices of value systems that offer possibility of improving traits that we value human life. Despite all of the above progressive strategies, however, mankind is facing ethical and moral dilemmas.

Ethics in biosciences and biotechnologies starts up with dialogues during times of crisis. The ethical problems of biotechnologies always have social, legal, and economic aspects. We need the diffusion of scientific knowledge and ethical perceptions of different people from a variety of perspectives to deal with them sensibly. Medical research aims at relieving the suffering of people and restoring them to their normal health. Its focus on discovering the individual patient's causes of illnesses and their welfare is its primary concern (Munson, 1983: 246). The father of traditional medicine, Abu Ali Avicenna (980-1037) alludes to experiments on the human body, warning that patients should not be treated as mere means of experiencing for learning (Bull, 1959: 218). As we indicated before, in the eugenic system of donating gametes, in which banking is the dominant metaphor, sperm and eggs are naturally sorted by worth. We do not like to speak of eugenics anymore, but it is hard to not think of eugenics when people are actively seeking the very best genes money can buy (Rothman, 1999: A52). There are two objectives in eugenic biotechnologies:

- Positive perspectives of the eugenic sciences and biotechnologies. These positive perspectives call for increasing the number of favorable genes in the human population in order to move towards an excellence of the species super man or super woman.
- Negative perspectives of the eugenic sciences and biotechnologies. These negative perspectives call for decreasing the number of undesirable or harmful genes and/or cells in order to eliminate or reduce the number of those genes and/or cells that are responsible for various kinds of birth defects and sex-linked diseases (Munson, 1983: 378).

By viewing the above positive and negative objectives we may ask: What modes of genetic control by biologists might be possible? Biologists should recognize that the questions involved in biopharmaceutical and biotechnologies are more sociological than biological. Taviss (1971: 28) stated that there are three general types of genetic control that might be possible:

Euphonic: The treatment of genetic maladjustments in individuals by alteration or control of the expression of the existing genes.

Genetic Engineering: The change of undesirable genes through chemical or surgical intervention.

Eugenic: The recombination of genes already existing in population, either by encouraging the reproduction of favorable genes and gene combinations or by preventing the reproduction of defective or undesirable genes.

Of the above three genetic controlling systems, the eugenic seems to be most objectionable. As we said above there are two objectives in eugenic biotechnologies: (1) positive eugenic and (2) negative eugenic. The positive eugenic calls for increasing the number of favorable genes in the human population in order to move them towards an excellent species. Edward Tatum (1966: 60) has pointed out: "The simplest form of *euphonic engineering* is already standard human therapy... It should be pointed out that replacement of a missing or defective gene product also constitutes *euphonic engineering*." The positive eugenic calls for decreasing the number of undesirable or harmful genes in order to eliminate or reduce the number of those genes that are responsible for various kinds of birth defects and sex-linked diseases (Munson, 1983: 378). Nevertheless, both types of genetic controlling systems are exposed to serious technical problems. Technically, the eugenic is a difficult task because it would require the ability to single out the exact identity of the presence of undesirable gene.

It is peculiar to the fast pace of eugenic development, that bioscientists have assessed the effects of the *Book of Life*. Fisher (1996: D1 & D4) said: "In 1996, two billion of an estimated three billion base pairs connecting DNA's double helix have been sequenced by bioscientists. These code sequences are grouped into estimated 100,000 genes." Edmondson, Carey, and Hamilton (1996: 86) announced that: "These genetic markers are the signposts necessary to find genes involved in diseases. From a business point of view, each of these markers is a clue which might lead to a marketable drug."

The discovery that there are only 30,000 genes, instead of the 100,000 or so previously estimated to exist in humans made it clear that the new research frontier is not genes but proteins. This was the turning point in eugenic development that indicated that, until the completion of the human genome project, many scientists believed that there was a one-to-one relationship between genes and proteins. The new path of biological research discovery indicates that if researchers can precisely understand how proteins work, they may be able to control all of the body's functions. Although genes provide the basic script for life, scientists now acknowledge that they are too few in number to run the whole biological show.

Proteins are more enigmatic than genes. Genes are static; individuals carry the same set throughout their lives. Proteins are fickle; they may appear in the morning and disappear at night. Genes are natural sources of existence, while proteins are nurturing sources of existence. Cataloguing proteins would simply be a matter of getting each gene to express itself biologically (Griffith, 2001: 11).

IS BIOETHICS JUST A MYTH
OR A REAL LOGIC?

Since the ruling of the United States' Supreme Court concerning patents of genetic codes, it has been decided that although the knowledge of biotechnology is primarily knowledge of codes contained in human and animal cells, this is no reason to refuse a patent. Every year the United States issues thousands of patents on parts of the human genome. There is a fundamental question in bioethics as to whether it is ethical to effect a cure in such a way that the cure is passed on to the offspring of the people cured.

In the pre-modern world culture, people had two separate ways of perceiving, speaking, and acquiring knowledge. Greek scholars have called these views *mythos* and *logos*. *Mythos,* or myths, are specific types of descriptive stories that are involved with the realm of supernatural beings and are designed to explain some of the big issues of human existence, such as where we came from, why are we here, and how we account for the things in our world. They are, in other words, stories of our search for significance, meaning, and truth (Ferraro, 1995: 321). Myths deal with timeless truths and meanings as an ancient form of psychology (Gates, 2000).

The bioscientific and biotechnological innovativeness in American society is primarily concerned with profitability. On the other hand, profitability is a social contract. It is a contract between workers and capital holders or between bioscientists and biopharmaceutical and biotech corporations. On the other hand it is a legitimate agreement between society and organizations, whose mandate and limits are set by legal systems. If people believe in a universal cause for existence, then international moral rights exist without the need for legal fortification.

International bioethical law faces a number of problems that stem directly from the simple fact that sourcing carries a suspicious motive to be justifiable for a pluralistic gain. It carries a partisan message of distrust among ordinary people and technologists. Such a lack of confidence in its inherent ability gives little reason to provide international support by all involved parties.

The contemporary community of international bioresearchers and bioscientists are more than legal entities engaged in conducting research projects for profit. They are holistic embodiments of the multi-resources of the different nationalities who shape their existence. Many bioscholars, bioresearchers, biotechnologists, and bioscientists from all over the world invest their time and efforts in order to discover the mystery of life. According to the amoral myth of business, people are not explicitly concerned with moral and ethical transactions. They are not unethical or immoral; rather, they are being legal. The prominent business advisor Peter Drucker (1980: 191) has written: "Ethics is a matter for one's private soul." Biopharmaceutical and biotech investors believe business is business and since the nature of business is concerned with exploitation of profitable resources, there is no room for ethical and moral standards. However, a 1987 Conference Board survey of 300 companies worldwide provided alertness for the global market economy by addressing the international code of conduct for multinational corporations, specifically for biopharmaceutical corporations. This survey reveals several items as having widespread agreement (80 percent or more saying yes) as being ethical issues for global businesses: unauthorized payments; affirmative action; employee privacy; and environmental issues (Brook, 1989: 117; and Berenheim, 1987).

THE LOGIC OF BIOETHICS

Regardless of the different views on bioethics, in the postmodern culture, *logos* or logic deals with pragmatic realities. Logic or reason as a scientific type of realism deals with a dominative form of the modern cognitive study of human intention, objectives, and processes through six major stages: (1) acquisition of knowledge, (2) comprehension of problems, (3) analyzing factorial interrelated processes, (4) Synthesizing theoretical and pragmatic solutions, (5) formulating, selecting, and applying the viable and reliable solutions, (6) evaluating the consequential results of thinking and acting. The objectives in one stage are likely to make use of and build on the behaviors found in the preceding stages. While we are primarily concerned with the cognitive domain of conscience, we have done something to reveal the connectivity between the cognitive and pragmatic knowledge. This is the exact meaning of ethical behavior., Ethical logic is concerned with cognitive causes, pragmatic processes, and synthesized effects. Thus, the bioethical perceptions of biopharmaceutical and biotech corporations in the diffusive cognitive-pragmatic domain are largely characterized by a rather high degree of consciousness on the reality.

PHILOSOPHICAL AND SCIENTIFIC VIEWS OF HUMAN NATURE

People have always searched beyond their ages, probing the real and the universal image of finality. Their world-view helps them shed light on a variety of images in order to understand their natures and the entity in which they are living, perceiving, and proceeding. James Drane (1972: 99) stated: "Every ethic is founded in a philosophy of man, and every philosophy of man points toward ethical behavior." It is the conviction of human beings to integrate their holistic knowledge of humanity in order to discover their nature. Scientific trials without meaningful philosophical germination of moral and ethical convictions can end up with self-destruction. Any scientific intervention can change the nature of the human species. They can lead us either to enhance or to repress the human potential and human dignity. Eisenberg (1973: 214) states: "The planets will move as they always have, whether we adopt a geocentric or a heliocentric view of the heavens... But the behavior of men is not independent of the theories of human behavior that men adopt."

Although bioscientific and biotechnological discoveries have provided us with the ability to be able to discover the nature of our genes, ethics and morality are needed to provide us the real meaning of human identity. Human identity cannot be discovered in ignorance or prejudice, whether we believe that the universe is run by an absolute power (moral law of God), or by a natural force (universal law of cohesive entropy). The natural and cultural identity of human beings are conceived as:

- Somatic Identity
- Sensible Knowledge
- Emotional Expression
- Rational Behavior
- Intellectual Deliberation
- Informational Acquisition

Regardless of peoples' age, gender, marital status, and ability, all people do share similar somatic characteristics. The following descriptions will clarify the above characteristics.

Somatic Identity

The main ingredient of the formation of human identity starts with somatic cells that take part in the formation of the body. Through normal mutation, somatic cells become differentiated products into various tissues and organs (see Figure 1.4).

The concept of a somatic tendency view of human nature refers to the biological foundation of human consciousness that creates a derivative power to explain our experiences. Somatic tendencies manifest the individual's "selfhood." In other words, the somatic tendencies dictate the maleness or femaleness into the human mind to conceptualize the concepts of manhood and womanhood. Psychosocial tendencies through cognitive cultural value manipulation manifest self-worth. Cassirer (1956: 43) stated: "Man is... no longer in physical universe, man lives in a symbolic (self-worth image) universe."

A comprehensive analysis of peoples' lives must account for their physical nature, as well as the variety of their intellectual competencies. Although the ideas of *contextualization* and *canalization* echo that the physical body reflects a general materialistic trend within which an individual begins to develop, it also focuses on the relationship of the person to the things/objects in the immediate environment. *Contextualization* refers to being in a physical body in a contemporary post-industrial society, which is not different from being an individual during the early stage of the human culture on this planet (e.g., Neolithic or Homeric eras). *Canalization* refers to the tendency of interconnectivity of any organic system (e.g., the nervous system, the digestive system, the blood system and etc.) to follow certain developmental paths of behavioral patterns rather than others. In other words, a component of learned behavior can be channeled or influenced by biologically based pain and/or joy reflexes. All these characteristics can be affected by physiological and psychological needs.

Human somatic identity is made by the proper organization of atoms, molecules, cells, tissues, and organs during an individual's wet life span. The somatic wetness of human existence is the essence of the dynamic consciousness of human organs that is characterized by the synthesization of oxygen and hydrogenic molecules. Nevertheless, all human organs are constantly changing to revitalize their survival objectives through responding to their need-dispositions.

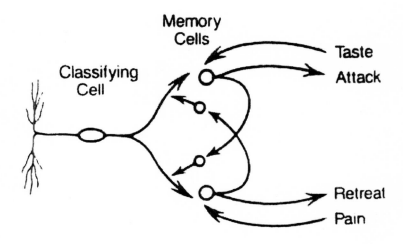

Figure 1.4: Development of Somatic Cells

Source: Trosko, J. E. (1984). "Scientific Views of Human Nature: Implications for the Ethics of Technological Intervention." In D. H. Brock and A. Harward (1984). *The Culture of Biomedicine: Studies in Science and Culture.* Vol. 1, Newark: NJ: University of Delaware Press: 76.

Needs are *deficiencies* of human organs. Needs are created whenever there is a physiological and/or psychological imbalance. Within the cybernetic nature of human beings, there are hierarchies of needs. There are two different perceptions concerning the cybernetic nature of human beings: (1) Skinnerian, (2) Wilsonian.

The Skinnerian approach leads rational planning ahead of time to adequately respond to the need disposition. In order to do that, it requires the establishment of psychosocial controlling systems in order to respond to spontaneous consequences (Skinner, 1953).

Wilson's (1978) sociological concept implies that the genetic information controls the potential human consciousness. Nevertheless, the natural dynamic properties of somatic identity (Parental differentiated DNAs) of a human being organize all somatic subunits (brain tissues, cells, enzymes, and so forth). The nature of human beings is a hierarchal structured system. Somatically, an individual is a collection of natural operative systems first, living things second, human beings third, members of a society fourth, and culture fifth.

If we think about ourselves, the majority of conscious behavior is acquired through learning and interacting with other members of our culture. Even those responses to our biological needs (e.g. eating, coughing, and digesting) are frequently influenced by our culture. In fact, the natural biological process of digestion is influenced by our behavioral perceptions.

Sensible Knowledge

Behavioral scientists such as Berelson and Steiner (1964: 87) generally acknowledged that: " (1) All knowledge of the world depends on the senses and their stimulation, but (2) the facts of raw sensory data are insufficient to produce or to explain the coherent picture of the world as experienced by the normal adult." The physical senses are considered to be seeing, hearing, touching, smelling, and tasting. There are many other so-called sixth senses, or we what have called them kinesthetic senses. The intuitive sensors pay attention holistically to the synergistic *contextualization* of the five senses and to what could be rather than to what actually exists.

The five senses are constantly interactive with numerous intrinsic and extrinsic forces of the physical body. However, the sensations deal chiefly with very elementary behavior that is determined by physiological functioning. Such a holistic deterministic bodily movement can be called *kinesthetic* sensation. In an individual's body the senses prefer to respond to the specific *canalized* needs and can become frustrated with vague instructions from the brain. It is relevant to add that a new integrated form of sensation is composed of the essence of all senses within the contextual boundary of the five senses with respect to the holistic movements of the physical body. Therefore, the *kinesthetic* sensation is the holistic (synergized) functional motions of human senses within a dynamic and intelligent environment. In this way, people use their somatic senses synergistically plus the cognitive potential of their brains (minds) to experience color, brightness, shape, loudness, pitch, heat, odor, taste, lightness, and weightless (in a kinesthetic sense).

Emotional Expression

Emotion is an experience of an affective state of consciousness in which joy, sorrow, fear, hate, love, and sympathy, or the like are manifested in human behavior. It is distinguished from cognitive and volitional states of consciousness. In addition, emotion is viewed as an agitation of the feelings which are actuated by experiencing certain emotive conditions and are usually accompanied by certain physiological changes, such as increased heartbeat, and respiration, and often overt manifestations, such as crying, shaking, laughing, and crying-shouting-laughing together. Emotion can be manifested as sadness, happiness, or a mixture of both.

Emotion is a vast magnitude of dimensions ranging from anxious, depressed, anger, insecure, and excitable at one end, to calm, enthusiastic, poised, and secure at the other. People in different cultures carry different connotations of emotion. Sociologists and psychologists have studied people on the basis of their race, ethnicity, age, and gender.

The term *emotion* is used to express feelings about certain objects, but not to make any assertion about them. Therefore, we can categorize people into two groups: *assertive* and *expressive*. *Assertion* is referred to the "cognitive" elements of thinking, and *expressive* is reserved for the emotive manifestation of feelings. However, ethical terms may not only express feelings, but they may also evoke feelings in others (Ayer, 1950: 107-108). In addition, the distinction between "expression of feeling" and "assertion of feeling" manifests two major states of group behavior: (1) *thinkers* and (2) *feelers*. The *thinker* views events in a quantified logical, objective fashion, whereas the *feeler* perceives events in a personal and value-oriented mission.

Rational Behavior

Human beings exist as an end in themselves, not merely as a means to be arbitrarily used by this or that will, but in all their actions, whether they concern themselves or other rational beings, must be always regarded at the same time as an end. Human beings, by their very nature, are very well organized. By the same token, they are organizers. They are called *persons*, because their very nature points them out as ends in themselves, which is something that must not be used merely as means. Human beings are *objective-ends* an end moreover for which no other can be substituted. The foundation of this principle is the rational nature of human beings.

Human beings by their very nature have always placed themselves as an end within nature. Such a maximal perception is consciously oriented because they have involved themselves in a universal cause of existence that carries the validity for every rational being. Therefore, human beings by their very nature never conceive themselves as a means, but as the supreme rational objective to achieve their survival ends.

Intellectual Deliberation

It is proper to speak about human intellectual proclivities that are part of our culture. Human beings are born into cultures that house a large number of domains such as discipline, crafts, and other pursuits in which one can become encultured and then be assessed in terms of the level of competence one has attained. There is a relationship between domains and intellectual abilities of human beings. More generally, nearly all domains require proficiency in a set of intellectual capabilities; and any intellectual ability can be mobilized for use in a wide array of culturally available domains. Socialization is one of the characteristics of *acculturalization* of human beings for acquisitioning of societal cultural wisdom. Intellectuality should be thought of as emerging from the interaction of three nodes:

- The individual with their own profile of intellectual capabilities and competence
- The domains (e.g., music, artistic, scientific and craftsmanship) available for study and mastery within a culture
- The judgments rendered by the societal cultural wisdom that is deemed competent within a nation

Human beings possess considerable intellectual potentials to be creative and innovative. Where is intellectuality? The answer is that intellectuality should be thought of as inhering principally in the brain, the mind, or the personality of a single individual. Specifically, an intellectual person is one who *regularly* uses effectively his/her intelligence to solve problems or fashion products in a *domain*, and whose work is considered both novel and acceptable by the community of scholars and scientists (Gardener, 1993: xvii).

For the purpose of understanding the fifth dimension of the human nature, we should identify two distinctive domains of knowledge: (1) *doxa* (what is believed to be true), and (2) *episteme* (which is known to be true). Knowledge, which is considered, as the main ingredient in human intellectuality, should be acquired it is more polemical. Therefore, an intellectual person is one that virtually searches for any scholarly attempt at acquiring knowledge to construed towards his/her scientific potential. However, some people use their potentials and others do not.

Informational Acquisition

In a sociological perception, informational systems have provided human beings superiority over the other five characteristics of human beings. It is human beings' conviction that each person must learn how to conceive of himself or herself and perceive others from both past and present. Human beings through their cross-cultural understandings have learned how to discover their real potential, but not to conceptualize their identity beyond finality. Human beings are committed to their survival cause of existence in order to adapt all perceptual aspects of their understandings to a meaningful conceptualized life style in days to come.

Almost all things that appear in a human's conceptual forms of understandings; metaphysically, epistemologically, axiologically, and aesthetically, are relative and comparative in humans' minds, because our world is pluralistic. Consequently, our cultures are becoming highly integrative. Human beings are living in a physical world where their priority objective is to understand its propensities. They can come to know these propensities well through long familiarity with real identities through *multiculturalism*. They sense an involvement with their physical world, which gives them the ability to predict which objects will fall, how well-known shapes look from other angles, and how much force is required to push objects against frictions. However, they lack corresponding familiarity with the forces on charged particles, forces in non-uniform dimensional forms, the effects of non-forecasted geometric transformation of high inertia and low-friction motion.

Human gene therapy, gene engineering, transgenetics cloning, and eugenic technologies are among many manipulative bioscientific and biotechnological endeavors. Biosocial scientific progress reports indicate that the potential use of animals as donors for human transplant has been a subject of controversial issue. Bioethicists indicate that putting animal organs into a human body raises the fear of the emergence of new diseases that could infect human cells. The concerns are real. A group of researchers recently demonstrated that the human cell infection in vitro with porcine endogenous retrovirus (PERV) has raised safety concerns for new therapies that involve the transplantation of pig cells or organs into humans. Dinsmore, Manhart, Raineri, Jacoby, Moore, and Diacrin (2000: 1382) have conducted studies to determine whether there is evidence for in vivo or in vitro transmission of PERV from fetal pig neuronal cells to humans. They found no evidence of PERV provirus integration in the DNA from PBMC of 24 neuronal transplant recipients. They confirmed that the results, demonstrated by both examination of transplant patient blood samples and in vitro studies, that there is no evidence for transmission of PERV from porcine fetal neural cells to human cells. Nevertheless, the side effects of such attempts in the long run are unclear. The HIV virus that has afflicted millions of people worldwide almost certainly originated in monkeys where, like PERV, it produced no ill effects in monkeys. Somehow, in crossing species, HIV became pathogenetic, setting off a deadly epidemic (Pilling 1999:3).

Juengst (1997: 125) summarizes bioscientific and biotechnological innovations this way:

> In the discussion of ethics of human gene transfer, two distinctions have become standard rhetorical tools. The first distinction separates interventions that will only affect somatic cells from interventions aimed at modifying human germ-line cells. The second distinction contrasts the

use of human gene transfer techniques to treat health problems with their
use to enhance or improve normal human traits.

Historically, from Hippocrates time until the early part of the Twentieth
century, biosciences and medical practices were not clearly distinguished from
experimental research. Biosciences and medical practices consisted primarily of
observing the causes, incubation, duration, diagnosis, treatment, prognosis, and
therapy of diseases through synthesized herbal medicine. Through careful
observation, scientists and physicians have experienced the efficacy, efficiency,
and futility of their attempts to generalize their positive efforts to have provided
adequate care to cure patients. However, bioscientific experiments in the
Twentieth century started to assess practical results of findings on the basis of
philosophy of benefit and do not harm. This new direction urged most
bioscientists and physicians to express their findings for the welfare of the future
generations (Jonsen 1998: 125).

CHAPTER 2

COMPARATIVE ANALYSIS OF MORALITY, ETHICALITY, AND LEGALITY*

CHAPTER OBJECTIVES

When you have read this chapter, you should be able to do the following:

- Define morality, ethics, and legality.
- Identify differences between ethical and moral definitions.
- Explain the ultimate objectives of moral behavior and codes of ethical conduct.
- Identify component parts of moral, ethical, and legal intentions and actions.

---

* This chapter is adopted from K. D. Parhizgar and R.R. Parhizgar (2006). *Multicultural Business Ethics and Global Managerial Moral Reasoning*. Lanham, MD: University Press of America, Inc.

- Describe speculative and practical moral, ethical, and legal knowledge.
- Understand the meaning of commitments.
- Know the meaning of ignorance, appetite, deceit, and greed.
- Analyze conscience awareness and cognitive judgments.
- Know the difference between choice and force.
- Know bioscientists and biotechnologists' rights and duties.

PLAN OF THIS CHAPTER

The primary concern of this chapter is to first define biomorality, bioethicality, and biolegality. Second is to identify bioethical ordinations in terms of two fundamental distinctions: (1) whether these phenomena are speculative understanding or (2) they are pragmatic knowledge. Speculative understanding of bioethics, which refers to a phenomenon or an object in which nothing is directly effective, and hence the phenomenon or object is placid; and pragmatic bioethical knowledge, on which the contrary, is concerned precisely with a phenomenon or an object insofar as it is dynamic and tangible. In addition, speculative understanding and pragmatic knowledge of bioethics are either for the sake an individual's *conscience awareness* and *cognitive judgments,* or for the sake of *formative* and *summative* knowledge applications to ordinate bioscientists, biotechnologists, bioinformationalists, and biomedical practitioners and their societal commitments. Striving for such judgmental perceptions mandates that people be involved within the context of intellectual deliberation, time, and often-legal costs. Such an ordinal judgment varies from person to person and culture to culture. Therefore, our initial concern in this chapter is to identify precisely what kinds of speculative bioinformation or biopragmatic knowledge are moral, ethical, and legal.

THE EFFECTS OF AWARENESS AND COGNITION ON BEHAVIOR

Conscience Awareness

For a long time emphasis was placed on the separation of bioethics from bioresearch. The assumption that bioethics was not a valid instrument for regulating bioresearch activities was based on a number of reasons. The first of these was the novelty of these kinds of problems and the speed of bio-techno-scientific advancements and developments. A second reason was that bio-techno-scientific research emerged in concrete situations, which made it difficult to solve particular somatic cases within the framework of general politico-economic norms. A third and final argument was the difficulty of integrating religious faiths, political doctrines, and cultural values to unify divergent moral and ethical conceptions concerning the present and future destination of humanity. These and other perplexities have emerged in the last few years through the recognition of serious problems caused by the lack of conscientiousness.

Conscience awareness in bioethics merely says that a scientist ought to fulfill universally worthy objectives. This type of commitment is contingent upon the affordability and solvency of those who are knowledgeable to deliberate their views without fear of retaliation by those who hold power. For example, Latif (2001: 132) indicated:

> The pharmacy profession is presently undergoing a paradigm shift from a product-focused profession, whose primary function I s prescription dispensing, to a more patient centered one, one which emphasizes a "shared" responsibility between the patient and pharmacist for optimal drug therapy outcomes. Pharmaceutical care reflects this shift and is defined as the responsible provision of drug therapy for the purpose of achieving definite outcomes that improve a patient's quality of life.

Such a new professional role mandates that pharmacists consider two important phenomena: choice and force. The relationship between a pharmacist and a patient is based upon a conscience awareness to acquire appropriate medical and health care knowledge from pharmaceutical companies and to provide patients' sufficient advisement and awareness concerning the positive and negative effects of prescribed drugs and/or over-the-counter pharmaceutical products. The connection between choice and force of the "will" is usually so close that the two seem to be one in the end. Since the choice is an intrinsic, deliberative voluntary will, it requires an individual to conform to conscious commitments. On the other hand, force is an extrinsic involuntary commitment to fulfill psychosocial demands. Therefore, a situation at the stage of complex moral, ethical, and legal decision and acts is based on the following conditions:

In relationships between pharmacists and patients both parties must, at a minimum, respect the universal moral rights for dispensing and consuming drugs. For the purpose of these purported rights, there are at least three conditions that must be considered:

- The rights must protect something of great mutual importance to both pharmacists and patients.
- The rights must be subject to substantial and recurrent opportunities and threats.
- The obligations or burdens imposed by the mutual rights must satisfy a fairness affordability test for both parties (Parhizgar and Jesswein, 1998: 141).

Within contextual analysis of the above conditions, many pharmacists are employed by business ventures. There often exists an inherent conflict between professional codes of ethics and business profitability demands. For example, the primary remuneration in the community setting comes from prescription dispensing. Because more time is required to perform patient-focused care activities (time that may take away from the revenue activities of the employer, prescription, dispensing), an ethical conflict may arise between professional and occupational commitments. Thus, the present reward system inherent in pharmaceutical practice may result in ethical ambivalence (Jensen and Von Glinow, 1985: 814).

In the field of the medical and health care industry, there are certain professional commitments such as diagnosis, treatment, prognosis, and therapy. Within such a process patients will be exposed to professionals, paraprofessionals, and occupationals; some of whom like physicians are under "professional codes of ethics" and others who are under "occupational codes of conduct," and "codes of behavior." What makes the difference between the three are the conscientious awareness and commitments to their professions and/or their occupations.

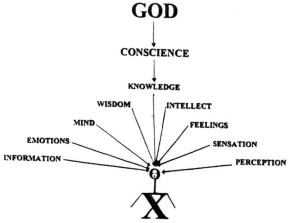

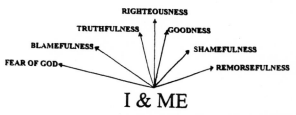

Figure 2.1: Theological Conceptions Concerning Understanding

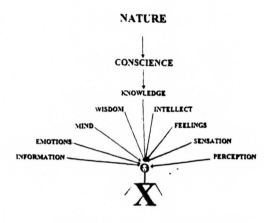

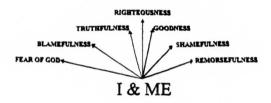

Figure 2.2: Existential Conception Concerning Understanding
Moral Codes of Behavior

By looking at Figures 2.1 and 2.2, we find that generally there are two groups of people: (1) those that who are religiously oriented and believe in "creation," and (2) those that who are known as existentialists and believe in "evolution." Both groups believe morality is a cognitive judgment between "I' and "Me." They base their judgments on conscience conception through acquisition of knowledge, intellectual deliberation, feelings, sensations, perception, emotions, information, mind setting, and wisdom for enhancing their moral codes of behavior through the fear of God, blamefulness, truthfulness, righteousness, goodness, shamefulness, and remorsefulness.

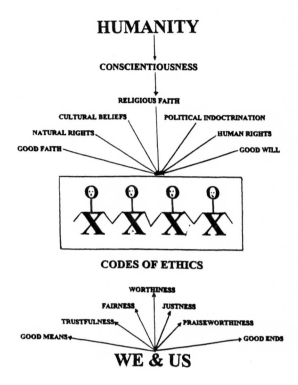

Figure 2-3: Cognitive Professional Codes of Ethics

Cognitive Judgments

Cognition is the insightful knowledge by which people express their judgments about conceiving an object or an event in a rational way. The cognitive, rational, or intellectual component of an attitude is what most people understand to be the reason for an expression of self-behavior based upon conscious awareness, knowledge, and understanding.

Attitude is the positive and free will aspect of human behavior. An attitude utilizes conscious awareness such as expectancies, demands, and incentives. Since cognition is based on conceptual rational judgments, an attitude is based upon holistic feelings, thought, and behavior. Attitude is differentiated from the reality of past experiences.

By looking at Figure 2.3 we will find that codes of professional ethics are based upon conscientious commitment to truthful judgments. It is based upon acquisition of goodness for the sake of humanity. Professionals follow the path of altruistic commitments to serve humanity beyond of their self-interest. A professional individual's cognitive professional judgment is based upon holistic perceptions of good faith, natural rights, human rights, civil rights, cultural beliefs, and in some cases religious faith through implantation of good means, good ends, trustfulness, fairness, worthiness, justness, and praiseworthiness.

Cognitive information is based on truth and reality. Cognitive perception is a purposive behavior that is directed toward understanding the real nature of an object, a phenomenon, or an event. For example, in the field of biomedical practice, specifically in the field of forensic research; the cognitive judgment concerning negligence, dishonesty, and perjury depends on conditional situations and purity of samples and information, which creates a problem with cognitive perceptions, in that cognitive perceptions are based upon socio-scientific conditions, cultural orientations, and psychological understanding of the cause-effect of some attributions. This variation in cognitive perception is based upon perceptual judgment and becomes very subjective. Nevertheless, the cognitive perceptual component of an attitude may be logical or illogical, rational or irrational, and/or relevant or irrelevant to an object. This perceptual knowledge may be true, partially true, or totally false. For example, pharmaceutical companies are committing more resources to promoting prescription drugs to consumers. Most notably, they hold thousands of educational meetings each year and invite physicians to attend such meetings to listen to lectures about specific drugs and their uses. Do you find any ethical and moral dilemma in such programs? Findlay (2002: 23) reported:

> Drug companies hosted an estimated 314,000 educational events in 2000 at a cost of 1.9 billion, up from 280,000 in 1999 at a cost of $1.68 billion and 70,000 events (at unknown cost) in 1993... A 1999 FDA telephone survey of 1,081 consumers found that three-quarters remembered seeing a prescription drug ad in the previous three months, mostly on TV. About 25% who had seen an ad said they had asked a doctor about a condition or illness referred to in the ad; 13% asked for a specific drug and about half got it.

BEHAVIORAL ORDINATIONS

Getting ourselves intellectually out of the state of nature is simply a matter of good sense and reason. Hobbes (1588-1679) said the state of nature is the beginning point for our development. The ending point is our intellectual deliberations. There are three major behavioral *orders* of reasons for people who strive to achieve a common good through a common good cause: (1) constructive ideas, (2) valuable contents, (3) cultivation of a sense of commitment. Ordination of reason signifies the establishment of cognitive and pragmatic orders to search for proper ends through good means. Not all ordinations can establish practical patterns of expected worthy intentions and actions. One kind of ordination gives you "constructive ideas," another kind offers you "valuable contents," and the other one binds you with "decisive commitments." These are rooted in variations of generalization, understanding, defining fundamental principles, and the distinctive outcomes of our natural life. The various ordinations for the bioscientists and biotechnologists' behavioral ethical, moral, and legal means and ends are the three major topics in this chapter. In addition, the notions of sensational and emotional achievements, rational happiness, and the means and ends in bioethics will be discussed in the following pages.

Constructive Ideas

We are what we either positively and/or negatively think. Whatever we conceive and perceive is determined by our ability to think critically. If our thinking is overly unrealistic, our cognitive judgments will lead us to a fantasized world. If our thinking is overly optimistic, it will enhance our intellectual ability to recognize the real characteristics of things in which we should properly rejoice. If individuals think about their life positively, they will feel positive about it and they will be able to pursue a fruitful life. The most important source of critical thinking within the contextual domain of our identity is conscientious awareness. It explicitly puts our intellectual ability into words, phrases, and ideas.

Conscientious awareness provides us with a psychological reinforcement within our personality in order to express our identity and autonomy. Also, conscientious awareness facilitates critical thinking to make corrections in our judgments. The truth is that since very few people realize the powerful role of critical thinking, they can gain a significant command over their independent thinking. Such a superlative spiritual characteristic allows an individual not to be victimized and/or harmed by ignorant, greedy, and selfish people.

Valuable Contents

Life is swiftly changing. With each passing day, we care confronted with new challenges. The pressure to cope with those challenges is very intense. New global realities are deeply affecting our lives. We need to think first and then act, not act first and then think. Critical thinking inspires people to move towards novelty through learning, analyzing, and experiencing new things.

Ordinary people are accustomed to habitual, automated, and fixed procedures. They are afraid to change, because they do not desire to progress and develop their intellectual abilities. They are satisfied with what they have learned and are accustomed to doing them over and over. These types of people are viewed as imitators, because they do not convince themselves to think critically. On the other hand, there are exceptional critical thinkers, bioscientists and biotechnologists; who strive to reveal the truths. They are curious to discover novel truth. These scientists are innovators. Nevertheless, these groups' of codes of conduct are based on constitutional law of their nations that are conducting their research projects.

By looking at Figure 2.4, we will find sources of codes of legal conduct through human rights, civil law, criminal law, common law, code law, statutory law, executive law, reward and punishment law, and institutional promotion and demotion.

Critical thinking is very complex. It requires a periodic radical revision in adaptability to divergent points of view. The world in which we now live requires us to continually and rapidly reevaluate, reanalyze, and relearn innovative techniques. In short, there is a new world facing us everyday. In order to be able to digest new changes, we need to critically and periodically enhance our judgments with the power of the mind to command it, to process itself, and to determine how to increase the quality of our work and our lives.

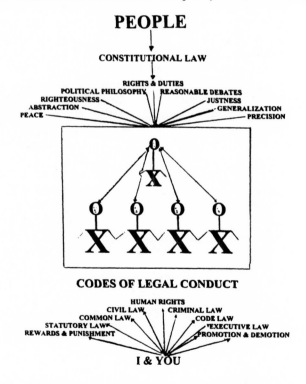

Figure 2.4: Occupational Codes of Legal Conduct

Cultivation of a Sense of Commitment

The ability to define and to set priorities concerning the ethical and moral mandates in the field of bioethics requires the cultivation of a sense of commitment. Bioscientists and biotechnologists need to establish commitments in their behavior during the decision-making processes and actions and to quickly analyze their research projects' outcomes rationally rather than just sensationally or emotionally. Commitment to ethical, moral, and legal principles in the scientific community is as old as human civilization (e.g. the Socratic Oath in medicine). However, including ethics in biosciences and biotechnological curriculum programs and practices is new. Ethical philosophers advocated measuring each ethical transgression against a universal ethics of sincerity; actions which are appropriate to the spirit of interdependence and, hence, promote harmony in specific relationships are right behavior.

In the modern cosmocratic societies, power would follow professional functions rather than property or the consent of the governed. In supporting this proposition, Lilla (1980: 5) urged that pragmatic ethics should be taught to professional students in order to do the right things through the duties and virtues of democratic moral behavior. For Lilla, the correct behavioral virtues are rather obvious: courage, tenacity, and prudence. Lilla would have ethics instructors be, first of all, good human beings who preach, witness, and exemplify what is moral.

In order to be committed to the ideal of professional knowledge, we need to understand the nature of professions. Scientifically, all professions do not follow a generic methodology to learn and perform their jobs. They require the theoretical and pragmatic acquisition of different levels of data, information, and knowledge. They require different types of searching, learning, and applying data, information, and knowledge when they make the best sense to acquire them. What all professions have in common are ethical and moral responsibilities and commitments to preserve their professional integrity. Professionals need sincere commitments to preserve the sanctity of their professions. They need commitments to fair-mindedness in order to minimize human suffering. They should be committed to a more just world and serve rational rather than irrational ends. In the field of bioethics, we have observed how some bioscientists, through the manipulation of interest groups, converted their intellectual career to crime. Those bioscientists, and biotechnologists who have developed and promoted biological and chemical warfare have betrayed their professional ethical and moral commitments and become criminals against humanity. Such criminal practical unprofessional activities were due to a lack of intellectual virtues and to a tendency to violate the public trust and to betray the sanctity of their intellect. These indicators should make us worry about where we look for probable weaknesses and how to recognize likely strengths in all professions. Also, we need to understand the differences between the ideal of professional commitments and the manner in which professionals practice their professions in the real world.

SEPARATION OF MORAL AND ETHICAL BEHAVIOR

Let us first begin our discussion with how we perceive morality and ethicality. Then we can link morality and ethicality to legality. By looking at Figure 2-5, we may understand the differences among the terms and processes of these phenomena.

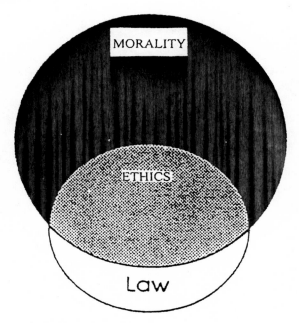

Figure 2.5: Interrelatedness of Morality, Ethics, and Law

Within the analytical domain of this chapter, we have raised some questions concerning the main domain of moral, ethical, and legal understanding as follow: Do we perceive the common understanding, of moral, ethical, and legal ordinations primarily as *speculative* understanding or do we view them primarily as the *pragmatic* knowledge of how to behave according to the commonality of our cultural beliefs? In other words, are moral, ethical, and legal contemplations serving the intellectual means for our behavioral ends, or are we examining the people's behavioral manifestation of their thoughts and emotions as the prime objectives for achieving our ends? These questions are not simple to be answered. If we presume that moral virtues, ethical values, and legal principles are practical in the sense that they are considered, then how should people's intentions and actions be coordinated. In general terms, we are examining the nature of moral, ethical, and legal intentions and actions (see Tables 2-1 and 2-2).

Table 2.1: Analysis of Positive Perceptual Attributions of Religious
Faiths, Moral Judgments, Ethical Behavior, and Legal
Actions

Perceptual Attributions	Positive Attitudes	Expected Consequences (Earthly)	Expected Consequences (Heavenly)
Religious Faith: Family Orientation	Virtuous intentions	Conscious awareness	Spiritual revelation
Moral Judgments: Individualistic Orientation	Conscientious normative judgments	Syllogistic reasoning for philanthropic helps	Universal order of goodness and tranquility
Ethical Behavior: Pluralistic Orientation	Conscious cognitive behavior	Social praiseworthiness and honorable reception	Blessing wishes and solemn ritual happiness
Legal Decisions and Actions: Collectivistic Orientation	Meritorious compliance, jurisprudence, sociological jurisprudence, and legal realism jurisprudence	Material goodness; peace of mind; advocacy for just, fair, and right decisions and actions	XXX

In order to understand the holistic means and ends of bioscientists and biotechnologists, we need to define morality, ethics, and legality, and their applications in human relations. Understanding human thoughts and activities is impossible without defining their theoretical and practical boundaries. This is true of bioethics and biomorality. Whatever the advantages are, a shared meaning does two things. First, it allows us to insure that all meanings and attributes mean the same thing when discussants and practitioners use a term or refer to an idea. Second, we closely ally this to the first so that discussants and practitioners can pursue carefully defined terms. Therefore, many philosophers and social scientists expend much effort analyzing and defining ethics, morality, and legality. These phenomena address what are truthfulness and falsehood, goodness and evil, rightness and wrongness, justness and unjustness, honestly and dishonestly, responsibility and irresponsibility, fairness and unfairness, worthiness and worthlessness, and the like.

Table 2.2: Analysis of Negative Perceptual Attributions of Antagonistic Beliefs, Immoral Judgments, Unethical Behavior, and Illegal Actions

Perceptual Attributions	Negative Attitudes	Expected Consequences (Earthly)	Expected Consequences (Heavenly)
Antagonistic Beliefs: Family Orientation	Sinful and Filthy intentions	Conscious remorse and condemned intentions	Godly Dissatisfaction and forbidden intentions
Immoral Judgments: Individualistic Orientation	Shameful, improbable, and faulty judgments	Damned reactionary vindication	Psychological exonerated punishment
Unethical Behavior: Pluralistic Orientation	Blameworthy and condemned reactions	Social hatred and abhorrent abominations	Presumption of eternal painful, distressful,\ and miserable life
Illegal Decisions and Actions: Collectivistic Orientation	Chaotic, anarchic, terrorist, fraudulent, criminal, defaulted, deceptive, and corruptive conducts	Punishment, imprisonment, fine, torturous, exoneration, and execution	XXX

The distinction between conscientious objectives marks the prevailing virtue of the intellect and wisdom of human beings over the mind and conscious behavior of the body. Both make morals and ethics different. In making a distinction between morality and ethics, we discover that the challenge of morality consists of intellectual generalization in universal reasoning, and that the challenge of ethics exists more in the stimulation of its question than in the finality of its answer. Moral absolutism, which assumes that all moral issues can be measured by one universal standard regardless of cultural, religious, and political differences, has been offered as an alternative view to ethical relativism.

Etymologically, religious faiths, political ideologies, and cultural values are the three foundations of moral and ethical views among people. They have different meanings and perceptions concerning what is the common good for individuals and groups. Most writers have stated that the term *moral* is essentially equivalent to the term *ethical*. Albert, Denise, and Peterfreund (1984) state that: "Etymologically, these terms are identical, the former (moral) being derived from the Latin word *mores*, the latter (ethics) from the Greek word *ethos*, both words are referring to customary behavior." Both terms may be used with two different antonyms. Ordinarily, the opposite of moral is taken to be immoral, so that we mean by a moral person, one who is good and does what is right, and by an immoral person, one who is bad and does what is wrong. However, moral may also be used in a wider sense to refer simultaneously to right and wrong thoughts and actions. Then, morals' antonym is *amoral*. In this usage, people are moral in the sense that certain of their actions are subject to judgments of right and wrong. The same analysis may be used with the term ethical: Its antonym may be either unethical; that is, it may refer to what is wrong, or it may have as an antonym unethical, in which case it would apply to objectives that are not subject to moral or ethical evaluation.

In some cases people believe in *amoral* behavior. An amoral behavior relies on a partial truth while it conceals a good deal of the whole truth. According to this philosophy, people are not explicitly concerned with ethics. They are concerned with law. They do not consider themselves as unethical or immoral; rather they are *amoral* as far as they feel that ethical considerations are inappropriate in their activities (De George, 1995: 5).

There is still another sense of understanding in that the words ethics and morals are used differently in other cultures. For example, in the Persian culture the words *Akhlagh* for ethics and *Khooy* for morality have been perceived separately through the philosophy of *Eshragh*; illuminationism. Illuminationism means that the intellectual enlightenment should search for revelation through truthful scriptures. This behavior is based upon the divine inspiration of truth and the observation of rational and logical reasoning for the blessing in earthly life and revelation in eternal life after death (Parhizgar, 2002: 297). Therefore, discovering the intellectual truth and acting on the whole truth can provide soundness in behavior.

The Buddhist cultural value system involves paying attention to *mundane* (such as earthly refinement) and individual problems (such as health), to salvation, and to morality. There are many facets related to such an ethical and moral goodness. Seen from this perspective, the dominant view in the Asian culture is *monistic*. *Monism* is a doctrine in which moral and ethical behaviors are considered as ultimately one unit of reality. Therefore, in such a cultural perception, there is no separation between morality and ethics (Yinger, 1970: 45).

Shaw (1996: 4) stated:

> In everyday parlance, we interchange 'ethical' and 'moral' to describe people we consider good and actions we consider right. And we interchange 'unethical' and 'immoral' to describe what we consider bad people and wrong action.

French and Granrose (1995: 9) stated:

> We use these terms (ethics and morality) interchangeably between the words ethics and morals are that the first is derived from Greek word, the second from a Latin one. Both words originally referred to the customs or habits of a society or an individual.

As we have seen, there is no agreement among philosophers and scholars in regard to a unified and generalized definition concerning the phenomena of morals and ethics. Some people object to the term ethics and prefer to characterize ethical problems as religious problems. For example, in the American culture, the subject of business ethics refers to legal market liability, business and external environment, and corporate responsibility. The Germans prefer to call it *"Wirtschaftsethik,"* which exactly translated means the ethics of relationship between economics and society.

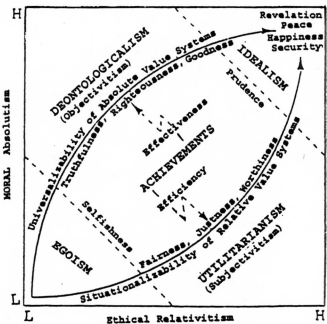

Figure 2.6: Taxonomy of Moral and Ethical Achievements

On the other hand, some philosophers and scholars make a distinction between morality and ethics. They define "morality" as referring to human conduct and values and "ethics" as referring to the study of those areas. Walton (1977: 6) defined ethics as a critical analysis of human acts to decide their rightness or wrongness in terms of two major criteria: truth and justice. De George (1995: 19) perceived:

> Morality is a term used to cover those 'practices and activities' considered importantly right and wrong; the rules that govern those activities; and the values that are embedded, fostered, or pursued in those activities and practices... Ethics is a systematic attempt to make sense of our individual and social moral experience, in such a way as to determine the rules that ought to govern human conduct, the values worth pursuing, and the character traits deserving development in life.

Oesterle (1957: 5) defined: "Ethics is the science which deals with those acts that proceed from the deliberative will of man, especially as they are ordered to the end of man." As ethics is formally practical knowledge, morality is the sound knowledge of what constitutes good or bad actions.

Through a spiritual aesthetic view, morality is the very delightful, intelligible, and beautiful conscious awareness. It is an individual's knowledge. Many people feel that morality is personal and that no one should force their views on others. According to this position, people are entitled to their own personal moral understandings and judgments. In contrast, many people hold another position with respect to different countries and cultures, and believe that all members of a society must abide by their cultural values. This view is another popular form of ethical relativism. They deserve careful attention in defining and applying these terms. We need to clarify moral as a matter of an individual's choice and ethics as a matter of the popular cultural valuable force that determines what action is right or wrong. Furthermore, are morals and ethics culturally determined by an individual and/or by a group? Is there a universal morality to be applied to all people in different places and times around the globe? For the clarity of these positions we need to define carefully the terms of morality, ethicality, and legality (see Table 2.3).

WHAT IS MORALITY?

Before we consider specifically what makes an action good or bad in a moral sense, we should have a precise picture of the notion of morality itself. How we can define morality? Ernest Hemingway (1932: 4) once said: "What is moral is what you feel good after and what is immoral is what you feel bad after."

Table 2.3: Analytical Comparative Description of Moral, Ethical, and Legal Perceptions

MORALITY	ETHICALITY	LEGALITY
Psychosocial concern for excellence	Sociocultural concern for goodness	Econo-political concern for peace and harmony
Morality is the matter of an individual's choice	Ethics as the matter of cultural valuable norms	Legality is the socio-political mandated enforcement
Spiritual concern for happiness	Passionate concern for social satisfaction	Prudential concern for a secured life
Conscious concern for self-enhancement	Conscious concern for self-refinement	Citizen concern for social development and growth
Religious concern for revelation	Humanitarian concern for community welfare	Obligatory concern for community ordination
Fear of God and shameful self-blame	Fear of social group condemnation	Fear of court's punishment and fines
Conceptual faith for mental synergy	Societal beliefs for behavioral energy	Legal expectation for profitable prodigy
Universal concern for intellectual power	Natural concern for appetitive power	Legal concern for legitimized power
Searching for the ends of self-excellence	Searching for the means of self-confidence	Searching for the minimal means and ends of goodness
Building individual dignity and loyalty toward trustfulness	Building collective integrity and loyalty toward worthiness	Building personal records of decriminalization
Developing and maintaining emotional virtues	Developing and maintaining intellectual values	Developing and maintaining the notion of common interests
Humanitarian sensibility for goodness	Humanitarian concern with intrinsic fairness	Citizenship concern for extrinsic concern of common justness
Qualitative assessments of self behavior with heavenly rewarded expectations	Quantified assessment of self and others' behaviors with respect to human dignity	Quantified assessment of an individual's rights with human rights

In a narrow sense, morality refers to a particular personal judgment concerning right in contrast to wrong, conveying a strong sense of assertion or rejection. Frankena (1963: 6) defined: "Morality is a social institution of (personal) life, but is one which promotes rational self-guidance or self-determination." Biomorality means that an individual's conscious is an intrinsic potential power to serve humanity beyond self-interest; altruism. An individual who continually violates the moral standards of his or her consciousness can weaken the bond of reciprocal altruism, and such behavior cannot be tolerated indefinitely.

What is the basis of morality? Does morality have a distinctive foundation or is it merely a matter of social convention and tradition, or a matter of an individual's taste and opinion? Any moral definition or principle contains cognitive elements in conceiving and supporting reasoning. This is what we are dealing with. Moral reasoning is an appeal to establish moral principles. Both moral reasoning and moral principles are involved in determining moral character and action.

The term morality signifies primarily a certain relation of an individual's acts that have some ends, as to a standard or principal of action. Morality, therefore, is an abstract signifying the moral order of an individual's acts. Is morality considered the same as prudence? The answer is no. Whately (1859: 68) defined prudence as whatever is done wholly and solely from motives of personal expediency; the calculation of individual loss or gain is always accounted a matter of prudence, and not of morality. When someone submits himself or herself to the will of another person merely because it is in his or her interest, or because they dare not to resist, we never call it morality, but merely prudence. For example, if you were offered good wages for doing something in favor of your employer, and against your subordinates, you might think it expedient to accept the offer, but you would not account it as a moral duty. Newton and Schmidt (1996: 3) have defined morals or morality as: "The *rules* that govern our behavior as persons toward other persons; also, duties."

As indicated before, the term moral is derived from the Latin word *mores*. *Mores* means the embodiment of fundamental individual values. There are two main traditional fields of value inquiry: *morals*, which is concerned with the problems of truthfulness and falseness, worthiness and worthlessness, and goodness and badness, and their bearing on moral conduct, as opposed to which *ethics* we have already defined as being concerned with the problems of justness and unjustness, fairness and unfairness, and righteousness and wrongness and their bearing on societal ethical decisions and actions.

Morality means conformity to the rules of universal right conduct. For example, the term honesty is a universal phenomenon. In all cultures, honesty means to be truthful. An honest individual has been praised in all cultures. Therefore, there are some values among all people around the globe, which are universal, and these universal values are considered as the foundational principles of humaneness. In addition, if we are judging bribery as a moral term, we arrive at the same conclusion: bribery corrupts an individual's character, defects the group's cultural value systems, and is wrong. However, if bribery is a common practice in a given culture, then is it proper to engage in bribery in that country? This raises questions about the distinction between ethics and morality.

Morality is a term used to manifest humanity's universal virtues. ·Virtues refer to the excellence of intellect and wisdom and to the disposition of the cognitive mind to perform its proper function effectively. Moral virtues are concerned with the habitual choices of rational thoughts in accordance with universal logical principles. The contemplation of absolute truthfulness and the discovery of the rational principles that ought to control everyday actions, have given rise to the intellectual virtues. The distinction between goodness and badness, truthfulness and falseness, and worthiness and worthlessness is called moral consideration. For example, moral people may consider goodness if they habitually think, value, and act in accordance with their intellectual conscience.

Sincerity in continuity of moral thoughts and acts is the keynote for morality. In other words, the meaning of moral is one to which a moral individual aspires (De George, 1995). Morality denotes the total characteristics of intellect and wisdom of an individual. The maxim of the intellect and wisdom is a careful calculation of virtues in the mind or a description of the essential features of righteousness, truthfulness, and goodness in the character of a human being. Thus, when we speak of morality, we refer to a human's personal virtue through their intellectually excellent choices.

As human beings, we can make a distinction between true and false, and right and wrong. Therefore, we can make a distinction between the end results of morality and ethics. Morality's end result through intellectual truthfulness, righteousness, and goodness of thoughts and actions is revelation and happiness.

Wisdom and the intellectual ability of the mind and passionate activities of the body that can be considered right and wrong is the main contextual domain of morality. The rules that govern an individual's thoughts, and the values that are embedded in intellectual and rational virtues are the subject of morality. Therefore, morality is a universal, general, and intellectual characteristic of humanity.

Distinct from both the real (natural) order of existing things and the logical (intellectual) order formed by human reason is the moral order. Both orders are caused by reason. It is within this context that the term morality is introduced as understanding formally an orderly thought which wisdom has established as a rational reason in human acts. However, an individual's tendencies toward pleasure can change such rationalized thoughts and behaviors and divert them into passionate desires.

An individual's passion depends on a variety of circumstances and conclusive end-results. *Passion* is a motivational principle and tendentious operational factor in an individual's daily behavior. We act because of joy or sorrow, love or hatred, and success or failure. It is obvious that an individual's behavioral effects are accompanied by pleasure or pain, joy or sorrow, happiness or unhappiness, and courage or fear. All of these consequential motives are related to our intentional and tendentious attainment of personal objectives.

For behavior to be ethical and moral, individuals need to strive for excellence. Excellence in behavior is a virtue. Virtue is a positive derivative of the power of the mind toward happiness. Virtue is neither a passion nor a power. It is an extreme of excellence, rising above excess and effect. Virtue regulates behavioral pleasure. It is the disposition of the intention toward good actions in a regular manner. For example, when we avoid good behavior pain follows, or when we strive for happiness, a satisfactory end-result follows.

What is morality, given that it occupies such an unchallengeable place in our "mind?" Simply stated, morality consists of those family virtues that enhance all family members' activities. Such enhancements are the boundaries of sacrifice, tolerable efforts for children's security, and guarantee prosperous happiness for their future. Whatever it may be, morality is at least the following:

Morality Is Defined: Morality is a means to cope with surrounding deficient social behavior by providing enhanced advisory methods for understanding and behaving toward a virtuous end. When moralists try to define morality, they include all excellent human characteristics toward a happy life. The ultimate objective of morality is achieving excellence in mind and behavior, in an individual's societal life, and revelation after an individual's death.

Morality Is a Conscience Living Phenomenon: Our primary perception of morality is based upon self-trial within an individual's intellectual mind-body court system presided over by our conscience. It is an individual's defense in deciding for himself or herself what is true and what is false, what is right and what is wrong, what is worthy and what is worthless.

Morality Is What One Learns: Morality is not genetic or biological, it is relatively perceived as foundational learning objectives and as permanent virtuous objectives in an individual's thinking and behavior resulting from understanding and experiencing what happiness is. Most moralists agree that human beings are moral in nature because of the inherited intellectual wisdom of the human species. The most widely studied determinates of human intellect are biological, social, and cultural value understandings. Biology influences certain intellectual characteristics in a number of ways. Our genes help determine many physical righteousness characteristics, and these may in turn affect our intellectuality. It is very difficult to separate nature from nurture. The term nature denotes all genetic characteristics that people acquire from their parents and environments through their physical identity. The term nurture means all parental affection, protection, and attitudes towards happiness for themselves and their children. Children learn from their parents how to value, how to believe, and how to behave towards themselves and others. Although learning from parents does not necessarily imply a positive or negative attribution in an individual's behavior, you may learn, for example, through your family behavior to be a straight-faced truthful person or a straight-faced liar, or a pathological altruistic person or selfish liar. The changes resulting from family moral orientation is viewed as a life long process.

Morality Isn't Accidental: Morality is a continuous intellectual deliberation concerning the achievement of a state of excellence. It is not what one does that counts, but what one does *conscientiously* in thinking and behaving towards excellence. Promoting an individual's excellence by mistake isn't being moral. Giving money through corrupted people to charity isn't charity. In reality, it is deception.

Morality Requires Intellectual Deliberation: Judgmental perceptions on successful or unsuccessful conclusions within the environmental conditions without intellectual deliberation on life events are not sufficient. Conscientious experimental trials can provide people with virtuous solutions. We all are born as unreflective thinkers, fundamentally unaware of the role that intellectual thinking is playing in our lives. Gradually, we learn how to think and act. Paul and Elder (2002: 47) believed that development of thinking is a gradual process requiring plateaus of learning and hard work. They believed thinkers should pursue their life-long journey through six stages:

- Unreflective Thinking (we are unaware of significant problems in our thinking)
- Challenged Thinking (we become aware of problems in our thinking)
- Beginning Thinking (we try to improve, but without regular practice)
- Practicing Thinking (we recognize the necessity of regular practice)
- Advanced Thinking (we advance in accordance with our practice)
- Master Thinking (skilled and insightful thinking becomes second nature)

Morality Is a Manifestation of Self-Identity: We are living in a cryptomoral environment in which some groups of people admire smart criminals and charming cons or corrupted persons for fun not only in movies, but also on TV news shows. In addition, we are tempted to be attracted to people who break the virtuous rules. People should know consciously what is going on in their personal lives and surroundings. To be moral is an unquestioned good. What makes our moral identity is the line between purity and arrogant egocentrism. We need to understand the consequences of the self-motivations concerning self-deception, self-contradiction, and self-interest.

Figure 2.3: Stages of Critical Thinking Development

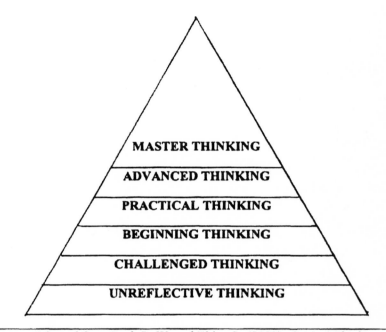

Source: Adapted from Paul, R. W. and Elder, L. (2002). *Critical Thinking*. Upper Saddle River, NJ: Prentice Hall, (2002), 48.

SPECULATIVE MORAL UNDERSTANDING

Purely speculative understanding of the right things through good will on the part of an individual depends on knowing the natures of the goodwill and the good people. This means that moral virtues, and ethical valuable thoughts and behaviors, are sought on the part of both the domains of a phenomenon and/or an object as "*known* in reality and as *knower*; an ethical and moral individual. In the field of medicine for example, cancer is a killing disease. Pathologists, who are morally, ethically, and legally responsible for examining the biopsy tissues of a patient, need through their good will and intentions to reveal the truth. If they neglect and/or intentionally ignore the known degenerated symptoms of tissues, then they are not performing their jobs with professional good will and intention as knowers. The nature of the cancer (as a killing disease) is not good, but the task of pathologists (as knowers) is good because they do have good will and intention to reveal the truth in order to save lives of patients. Therefore, if pathologists inform the patients' of the bad news, this does not mean that pathologists have bad will and intention. However, in other cases such as in *euthanasia* and physician-assisted suicide the actions of physicians are based on bad faith, bad intention, and bad will. Euthanasia is the administration of a lethal agent by another person to a patient for the purpose of relieving the patient's intolerable and incurable suffering. Physician-assisted suicide occurs when a doctor facilitates a patient's death by providing the necessary means and/or information in order to enable the patient to perform the life-ending act. Permitting physicians to engage in either euthanasia and/or assisted suicide is immoral, unethical, and unprofessional. These physicians are called doctors of death.

There are serious moral, ethical, and legal debates concerning the outcomes of euthanasia and physician-assisted-suicide intentions and actions. Both intentions and actions would ultimately cause more harm than good because euthanasia and physician-assisted suicide are fundamentally incompatible with the physicians' role as healers (Council on Ethical and Judicial Affairs, 1998-1999: 61). Both the object as lethal suicide injections and the doctor as the agent are not good, with reference to ill intentions and actions. What is the relationship between these intentions and actions in the fields of health and insurance? There are several parties involved in the analytical domain such as the patient, the life insurance policy, the malpractice insurance policies, the manufacturer of suicide machines, pharmacies, the home mortgage companies of the suicide occurring in their client's home, and the patient's relatives. In assessing the outcome of such an action, some insurance companies are viewed as winners. Insurance companies and health care insurance companies will save some money by not paying any more medical expenses and/or benefits for an insured. On the other hand some insurance companies such as mortgage insurance companies are losers because they should compensate for the suicide incident in the home. Nevertheless, it should be noted that through pure *speculative amoral knowledge,* the intention and behavior of the doctor of death is pro-business, because the doctor is marketing and promoting the suicide machines for a company. In addition, the doctor is assisting insured patients in terminating their lives in order to reduce costs for the health care insurance companies and/or Hospital Managed Organizations (HMOs). Therefore, doctors and the doctors of death's intentions and actions are not in accordance with the professional codes of ethical and moral commitments. The doctor of death's intention and behavior is based on an *amoral* business. It is clear from this explanation of speculative understanding that morality and ethics are not speculative understanding, but in reality they are pragmatic knowledge. Ethical and moral bioscientists are known by their decisions and actions, not by their deliberation without action.

PRAGMATIC ETHICAL KNOWLEDGE

Let us view the second ordination, *pragmatic knowledge.* In the experimental stages of research, we are faced with major problems through the examination of knowable ethical, moral, and legal information. What is knowable depends on the different ways in which people can make their intentional and behavioral means and ends known. Adding to this problem is the fact that moral virtues, ethical values, and legal principles in different locations around the world are different. Hence practical knowledge is an operative dynamic action; therefore, intentions and manners of knowing will be pragmatic phenomena. Thomas Hobbes's moral philosophy is related to his psychological theory, in which he constructs his mechanistic conception of motivation. He opposed the prevailing notion of his time that the mind and body are different substances; maintaining, *mental phenomena are nothing but physical motions.* He believed that any action is traced to a predisposition to that act in a certain direction. Desires move one to pursue objects, and aversions move one to avoid objects (Albert, Denise, and Peterfreund, 1984: 128).

The question arises here, what type of moral life does an individual prefer? Most moral and ethical issues are the result of more attention being paid to the knowable means and ends of an action. In some cases, they are more than conventions and consensus. They are arbitrary decisions and actions. Legal decisions and actions are known as the result of logical tests of consistency either through consensus or by some logic of relationship. Therefore, pragmatic knowledge is the result of some historical, experiential, or deliberated tests. While morality and ethics cannot tell you how to act at a given time and in particular circumstances, legal principles dictate in all situations what you should do because the law is a practical knowledge of what to do in defined situations and conditions. Nevertheless, moral and ethical ordinations provide knowledge that will serve as general guidelines for actions.

THE LIMIT OF SELF-INTEREST
AND MORAL CHARACTER

We all know that all people are to some extent, egocentric. They seriously pursue their objective lives. In the domain of survival, there are two connotations: *selfishness* and *prudence*. Since *selfishness* is defined as acting solely with a view to one's self- advantage without due regard to the interest of others, prudence is not same as selfishness. A prudent person is not necessarily selfish, and neither is a selfish person necessarily prudent. However, selfishness always involves a reference to self-interest, self-needs, self-wishes or self-desires. Prudence involves the self as well as the interests of a person or an organization that an individual is representing. However, it should be noted that prudence is the exercise of intelligence or forethought with respect to the mutual interest of self and others. To act imprudently is to think and act stupidly or irrationally from the mutual point of view of self and others. Finally, prudence is thinking and acting with a more rational or enlightened self-interest. Selfishness is immoral, while prudence is ethical. If we want to examine selfishness and prudence in relation to an arbitrary judgment, we must consider their effects on the agent and others. For example, suppose two professors that apply for promotion and tenure in a university system are concurrently serving as members of the promotion and tenure committee. Also suppose one of these professors is highly qualified and the other is unqualified. At the time of deliberation and judgment, the unqualified professor casts his/her vote in favor of the qualified professor, and in return, the qualified professor casts his/her vote as an abstention (neither in favor nor against) the unqualified professor. Such a judgment is called prudence. It should be noted that there is a distinction between prudence and morality. Such a distinction creates a borderline between prudence and morality. Morality by all means and ends relates individual's judgments to the truth and denies selfishness and prudence. Prudence in return relates judgments to the pluralistic interests of a group of professional specialists.

In order to fulfill the maximum of self-interest, an individual needs to benefit the self and may injure other(s). This means that survival is like playing a game. If you do not try hard to compete, you will soon be a loser. There are two types of competition: fair and unfair. A fair competition is based upon an equal opportunity at the beginning of the race with impartial judgment by the referees. Competitors inevitably need to express and manifest their volitions to the point of equilibrium, and then they accelerate them to proceed from that point to the ultimate succession. In doing so in moral competition, parties achieve three objectives:

- Competitors need to exercise their legitimate power in a way that competition proceeds with perfectly equal rights.
- They maximize the utility of their inherent power to lead other parties to admit their weaknesses and voluntarily relinquish their interest.
- They bring about these achievements in such a way that cell parties respect the right of the free consent.

Since people's behavior is based on voluntary or involuntary intentions, their achievement is also based on good and evil consequences. However, both good and evil actions are related to moral, ethical, and legal intentions and consequences.

Evaluating competitors' objectives and behaviors as good or evil depends upon no other basis than desires and aversions. One of the most moral duties is the duty to self. An individual carries the burden of two duties: to oneself and to others. It is a moral duty to preserve one's own life and self-respect. It is a moral duty to preserve others respect within the obligatory context of self-respect. This is especially true of moral virtue.

A moral virtue is the kind of personal habit whose proper means and ends are consistent with choosing alternatives as a mean between two extremes: (1) duty to self and (2) duty to others. This is precisely what we mean by an act of choice or force. We are now in a position to distinguish choice from force.

Indeed, the moral intentions and actions of an individual depend more upon what a person chooses than upon any other type of act they perform. Let us begin with self-interest perceptions and choices. While every forced action is involuntary, every voluntary action is strictly a free action of choice. Therefore, every act of choice refers to one specific kind of action performed and controlled by the will.

Egocentrism refers to an individual's inability to perceive perspectives other than his or her own. When personal objectives, motives, drives, and strongly held attitudes get in the way of the systematic analysis of causes, the attributive bias is known as a self-serving bias. This means that people tend to take credit for their successes while denying responsibility for their failures. Self-serving biases are quite robust, occurring in many situations for most people and even across cultures (Flecher and Ward, 1988: 230).

THE LIMIT OF SELF-CONTROL

One of the issues of today's societal life is the *promise*. A promise is a self-obligatory intention to fulfill duties within a specific short or long period of time. A promise carries two sides of moral and ethical obligatory duties: (1) to oneself, and (2) to others. Can one promise oneself to do something? Promises to oneself would be considered a form of self-control from which one could release oneself at will. The language here must be metaphorical. For example, to say: "I have promised myself not to gamble any more," is to say: "I have strongly resolved to control my greedy appetite by not gambling any more." Self-control is the stream of expression and action that is needed to resolve or settle an immoral and unethical habit. Although a promise to oneself is in some respect like a promise, it is not a genuine, or in any literal sense, a promise. To promise oneself to do something is to just be intentionally resolved to do it.

A promise to others is characterized by duties arising out of both written and oral contracts. In ethical contracts parties promise each other to fulfill their reciprocal duties during a specific period of time with specific terms of intentions and actions. If the parties do not fulfill their obligatory contracts, then one or both are in default. This rigid rule sometimes fails when the contract is not in writing with specific reciprocal obligatory duties. Then, conflict and dispute arise between parties whose expectations of each other are not fulfilled. One such equitable concept in the law of contract is called promissory, equitable, or stopple duty. The ethical doctrine of oral promissory duty is based upon an individual's cultural value systems within the boundary of self-moral control. Halbert and Ingulli (2000: 19) stated:

> In order for a promise to be enforceable under the concept of promissory stopple, there must be:

- A promise that the promisor should reasonably have expected to induce action of a definite and substantial character on the part of the promise
- Which in fact produced reliance or forbearance of that nature
- In circumstances such that the promise must be enforced if injustice is to be avoided

THE LIMIT OF SELF-DISCIPLINE

Perhaps most fundamentally, self-discipline has given way to an ethical, moral, and legal consciousness of the interrelatedness of an individual's behavior with others. Self-discipline is a cognitive controlled prudent intention and action through intellectual reasoning. It maintains self-dignity and integrity and prevents contradictions, frustrations, disappointment, and anger. Self-discipline, however, is important for a number of reasons: not only to manifest self-respect, but also to set the standard that certain behaviors are expected from others. Self-discipline for a scientist ensures that all possible pragmatic procedures have been followed. Research has provided us sufficient guidelines about the most effective ways to discipline one's self and others.

One of the immoral, unethical, and illegal problems threatening most bioscientists is sexual abuse in the workplace. Under federal law, sexual abuse includes such activities as posting pornographic posters, cartoons, and drawings at work, requesting sexual favors, unwanted sex, lewd remarks, unwanted hugs, touches and kisses, and retaliating against anyone who complains about sexual abuse. The Equal Employment Opportunity Commission initiated a guideline on sexual harassment as follows:

> Unwelcome sexual advance, request for sexual favors, and other verbal or physical conduct of a sexual nature constitute sexual abuses when:
>
> Submission to such conduct is made either explicitly or implicitly a term or condition of an individual's employment,
> Submission to or rejection of such conduct by an individual is used as the basis for employment decisions affecting such individual, or
> Such conduct has the purpose or effect of unreasonably interfering with an individual's work performance or creating an intimidating, hostile, or offensive working environment [The EEOC Guideline on Sexual Harassment, 29 CFR 1604.11(a)].

Traditionally, most organizations had been influenced by masculine power (Steiner and Steiner, 1988: 592). Men and women have considered their opposite gender's identity within two different emotional and submissive perceptions. In some cases, men perceived women (1) as enjoyable immoral and unethical lovers and lovely legal wives, (2) as virtuous and respectable mothers, sisters, and daughters. In return, women have considered men (1) as immoral and unethical pleasurable lovers and faithful legal husbands, (2) as virtuous fathers, brothers, and sons. Within the domain of moral virtues, ethical faithfulness, and legal doctrine, women and minor children have found in such settings a dilemma of abuses.

Today's organizational environments have been dramatically changed. Federal law has defined two types of sexual harassment: *Quid Pro Quo*, and *Hostile Work Environment*. *Quid Pro Quo* means that sexual favors are a requirement, or appear to be a requirement, for advancement in the workplace. *Hostile Work Environment* means that a worker has been made to feel uncomfortable because of unwelcome actions or comments relating to sexuality (Trevino and Nelson, 1995: 52). Barton (1995: 109) indicated that three primary requites must met for a claim of sexual abuse to be successful:

- The action must be sexual in nature, in a hostile environment, and unwelcome.
- The victim's clothing style, age, and position are irrelevant.
- Any statement, suggestion, or conduct (including physical, verbal, or visual activities) could be subject to a claim, including activities that one party considers to be merely playful, but others consider degrading.

Of course harassment involves more than just sexual, financial, and legal issues. It is also a moral one. Violation of the moral and ethical rights of patients, clients, peers, superiors, and subordinates may subject bioscientists, biotechnologists, and biomedical practitioners to civil or criminal liability. Expulsion from membership in a profession or loss of employment is the maximum penalty that may be imposed by a professional organization upon a scientist and/or a physician who violates ethical standards involving a breach of moral duty or ethical principles. In the field of medicine, medical societies have a civic and professional obligation to present to the appropriate governmental body or state board of medical examiners credible evidence that may come to their attention involving the alleged criminal conduct of any physician relating to the practice of medicine (*Council of Ethical and Judicial Affairs,* 1998:164). For example, three decades ago in 1968, 23-year-old G. Krist, M.D., a female accomplice abducted a student at Emory University in Atlanta at gunpoint from a motel and drugged her with chloroform. They put her in a wooden box with food and other provisions, and buried her in a remote area in Georgia. Police rescued her 3 days later, after her father paid a $500,000 ransom. Krist was later captured in Florida and was sentenced to life in prison for the 1968 kidnapping. After serving 10 years in prison, Krist was released and went on to study at medical schools in Grenada and the Dominican Republic. He earned his medical degree and returned to the United States and started to practice medicine in the state of Indiana. Indiana law does not prevent convicted felons from obtaining a medical license, although the state medical board put a number of restrictions on his ability to practice medicine. He is not allowed to prescribe certain drugs (*ABC NEWS,* 2002). There are those who think or from an ethical standpoint, one might think that the state of Indiana's Medical Council should have an ethical obligation of determining to disclose all facts about Dr. Krist's past criminal history to patients, whether or not disciplinary action is indicated.

WHAT IS ETHICS?

Thus far we have defined morality in terms of an individual's pursuing self-interest and/or searching for egoism towards virtuous excellence, but we have not seen what excellence is in terms of collective socio-cultural value systems. Ethics could be defined as both social habits as well as responses to perceived extraordinarily necessitated prudence in specific sociocultural situations. In conventional social behavior, ethics is defined as superior cultural behavioral values according to customs and traditions. In a narrow sense, ethics refers to particular superior social thought or behavior. It refers to a societal benchmark or instrument for the guidance of social behavioral niceties for individuals and groups. Nevertheless, ethics in social behavior differs somewhat in that it is coordinated with, but different from, science, technology, art, law, convention, and religion. All the above phenomena may be related to ethics, but they are not ethics. Ethics in this sense is a social enterprise into which an individual or groups of people are inducted. What is significant to note is the collectivistic aspect of the social enterprise, which we have called ethics. Thus, morality is defined as personal rational self-guidance and ethics is defined as a guided social enterprise (Park and Barron, 1977: 3-23).

Ethics involves a critical analysis of cultural values to determine the validity of their vigorous rightness or wrongness in terms of two major criteria: truth and justice. Ethics is examining the relation of an individual to society, to nature, and/or to humanity. How do people make ethical decisions? They are influenced by how they perceive themselves in relation to goodness and/or excellence.

In this section we will define ethics as a purely theoretical treatment of moral virtues in terms of speculative and practical collective cultural value systems. In the speculative and practical knowledge of goodness, righteousness, and worthiness, we are concerned with cultural value systems that are operable, in either intending to do something or actually doing something in the realm of goodness. Now, through these two alternatives, might seem to define what ethical life should be for bioscientists and biotechnologists, as a manner of reflection which will indicate that it is not the kind of intending or knowing goodness, but the complete practical execution of goodness through pluralistic scientific behavior.

The term *ethics* is derived from the Greek word *ethos*. In the Oxford English Dictionary (1963) ethos means the genius of an institution or system. It, also defines *ethics* as the science of morals and the area of study concerned with the principles of human duty. Ethics concerns itself with human societal conduct, activity, and behavior in that they are done knowingly and to a large extent, deliberately and willingly. Ethics is concerned with the construction of a rational societal system through the application of moral principles (virtues) by a group of people in a society.

Ethics is concerned with the nicety (not nasty) of psychosocial actions and can deal with good deeds in a society. Philosophers have identified ethics with one or the other of these extremes. Some have understood ethics to be speculative and demonstrative good of thoughts and behavior (deontological) and others have tended to identify ethics with completely the practical good end-results (teleological).

In Chinese culture, the word for ethics has been used as the word for etiquette, "li," which originally meant, to sacrifice. It refers to the idea that Chinese people should follow legally sanctioned etiquette, not to mention the knowledge of hundreds of correct forms of behavior. The Chinese eventually came to believe that their behavior was the only correct etiquette in the universe, and that all who did not follow the same meticulous rules of conduct were uncivilized barbarians (De Mente, 1989: 27-28). In the homogenous European and American cultures, the meaning of ethics is related to "The Love of God," and to "The Love of Wisdom." In the Greek tradition, ethics was conceived as relating to the social niceties. Social niceties could be considered as custom, convention, and courtesy. Later on a quite different orientation was introduced by the Judo-Christian ethics. In this tradition, the ideals of righteousness before God and the love of God and neighbor, not the happy or pleasant life, constitute the substance of ethical behavior.

As far as the term morality is related to the deliberation of an individual's intellectual characteristics through their conscientious awareness, ethics is the pluralistic social conscious awareness of a group of people. Thus, morality is related to the individual virtues, and ethics is related to the cultural value systems; society's fairness, justness, and worthiness as goodness. Hence, morality is the foundation of an ethical society, and it also relates to the existence of moral people who make the collective distinction of right judgments from wrong, and good behavior from bad. Ethics generally requires people to behave in accordance with valuable norms and standards of goodness that they accept and to which they and the rest of society hold others.

Ethics then can be defined as a systematic pluralistic attempt at social well-being in a society in order to make sense of our individual security and societal efforts towards peace in such a way as to determine the rules that "ought" to govern human social conduct, the values worth pursuing, and the character traits deserving development in life. In his foundation of the metaphysics of morals the German philosopher Immanuel Kant (1785) stated that: "Act only in accordance to that maxim by which you can at the same time will that it should become a universal law." In other words, human beings cannot adopt ethical principles of social actions unless they can do it with consistency, and it has to be adopted by everyone. Without an accepted universal morality (virtues) there would be no stabilized ethical society to keep the world in peace and security. Beliefs and faiths are important ingredients in ethical behavior. Different beliefs and faiths about moral and intellectual virtues can lead to differences in what is described as ethical relativism.

Ethics Promotes Humaneness: As mentioned before, the nature of human beings is viewed as having dual characteristics. Humanity's potentialities are multiple. Philosopher Sidney Hook (1946) stated that a human is like the egg which might develop into a chicken, but which might also, among other things, become an egg sandwich. Human objectives are pluralistic, and they may conflict with each other or even with themselves in different situations. Why is such a complexity inherited in human nature? The answer indicates that when a choice has to be made between an individual and a group need, different people will weigh values differently. People may agree about a word but the word may have different meanings for different individuals. Such a general disagreement is rooted in the nature of egoism and the selfishness of people.

Generally, people search for happiness and pleasure through the acquisition of the excessive power, wealth, reputation, sexual enjoyment, and luxurious life styles. Such an excessive acquisition is the result of *appetite* and *greed.*

There are two important connotations in regard to conscience awareness and the cognitive perceptions of: *appetite* and *greed. Appetite, as* a physiological term, is an intrinsic desire to supply any bodily want or craving. However, *appetite* as a psychosocial term is an inner drive or propensity to satisfy a want on the basis of acquired extrinsic demand. Appetite through physiological capacity contains limitation, but as a psychosocial experience is unlimited. These issues are manifest in the moral, ethical, and legal commitments of human behavior.

The term *greed* is an inordinate and rapacious desire, especially for wealth, power, sex, and reputation. It is denoted as an excessive and extreme desire for something, often more than an individual's rational share. Also, greed means avid desire for unethical, immoral, and illegal gain or wealth. Greedy intentions and actions are rapacious, ravenous, voracious, and gluttonous. Greed is simply what individuals want, then they immediately try to have them. Both appetite and greed are highly associated with an individual's intellectual, emotional, and sensational powers. Therefore, appetite and greed are highly influential in the field of bioethics as a drive discover more and patent more in order to make more profits.

Ethics Harnesses Power: *Power* is an almost absolute nicety and/or a dirty word. It may be associated with competence, or strength, and perhaps with legitimate authority. Much of the writings of philosophers, political scientists, and researchers in academia is concerned with the definition of power and with distinguishing among its types. Power stems from the Latin word *potere,* which means, "to be able." Benn (1967: 424) defined: "Power is the ability to get someone to do something that he/she otherwise would not do." Emerson (1962:31) emphasized the application of power: "Its operationalization rests on the interaction of two factors: dependence and goals." Within the bounds of power relationships French and Raven (1959), indicated several types of power: Coercive Power, Reward Power, Referent Power, and Legitimate Power.

Within the domain of bioscientific and biotechnological power, there are other kinds of power: Intellectual Power, Expert Power, Authoritative Power, Abusive Power, and Oppressive Power. Each of the above kinds of power has its specific consequences. For example, coercive power often combines selfish interest with some types of threatening consequences such as fear, wrath, retaliation, domination, and intimidation. Some bioresearchers hope that one day they will be able to capture the biochemical messages of stem cells and turn them into drugs. Bioethicists fear that regenerative medicine may go too far in the biopharmaceutical industry. If cells are over-stimulated and/or over-manipulated to reproduce, patients may face a battle with cancer: Some biologists believe that a limit on the body's ability to regenerate tissue is "mother nature's" way of preventing rampant cancer in humans. Bioethicists believe that humans are born with a natural biological clock power that tells us when our time is up.

Ethics Promotes Intellectual Choices and Prohibits Mandatory Forces:
When we speak of an ethical decision, we imply two different alternatives for its execution: 1) Free choice, and 2) Mandatory force. Free choice, in an ethical sense, is often taken to mean just " voluntary choice." Equally obvious, however, is that the distinction between choice and force is the degree of coercion. Ethics promotes intellectual voluntary choices to comply with power.

Choice and Definite Means and Ends:
There are two different behavioral directions within an individual's body-mind interaction: desire and will. Desires are emotional and sensational please appeals which meditate an individual to achieve an end-result (moral, immoral, or amoral). Desires pursue pleasure and enjoyment for favorable self-oriented end-results and to avoid pain and misery. The origin of desires is a mixture of emotional and sensational end-results but not can assessment of their causes. On the other hand a will, in its intellectual sense, is a dynamic moving drive, which guides an individual to be aware of the particular circumstance of the means and ends relationships. But the origin of a will is in its efficient and effective means and ends assessment (cause and effect assessment). A will is a conscience-deliberated awareness of a choice. A moral and ethical individual tends to choose pleasure or pain not merely because of pleasure or pain but in order to achieve a good end-result to avoid or an evil to be avoided.

Sometimes, individuals choose what is painful, not because it is painful but because of some good end-results that can be achieved through painful experiences. Therefore, people choose their intentional objectives as conscious expected ends in terms of good or evil rather than pleasure or pain. Being a self-willed individual means being very intent on one getting what is seeking. Acts of simple desires are not acts of choices. They are unconscious and on most occasions habitual behaviors. But the acts of emotional feelings spring from sensational will. Since a desire is always associated with pleasure, an intellectual choice is not necessarily connected with pleasure and/or enjoyment. It is related to happiness and satisfaction.

We have now distinguished desire, will, and choice in relation to means and ends or intentions and actions. We still need to understand more of the nature of choice and to analyze precisely what the intention and act of choice is in an individual's mind-body relations. Also, we must realize how an intention in the action of choice takes place in the mind. A choice is a presupposed act of decisive deliberation. Just as the emotional and sensational desires follow upon an individual's feelings, so a specific act of choice follows upon a specific act of the intellect. Therefore, the act of choice is following upon the intention of intellectual deliberation.

Deliberation is the essence of intellectual reasoning for deciding a preference among the final choices. Deliberation is the process of evaluating reasons for or against doing something. Consequently, deliberation is a conscience analysis about good and evil means. In moral and ethical reasoning, we cannot exercise a choice unless we deliberate the means of an action in terms of good and evil.

Command of Execution of Choice: Deliberated moral choices of good or bad, fair and unfair, just and unjust, and right and wrong in actions can be assessed in value terms as the subject of the execution of decisions. Execution of moral choices depends on reasoning and circumstances. They signify primarily certain cause-effect orders. We simply need to discover these orders, observe them, analyze them, formulate them, plan them, and execute them. There are several orders in an individual's life (e.g., moral order, ethical order, legal order, scientific order, systematic order, historical order, etc). All these orders are viewed as real and logical. All orders are caused by reasons and reasons, are the efficient causes of effects. Reasons construct choices to be implemented in actions by the "will" in seeking an end. In studying the command of the execution of choices, we need to analyze the "will" and the expected consequential results of actions.

Evidence suggests that a number of factors may need to be considered during the decision-making and implementation processes. When bioscientists and biotechnologists are faced with a totally new situation, they tend to immediately think about the future by looking at the present circumstances through a rear-view mirror. This mirror reflects their conscience awareness. In order to analyze the present circumstances and predict the future, bioscientists and biotechnologists need to go through a self-interrogatory process in order to discover the real choices and execute them. The guidelines below will assist you to clarify this self-interrogatory process.

Why Should the Choice Be Executed? This question concerns a holistic assessment in the mind of bioscientists and biotechnologists in executing rational decisions in action. They need to ask themselves: why are they doing what they are doing? Are their decisions rightly executed? Are their scientific techniques valid and viable in order to safely obtain their hypothetical goals? Are there other right techniques? If yes, why are these techniques being used and not others? Are these executed scientific actions meeting the bioethical motives for acting? Are these executed techniques matching their ethical, moral, and legal intentions? Sometimes, one can have a certain intention in mind and at the same time proceed on a course of action that will bring about the opposite of what one intends.

When Should the Choices Be Executed? Moral virtues, ethical values, and legal principles are the basic foundational milestones of human actions. The timing of the execution of choices is the matter of finding appropriate circumstances. The circumstance of the execution of choices in terms of timing can be assessed before, during, or after the transformation of the decision-making processes. This timing refers not only to dates and hours but also to special periods of time, such as day or night, weeks, months, seasons, or a time of war or peace. Timing can be managed through three periods: preliminary, concurrent, and post scientific operations. Nevertheless, the length of time involved in an action may carry relevant moral, ethical, and legal circumstances. For example, as part of pathologist's responsibility to act quickly to examine a specimen received from a surgical suite for finding cancerous cells, he/she needs very quickly to report his/her scientific findings to the surgeon. If he/she doesn't the surgical ends will not be fulfilled.

Where Should the Choices Be Executed? People behave differently when they are situated in different places. Sometimes people are performing some actions that are morally right in private, but the same action is considered immoral when done in public. The place of the act can change its nature from moral to immoral, ethical to unethical, and legal to illegal. The distinction between private and public is sometimes a relevant moral, ethical, and legal circumstance. For example, while nudity in a religious place during a sermon can be considered a sin, nudity on the stage of a theater during a play a shameful exposure, in a classroom during a lecture an unethical and illegal action, in the operating room of a hospital for a patient it is a moral, ethical, and legal act. Therefore, moral, ethical, and legal actions can be practiced in a way that leads to harmony rather than disharmony in different places.

By What Means Should the Choice Be Executed? It is proper to state that people need to pursue their objectives according to their intellectual reasoning. Reason is a powerful means to empower people's mind grasp what is good and what is evil. The moral and ethical choices are related to particular determinations between good and evil reasoning. These determinations are perceived as proceeding from what is right to what is wrong, what is fair to what is unfair, what is just to what is unjust, what is nice to what is nasty, and what is simple to what is complex. The measure of moral and ethical means consists of the conformity of the execution of good choices. That measure needs to be correlated with a "good faith" in the sense that reason is rightly to be stated according to the order of the execution of a decision. It also needs to measure what is meant by action. In moral and ethical decision-making processes people need to make decisions to decide from simple and ordinary reasonable experiences to the utility of a complex multiplicity of objectives. Therefore, moral and ethical reasoning consists of a correlated and integrated nature of good faith, good intention, and good means in action. The opposite, which is called evil, consists of departing from goodness to nastiness in reasoning and actions.

Should What Ends Execute the Choices? It is the peoples' responsibility to turn their potential into effective and efficient work. Effectiveness is the ability to set the right objectives and achieve them. In other words, effectiveness is the right way to do something. Efficiency is doing things rightly. Productivity is also to doing right things rightly. Efficiency is the relative amount of resources used to obtain effectiveness. Since effective and efficient people in production systems are viewed as good means to reach to good ends, they need to be constructively and productively motivated in order to be morally and ethically good. Therefore, to be moral and ethical in the workplace, employees and employers must behave in a reasonably good way.

Who Should Execute the Choices? Bioscientific decisions and actions need to be implemented through appropriate formal channels by qualified scientists. The scientists need to be aware of what has been taught and how to execute those scientific commands. The scientists should not be ignorant of themselves and of who they are. They need to be professionally knowledgeable in executing decisions. They are accountable for wrongdoing. Inexcusable and unconvincing reasons cannot preclude the rights of people. It is unethical, immoral, and illegal for an expert to hire unprofessional people to perform professional tasks. For example, the primary objective of a university is to render academic services to students by qualified professors. In some cases, it has been observed that in order to obtain financial savings, the university administrators combine graduate and undergraduate students in a classroom to be taught by a professor. In these circumstances, the instructors know that the level of instruction, the course contents, the breadth of knowledge, and the testing systems at both graduate and undergraduate levels are different. In the event that a conflict develops between the instructor's professional commitment and an administrator's responsibility for the institutional financial savings, the conflict must be resolved morally and ethically for the student's learning objectives.

How Should the Choice Be Executed? The behavior of decision-makers can affect the nature and consequences of an action for better or worse. Bioscientists and biotechnologists should believe in establishing a healthy research environment. It is important for both employees (lab technicians and staff) and employers (bioscientists and biotechnologists) to respect human dignity and integrity in the workplace. Working in such an environment is a "social nicety." Morality and ethics are significantly more important than etiquette in fostering the mutuality of social niceties. Courtesy, convention, and respect are related to behavioral etiquette and to biobusiness ethics. All parties expect to be treated equitably and well. For example, it is wise when firing an expert employee to consider and implement moral, ethical, and legal mandates such as *careful consideration*, and *due process*.

WHAT IS LEGALITY?

Since ethics is a behavioral ordination to harmonize conflicting psychosocial interest between an individual and other people, law is another practical and operative econo-political attempt to resolve the disputable issues between individuals and groups. Law is not viewed formally as an act of will. It is a practical reason that determines means in relation to some given ends. Oesterle (1957: 20) defined law as a certain ordination of reason for the common good, promulgated by those who have care of the community.

Law formalizes the socio-cultural and econo-political contracts under which the community limits the *harm* that members can do to other people, animals, and environments. Also as Ahmed (1999: 113) stated: "While it is recognized that the law is only setting the minimum standards for conduct, it is also assumed that competition shall keep raising that minimum level." As we understand, law resembles ethics in that both are social institutions that aim to improve human relations in various ways. However, law is an exterior principle of action in the sense that it establishes, in a universal and objective fashion, an order of action to be followed by people seeking a common end. If people do not comply with the law, they will be fined or sentenced to jail, and have an injunction against them.

Law, however, presents certain mandatory minimal standards of an individual's social conduct within the contextual boundary of group behavior. Legal standards regulate people's social actions with respect to what to do or what not to do. Also, law is a creative institution, an enactment of new statues of social general order. Of course, the law does not establish all expected standards of social orders and codes of conduct for a society. Therefore, law is an ordination pertaining to societal well-being reasons. It is the expression of what is reasonable to do under special circumstances and situations, by all people.

Nevertheless, it should be noted that two major concerns might be added to the above definitions. The first is that by designation of the common good as the necessary end of everything, we may distinguish a true law from a so-called law laid down by a tyrant. Suppose an authoritative ruler who is in control of a state, claims that in reality he/she enacts laws for the political common good. Such ordinances are directed at maintaining maintain personal power in order to rule over the state and they are not true laws and do not properly carry an obligation to be obeyed by all people. Second, while the common good is the necessary end of every law, the common good needs to be directly effective for the benefit of the community as whole, not as an egalitarian law for maintaining the interests of a partisan group.

Law Protects Individual and Group Rights: The law protects individual and group rights. A right is an entitlement and/or a privilege to act or have others act in a certain mandated fashion. The connection between legal rights and duties is that if you have a right to do something, the law mandates others to perform their duties in a certain way. One of the major issues in legality questions is: Why is legal compliance a must? Compliance follows the law, which is generally looking backward to past mandates. Compliant efforts reduce discretion, increase oversight, and tighten controls. Legal compliance has been viewed as a solid social floor for accepted behavior in a society. Since the law has to apply to everybody, therefore its standards are not so high as to inspire human excellence. Therefore, it is ethics that inspires people to search for excellence, not law.

Law Recovers Sustained Damages: Life is a challenge and people in their lifetimes confront misfortunes. If people suffer misfortune, they need to put up with it and find sources and resources to deal with it. If their misfortune is the fault of others, the law may step in and make violators pay damages. Through civil law, the public steps in and demands punishment, fines, and imprisonment for offenses that are serious enough to violate human rights. The law demands victims be compensated when offenders are found guilty of violating rules and regulations, ignoring human rights, not performing legal duties, not complying with ordinances, breaching contracts, alleged to be negligent, acting as proximate causes of injury, and possessing illegal properties and controlled substances (e.g., narcotics and some specified sedatives, methadone, and phedamine).

Law Maintains the Promissory Contractual Statues of People: Law is a dynamic process to create peace and harmony among people. It cannot stand still, yet in certain ways it appears clear-cut. It provides a set of rules for peoples' behavior and institutional operations. The creation of law and the delivery of sanctions for rule breaking are contested processes. How law is made, and how it is interpreted and enforced is always debatable. We may disagree ethically and morally with laws, but we should understand and comply with them. Law establishes expected behavioral standards and sets up a bureaucratic judiciary system for compliance with them. There is no free choice in legality. The only force is a mandatory compliance. While ethics and morality provide us with a menu of options, legality requires us to comply with those rules that are set in our society. One of the issues in human socialization is compliance with rigid and technical rules of promissory contracts.

CHAPTER 3

MORAL THEORIES: IDEALISTIC, REALISTIC, HEDONISTIC, EUDAEMONISTIC, AND AUTHENTIC*

CHAPTER OBJECTIVES

When you have read this chapter you should be able to do the following:

- Understand what we mean by a happy life.
- Analyze cultural influences on the moral character of individuals.

---

* This chapter was adopted from: Parhizgar, K. D. and Parhizgar, R. R. (2006). *Multicultural Business Ethics and Global Managerial Moral Reasoning*. Lanham, MD: University Press of America, Inc.

- Know what is the foundational basis of morality in human behavior by examining optimistic, pessimistic, and moderate views on morality.
- Know why people perceive morality differently.
- Develop conceptual skills towards a general agreement on the topics of pleasure and happiness.
- Establish foundational principles concerning how we perceive moral faith and beliefs.
- Develop a framework to examine different theoretical dimensions of moral theories.
- Establish a rational argument that places the components of morality into five major realms of deliberations: moral theories, moral principles, moral merits, moral intentions, and moral actions.
- Analyze moral theories in terms of their means and ends.
- Introduce the general characteristics of moral theories.
- Conduct a comparative study among moral theories: moral idealism, moral realism, moral hedonism, moral eudaemonism, and moral authenticism.
- Know what the Platonic moral idealism is.
- Know what the Aquinasian moral idealism is
- Know what the Hobbesian moral idealism is.
- Know what the Kantian moral realism is.
- Know what the Reidian moral realism is.
- Know what the Lockeian moral realism is.
- Know what the Spenserian hedonistic moral view is.
- Know what the eudaemonistic views of Jeremy Bentham on morality are.
- Compare hedonistic and eudaemonistic moral views.

PLAN OF THIS CHAPTER

The primary concern of this chapter is to first define moral theories. The second is to identify moral theories in terms of two fundamental distinctions: Whether these theories are speculative idealistic understandings or realistic pragmatic knowledge. Speculative understanding concerns a phenomenon or an object about which nothing is directly effective, and hence the phenomenon or object is placid. Pragmatic knowledge, on the contrary, is concerned precisely with a phenomenon or an object insofar as it is dynamic and tangible. In addition, speculative understanding and pragmatic knowledge are either for the sake of an individual's *conscience awareness* and *cognitive judgments,* or for the sake of *formative* and *summative* knowledge application to ordinate people's behavior or their societal interactions. We want to know what a pleasurable life is. What is a pleasant life? Is it the same through moral deliberations? How do different moralists view morality in terms of human beings' means and ends?

How can morality influence bioscientists and biotechnologists to be receptive to moral principles in their decision-making processes and actions? These and other issues are the main objectives for this chapter.

VIRTUE, MORALITY, AND HAPPINESS

People commonly speak of having peace of mind and a happy life within the contextual boundary of a sense of the fulfillment of their wishes. The problem of what peace of mind and happiness consists of and how they can be attained proves difficult to perceive. Since all human activities are differentiated from reason (rational deliberations, emotional expressions, and sensational manifestations), a life style could be moral, or amoral, or immoral. Nevertheless, the law of reasoning indicates that happiness is greatly influenced and formed by extrinsic virtuous measures of moral beliefs and actions. Accordingly, we need to search for virtuous means and acts to be more fully oriented towards virtue in general,

One might observe that emotional and sensational people sometimes end up with miserable outcomes. To understand virtuous decisions and moral acts, we need to distinguish between voluntary and involuntary means and ends. Such considerations enable us to recognize precisely which intentions and acts are morally good and which are morally bad. Such recognitions need to be coherent with syllogism reasoning as the fundamental intrinsic manifestation of morality.

It is evident that not all humans can lead a virtuous life or act according to the spirit of happiness. Searching for and solving the problems of humanity can generate good in one's character. Since human beings psychologically do not live in a solitary fashion within and beyond themselves, they possess specific intrinsic relations within themselves and their conscientiousness. Such a· quality in its perfect state presumes a virtuous intellect and/or the pursuit of goodness in a moral character.

As we have separated morality from ethics in Chapter 2, we defined *morality* as conformity to the universal right conduct. In addition, morality is a term used to manifest humanity's universal virtues, or intellectual excellence. Virtues refer to the superiority of intellect and wisdom and to the disposition of the cognizance of mind to effectively perform its proper function. Moral virtues concern the habitual choices of rational thoughts in accordance with the universal logical principles. The contemplation of absolute truthfulness and the discovery of the rational principles, which ought to control everyday actions, have given rise to intellectual virtues. The distinction between goodness and badness, truthfulness and falseness, and worthiness and worthlessness is called moral consideration.

It is possible to divide the phenomenon of morality into five realms. Here the interest is in what the perceptual meaning of morality looks like, and how it functions within the cognitive conscientiousness awareness of an individual. Therefore, the first level is *moral theory*. As moralists and ethicists study it, it may, for our purposes, be taken as the foundational floor for humaneness. The second level appears in the realm of *moral principles*. The third level is the realm of *moral merits*. The fourth level manifests the *moral intention*. The fifth level comes into the realm of *moral actions*. In the following pages we will examine five major moral theories: (1) Idealism, (2) Realism, (3) Hedonism, and (4) Eudaemonism, and (5) Authenticism.

As you can see in Figure 3-1, there are eight characteristics shared by five major moral theories within the contextual boundary of common moral sense. The common moral sense attributions are causal means, searching for ends, attributes, dimensional context, ideological views, prospective outcomes, psychosocial manifestations, and life-style orientations.

Table 3.1: Comparative Characteristics of Moral Theories

Common Sense	Idealism	Realism	Hedonism	Eudaemonism	Authenticism
Causal Means	Ultimate cause: God	Ultimate cause: Government	Ultimate cause: Self	Ultimate cause: All creatures	Ultimate cause: Conscience
Searching for ends	Excellence	Values	Satisfaction	Happiness	Virtues
Attributes	Aesthetic	Conventional	Sensational	Rational	Humaneness
Dimensional Context	Super-naturalistic	Intrinsic and extrinsic	Intrinsic	Holistic	Extrinsic
Ideological Views	Utopianism	Materialism	Humanism	Naturalism	Spiritualism
Prospective Outcomes	Exaggerated beautification	Desirable ownership	Standardized indoctrination	Objectiveity in oriented solutions	Intuitivism
Psychosocial Manifestations	Faith	Beliefs	Ideas	Opinions	Wisdom
Life-style Orientations	Religious	Econo-political	Sociocultural	Ecological	Peaceful and Harmonious

Through analytical perceptions concerning faith, beliefs, ideas, and opinions we need to identify the specific characteristics of each. Since faith stands above beliefs, ideas, and opinions, it is an invisible power in the human mind concerning immortal certainties in existence. Faith is not concerned with the material world itself, which is an object of knowledge; nevertheless, opinions are accompanied by doubt and fear, but faith is accompanied by certainty. Also, faith is firm and free from all hesitations, because it is a manifestation of spiritual power within the mind of an individual.

Table 3.2: Cultural Influences on Life Issues

Views	Pessimistic	Moderate	Optimistic
What is the character of human nature?	Human is evil	Human is a mixture of good and evil	Human is good
What is the Relationship of human to nature?	Human is subject to nature	Human is harmony with nature	Human is master of nature
What is the temporal focus of life?	To the past	To the present	To the future
What is the modality of human's activities?	A spontaneous expression in impulse and desires	Activity that emphasizes as a goal the development of all aspects of the self	Activity that is motivated primarily toward measurable accomplish-ments
What is the relationship of human to other humans?	Lineal: Group goals are primary and an important goal is continuity through time	Collateral: group goals are primary. Well regulated continuity of group relationships through time are not critical	Individual: The individual goals are most important

Sources: Adapted from Kluckhohn, F.R. and Strodtbeck, F.L. *Variation Value Orientations. Evanston.* Illinois: Row, Peterson and Company, (1961), 11. In Moran, R. T. and Harris, P.H. (1982). *Managing Cultural Synergy.* Houston: Gulf Publishing Company, (1982), 19.

In all of the above moral theories we are concerned with the nature of "goodness." How do we conceptualize goodness? With what courage and with what virtues can we pursue it? If we ask lay people on the street what their moral ground is, we are apt to gain an answer from a Judeo-Christian faith like: "The Ten Commandments." From Confucianism the answer is to be obedient to the rule of harmonious goodness. From a Hinduism belief, the answer is the tolerance of harsh conditions and the search for peaceful solutions. From a Moslem's view, the answer is to submit you to God's will; *Ensha-Allah.*

The moralists see human behavior in relation to the intrinsic nature of conscientiousness and the extrinsic nature of God's authority, or purposive excellent reason. The moralists define moral principles as a rule without exceptions. Finally, the moralists look at a human's good intentions and actions in all levels of life. There are different perceptions concerning happiness. Some people claim that wealth produces happiness while; others believe that wealth is identical with happiness, and there are some other people who seek wealth above everything, including happiness. It is uncommon to find people who sacrifice their health, honor, and beyond for the sake of wealth. Such a different perceptual array of beliefs concerning happiness has dominated today's world. For the clarity of such an important issue, we need to analyze cultural and behavioral stratification.

CULTURAL AND BEHAVIORAL STRATIFICATION

The perceptual relation of an individual to nature is based upon life their orientation. People place themselves and their possessions under the direction of the common natural and artificial value systems of their societies, and in return societies protect the rights and freedom of the individuals. People's qualities as individuals, their relationship to nature and to the world, their relationship to other people, and their orientation in time, place, and space are influenced by their moral virtues and cultural value systems.

Adler (1986: 12) raises several questions regarding six dimensions:

- Who am I?
- How do I see the world?
- How do I relate to other people? What do I do?
- How do I use space and time?

In addition to the above questions, there are two other important questions:

- How much money is an individual seeking to gain as the primary means in life?
- How can money make an individual's life happy?

Responses to these and similar questions vary from culture to culture and/or person to person. Some cultures are more synergistic than others. Some cultures are more materialistic and others are more spiritualistic. Table 3.2 helps us to understand how some of these factors might influence the behavior of human beings (Moran and Harris, 1982: 19).

In relation to the above cultural value systems described in Table 3.2, we will look briefly at the three major cultural dimensions: (1) optimistic views, (2) moderate views, and (3) pessimistic views.

OPTIMISTIC VIEWS

How Do People Perceive the Nature of a Human Being?

Some people basically perceive themselves and others as good; as reflected in a utopian cultural value system. There are some cultures that perceive human beings as the best products of nature or, in religious terms, as the best of God's creatures on the earth as compared to other creatures. They perceive good nature in human beings in order to trust each other with a great deal of reliance. In a highly respectful society, there is no secrecy about human affairs because people live in harmony with themselves and with the environment. People are open-minded and individuals enjoy liberty. The judiciary philosophy of these cultures is based upon this connotation: People are considered innocent until proven guilty. They freely share their knowledge and experiences and help each other by all means and end. They are very sincere and friendly. In these societies change is permissible toward betterment and progress with good faith. or example, the traditional American society represented this type of cultural perception in its attitude that the burden of proof is on the accuser. However, if we look at Spanish culture, we find that in such a society, people are suspicious of each other. For example, they believe they must constantly watch customers in stores. Shoplifting is a pattern of expected behavior in Spain.

What Are Individuals' Relationships to Their Institutions?

There is a general cultural pattern that indicates how people can dominate their social institutions and overcome obstacles. People perceive no real separation between institutional and individuals' boundaries. Their cultural beliefs allow them to live side by side with their institutions as their institutions grow, they are developing their capabilities too. In an optimistic culture, policies and regulations have been mandated to adjust the natural opportunities to the peoples' needs. People are allowed to alter and modify the nature of their institutions in order to enhance their lifestyles. Societal institutions help, guide, and assist people to search for better understanding. Change is possible because development, growth, and progress are the results of change.

What Are the Primary Relationships of Individuals to Others?

Human beings are not born with ready-made relationships with others. Individuals create contacts and relationships with others. However, one cannot achieve this state of existence unless he/she is free. Human beings exist to create their positions and relationships with others. This indicates the reality that human beings attribute to their value systems.

What Are the Primary Modes of Human Activities?

Cultural value systems in a society reflect the differentiated relationships among people. People are oriented with the mode of "will-er." The "will-er" culture is more oriented to the prosperous moral activities. The psychological and sociological "will-er" orientations speed up the process of change and specify the direction of change to themselves and their environment. Progressive assessment of individuals' achievement is not perceived inherently in the nature of the performers. The measurement is based upon the societal standards of expected moral behavior. Optimistic people are more motivated towards efficiency through hard working habits.

What Is the Temporal Focus of an Individual to the Society?

It is human perception that an individual should physically live in the present and metaphysically perceive the future. Future oriented cultures are more innovative in science and technology. Conservative cultures prefer to maintain their traditional value systems. They scarcely believe in drastic changes. They are very satisfied with the *status quo*. However, optimistic cultures evolve with new hopes and prosperity through progress and development, both individually and collectively.

MODERATE VIEWS

Americans traditionally see people as a mixture of good and evil, capable of choosing one over the other. They are neither moral nor immoral. They are amoral. They believe in the possibility of improvement through change (Adler, 1986:13). This notion brings to mind the idea that American culture is a balanced culture. We will examine the same connotations through the moderate view as follow.

How Do People Perceive the Nature of a Human Being?

Although many people do not hold the extreme position of saying that individuals virtually "can do no wrong or no right" at all times, they believe that the individual nature of a human being is a dualistic function of mind and body. At one time, religiously, the soul of human beings existed in the world of pure spirit and enjoyed the highest bliss, pure contemplation. However, because of some contact with evil in a world of pure spirit, at the same time, the soul of a human being had been condemned and became a part of a body and formed an organic unit to live on the earth. Since the soul of a human being has formed an organic unit with the body, it is then subject to weaknesses. The end result of such dualistic functioning does not have a heavenly existence. By viewing these types of beliefs, bioscientists and biotechnologists need to make corrections in their natures. Biomoral principles require them to be aggressive in finding out what harms would be (a) avoided, (b) prevented, and (c) caused.

Plato stated that a human being's superior faculty is attributed to the soul (e.g. mind, logic, and reasoning) and inferior organic existence is attributed to the body (e.g. evil, change, corruption, and the like). People with such a cultural belief tend to categorize individuals into two major categories:

- Those people with the highest intellectual abilities who can be considered as rulers, (rulers must be intellectual authorities that should be perfectly educated).
- Those people who have less intellectual ability and should be subordinate to the first group. If we consider the caste tradition in India, we see how the Indian people conceptually make distinctive class stratifications among themselves on the basis of their cultural family heritage.

What Are Individuals' Relationships to Their Social Institutions?

There are some cultures that strongly believe that life is the essence of conscience. Individuals should live in harmony with their organizations and be loyal to their institutions, both family members and organizations. In return, organizations should provide them lifetime supports. There shouldn't be a separated view between family members or employees and employers in such a society. Institutions should serve both organizational members and consumers as parts and as a whole. Preventing the violation of this moral rule by bioscientists, biotechnologists, and biomedical practitioners including physicians applies in critical situations, but it can be transgressed when they consider violating confidentiality in order to prevent AIDS patients from having unprotected sex with their spouses who are unaware of their HIV positive status.

What Are the Primary Relationships Between an Individual and Others?

Some cultures are more group oriented and strive to serve each other. In a general sense, while people share their views and help each other, individuals maintain and restore their privacy and independence. Mutual interest among professional groups facilitates harmony and helpfulness in these societies. These cultures are searching for and are proceeding toward unity through diversity. The surest path to the truth in these societies relies upon expert authorities and scientific findings. Lateral group membership includes all people who are currently part of an institution and provide opportunities for people who desire to join them. The prime criteria for the recruitment of organizational members are trustworthiness, loyalty to the group, and comparability with other co-workers. For example, French culture is perceived to be more individualistic and less synergistic than other cultures (Moran and Harris, 1982: 19).

What Are the Primary Modes of Human Activities?

Balancing professional priorities in a moderate culture can provide each member with adequate opportunities for growth and development. Institutional authorities within the contextual boundaries of a moderate culture tend to develop loyalty and normative ethics in their employees in order to better coordinate different organizational factions. Under a moderate cultural view, institutions maintain more autonomy and responsibility toward organizational stakeholders.

What Is the Temporal Focus of an Individual in the Society?

Under the moderate view of cultural value systems some cultures prefer to perceive the use of time within the present outcomes. These people like to live in momentum fashion. They react to short-term profits and make priorities to meet their short career path. In a general behavioral mode description, we call them "do-er" cultures. Many actions would be morally accepted in a society if there were not better alternatives, although morally unacceptable if there is. For example, the persuasion of spouses by bioscientists in a medical lab and/or by a physician in a clinic or hospital to tell their partners that they are HIV positive is a better alternative than simply violating confidentiality by bioscientists or doctors telling them themselves, even though, if the spouse is not persuaded, it may be morally acceptable for the bioscientists or doctors to tell the partners themselves.

PESSIMISTIC VIEWS

Although all human beings have distinctive cultural norms and values, it would be a mistake to judge any particular group and label them with a pessimistic value judgment. Geertz (1970: 47) indicated that: "We are, in sum, incomplete or unfinished animals who complete ourselves through culture." However, some cultures are more attached to past traditions, and others lean either to the present or future. By the same token, some cultures are more optimistically oriented and others are either more pessimistic or moderate. Pessimistic cultures view things with more emphasis on the negative and finally try to evolve positive outcomes. By viewing different studies of this direction, we can provide you with the following associations regarding pessimistic views:

How Do People Perceive the Nature of a Human Being?

Some cultures function negatively. People tend to view others as basically evil. They are unethical and immoral in the real sense. They should not be trusted, because they are selfish. They are very capable of turning themselves to tyranny, savagery, atrocity, and inhumane feelings. They suspect and mistrust each other. People in daily behavioral interactions are very cautious. Doubt and suspicion are the main bedrock of such a society. They resolve not to be open to each other. People don't change voluntarily, because of their cultural orientation. They are controlled through very rigid value systems. In these cultures, interpersonal change within their personality is very difficult. In the event some forced change happens, the end results carry some degree of personality degradation. In these cultures, the judiciary philosophy is based upon the concept that: people are considered guilty until proven innocent. Suspicion, resistance, and disloyalty to the cultural authorities are very popular in these cultures.

What Are Individuals' Relationships to Their Institutions?

Cultural obedience is one of the distinctive manifestations of normative behaviors in pessimistic cultures. In these cultures people do not trust each other. However, they need to rely on some forms of authority. These cultures give more credit to the rulers' power and lose a sense of individual liberty. People are expected to be obedient to the rulers' wishes in order to be cared for doing thing at a time of necessity. All members of a pessimistic culture are virtually dominated by elite ruling groups. Within such a cultural environment power plays an important role. Like wealth, it is more a means than an end. One seeks political power not really for its own sake but as a means for achieving pleasure, wealth, reputation or something else. Furthermore, it is evident that power can be used for good or evil, or happiness or misery.

What Are the Primary Relationships of an Individual and Others?

As indicated before, under the pessimistic cultural views, human beings are evil. They are not moral. Therefore, people under such conditions misbehave. People with this instructional behavior and these types of relationships with others must be constantly controlled. They believe that society should not provide maximum freedom for individuals, because if they are provided with liberty, they will revolt against authorities. Religiously, they stick with the cultural story of Adam and Eve who revolted against God in the Garden of Eden (Dupuios, 1985: 10). Therefore, organizational members should be obedient, silent, and controlled by authorities. Society should restrict individual freedom through rigid policies. High ranked authorities control societal members. They strongly believe in collectivistic judgment. If one person in the group is suspicious of another, other members of the group without question adhere to such a belief. They believe that all the others can trust organizational members, who are known by others the or vice versa. Under pessimistic cultures, the process of policy is less flexible, because it is less time consuming.

What Are the Primary Modes of Human Activities?

Human perceptions under pessimistic cultural views tend to be more passive. They are more attached to their past experiences. They like to minimize their activities, because they believe that they will not enjoy adequate profits from their efforts. They tend to be motivated to work fewer hours, because they believe that the generation of wealth will not provide them with happiness. People believe major changes will happen at their own often-slow pace. They do not need to push or to be pushed to achieve long-term objectives. They believe everything and everybody is subject to the process of birth and death and that fate and destiny migrate from one authority to another sooner or later.

What Is the Temporal Focus of an Individual to the Society?

Under pessimistic cultural views, people perceive future life as the extension of past experiences. We call these types of people "be-ers." Under this view, all cultural value systems should be evaluated according to past experiences. Innovations and creativity should be justified according to the past experiences. For example, like most Asians, the Vietnamese have a more extended concept of time than most Americans. Americans measure time and react by the clock, Vietnamese by the monsoon. Vietnamese are suspicious of the need for urgency in making decisions or culminating a business deal.

Traditional experiences of patience remain as the ultimate Confucian virtue in personal life as well as in business (Smith, and Pham, 1998: 174).

FOUNDATION OF MORAL THEORIES

Foundational Factual Problems in Morality

There are differences between moral and immoral intentions and actions. Those differences are related to means and ends in an individual's thoughts and behavior. There is an interest in having moral behaviors result in something constructive. Both moral and immoral people draw upon reasoning to justify their beliefs and actions. We cannot be immoral by accident, because it is a deliberative action. It is important that we stress here the possible problems that may be viewed by an individual as immoral. The moral opinions could be:

- The human's biggest problem is "themselves." Their natures are not certain, but in doubt (even about themselves).
- Morality inspires humans to be valuable as a criterion to measure all things. Therefore, they can be changed toward stages of good, better, best, and excellent and avoid bad, worse, worst, and vice in thoughts and actions.
- The primary purpose of morality is to create and maintain a dignified conscientious awareness within the boundaries of reasoning power. Such a fundamental belief is based upon how an individual views autonomy, rationality, and impartiality in their judgmental perceptions.
- Moral beliefs should not be imposed upon an individual by some authorities. They must be freely adhered to in order to be reasonable. Thus, morality is a product of reflective thinking.
- Individuals have the moral responsibility to develop their moral characteristics and reform and enhance them through virtuous work experiences.
- Individuals have the moral obligation to develop and maintain virtuous power for developing their enhanced social behavior.
- The moral social reforms in an individual's moral character must genuinely move society towards goodness.
- Moralists should be the symbols of leading forces to teach other people the truth about the construction and reconstruction of human personalities within the context of goodness.
- Reconstruction of morality in a society requires a virtuous doctrine based on behavioral excellence.
- Morality deals with human inner space, while ethics deals with outer human space.

Since the major theme of this chapter is moral theories, we will elaborate on this topic by reviewing different hypothetical assumptions of moral theories in the following pages.

DIFFERENCES AMONG MORAL THEORIES

Socrates, the first great moral philosopher, stated the creed of reflective individuals and set the milestone of the task of moral theories. Since then most philosophers and writers have perceived and treated human beings in relation to morality and ethics. Some philosophers, whose views are oriented towards theological doctrines, appear to believe human beings are situated in the kingdom of God and they have to be obedient to Him and follow the Lord's orders in order to have "revelation." On the other hand, non-theological philosophers such as existentialists, materialists, and naturalists conceive that human beings are situated within the general realm of nature with their own "free choices and volitions." They believe that if human beings want comfort and peace they should not disturb or violate the rules of nature. The latter philosophers believed that human beings possess absolute control over their minds and actions and that is why only they themselves determine them. In such a path of life, existentialist philosophers believe that human beings, through their decisive virtues, can discover the worthy means concerning the right way of life.

Both groups of philosophers agree that, in the kingdom of God or in the realm of nature, human beings through their emotional fickleness and sensational infirmities are exposed to the mysterious flaws of greed, bemoaning, revenge, fear, anger, savagery, cruelty, atrocity, and discrimination. However, both theoretical ethicality and morality focus their views on the nature of human beings. They perceive that humans possess means to overcome unpleasant emotional and sensational desires. These philosophers believe that human beings have to eradicate their sensational weaknesses, emotional absurdities, and dreadful desires.

In viewing and applying moral, intellectual, and necessitated virtues, many philosophers and researchers express their views through various types of reasoning. There are different schools of thought concerning moral theories such as idealism, realism, hedonism, eudaemonism, and authenticism.

IDEALISTIC MORAL THEORY

Idealism moral theory includes all views that hold that there is an independent world that is mental or spiritual in nature. Idealists are usually religious or at least sympathetic with religious outlooks. Opponents to idealism morality are materialists or existentialists, or naturalists. The materialists consider that all reality consists of matter (money) and its manifestation is a comfortable life. They believe that even moral consciousness is a manifestation of material or bodily processes. We may distinguish three basic meanings of the terms of *ideals*:

In the world of goodness, there are perfect ideals that can never be fully realized. Ideals are not static. Ideals are dynamic sources of urge. All ideals strive for self-identification and preservation. They struggle to rise to the threshold of consciousness. Thinking and willingness perceptions arise from the circle of intellectuality.

- Philosopher John Fredrich Herbart (1806) appeared to look upon goodness with favor in the so-called ideomotor theory of action that William James upheld. The theory of ideomotor action holds that ideas in the mind, which have reference to action, tend to produce actions. For example, we are inclined to think of perfect beauty as a physical term and excellence in character, not as attainable objectives, but as directions of aesthetic endeavors, which can never be realized as their final objectives – at least not in the form of earthly experiences. Biosceintists, biotechnologists, and biomedical practitioners seem primarily devoted to the moral ideals of discovering remedies to prevent death, pain, and disability. Genetic engineering, counseling, and enhancement may have as their primary ideal preventing the loss of freedom in their clients. They strive to find causes of abnormality and disability to prevent aging and death – eugenic biology.

- There is the ideal in the sense of something of *excellence* that can be realized by wisdom and/or intellect. For example, when we speak of "ideal weather," or "ideal life," we perceive it as a balanced term, neither severely cold nor very hot. Nevertheless, ideas are impulses. They are not separable from things. All ideas are impulsive. Morality involves approval and disapproval of judgments concerning those ideals. Aesthetics also deals with judgments regarding the beautiful and the ugly-judgments on appearances of things and phenomena. All moral judgments involve patterns of ideas, judgments that bear certain relations to each other. It is not important to decide how specific to make the moral ideals, for, normally, following any moral ideal is praiseworthy and rewarding. It is, however, important to distinguish moral ideals from other ideals to safeguard the sanctity and purity of human thoughts and behavior.

- Finally, there is an ideal in the derisive sense of something wholly visionary or quixotic. Within the contextual boundaries of the idealistic theory of morality, there are three basic moral ideas:

    o The ideas of intrinsic freedom and choice are viewed as a manifestation of moral judgments. These ideas state that the

intellectual deliberative "will" of the individual is in harmony
with an individual's inner conscientious convictions.

o   The ideas of extrinsic perfection and happiness are holistic in
    their nature. These ideas are harmonious relationships between
    the various striving powers of the self-will and the
    environmental orderliness.

o   The ideas of benevolence and altruism are viewed as the final
    cause of happiness. These ideas mandate individuals that help
    others in order to realize their worthwhile wills. For example,
    we are talking about medical responsibilities. This mandates
    that leading experts and specialists contribute their knowledge
    and experience for the goodness of society. Within such an
    ethical environment, not only patients will be cured,
    professionals also receive appreciation from the public
    because they are that they are service-oriented people.

Principles in Moral Idealism

This world is full of goodness and badness; it depends on how you perceive
them. Avoidance of goodness may cause sinful intentions (in religious terms)
and dreadful actions (in miserable earthly-life terms). Human beings should try
to stay within the domain of goodness. Nevertheless, separation of the human
mind from the godly ideal of goodness is considered in terms of good intention
and actions. It is the fear of bad intentions that tempts human beings to separate
themselves from goodness and join badness. They need to solve this problem by
"copying, following or imitating" knowledge. Like the installment plan of
buying, copying, following, or imitating knowledge can solve problems.

We may distinguish three basic meanings of the term moral idealism:

*   There is an ideal in the sense of excellent behavior that can be realized,
    as when we speak of "ideal friendship" or of "ideal weather." It is an
    idiom that states that: "A friend indeed is a friend in deed," or a friend
    in need is a friend indeed." This is the surest state of human mind that
    should pursue heavenly life without corruption and defectiveness.
    People need to live in harmony with each other and with nature in order
    to maintain peace of mind.

*   To search for goodness and beauty in our character is not an attainable
    goal, but a direction of our endeavor toward goodness. Goodness is not
    only viewed as a destiny, it also is viewed as a journey. This direction
    can orient a human's mind towards goodness. This means that we need
    not only to think and talk about goodness, but also to attend the
    pragmatic realm of goodness. Through mental goodness, we will be
    able to reach the portal of mental and moral health. Through the

pragmatic realm of goodness, we will be able to apply spiritual virtues in our deeds.

- Finally, there is the ideal in the derisive sense of something holistically visionary to pursue goodness as happiness. Moral idealists believe in happiness through attending to the process of goodness. They believe that we need to avoid blind-will, blind-fear, blind power, and blind-domination, because these kinds of actions, expressed as killing, causing unprofessional pain and suffering, deceiving patients, and breaking trustworthiness of professional promises, are against good will and good faith.

There is no doubt that "gifts of nature," such as intelligence, fortitude, courage, and perseverance are desirable, but they may be pernicious if the will directs them in such a way that they are not good. For example, *loyalty* in its moral term within a profession is not impressive as a virtue when we consider the loyalty of an auditor to an embezzler. Such loyalty is based on blind-fear. *Courage* may further evil as well as good ends, as the case of the intrepid patient abuser shows.

The global goodwill is not good purely good, because it may not achieve desirable consequences. The value of goodwill is based upon good means and good ends. Good will is reverence for duty and duty is founded on reason. Keeping one's promise or one's duty may require positive actions. Professional duty may require causing pain in patients, as in the case of a physician who, with the rational informed consent of a competent patient, performs some painful procedure in order to prevent or stop much more serious pain or death. Reasons seek universal principles for being ideally, physically, mentally, and socially good. There are three major schools of idealistic morality: Platonic, Aquinasian, and Hobbesian.

Platonic Moral Idealism: Plato (427-347 B.C.) supposed that there are permanent good ideas that maintain their own existence irrespective of the existence or nonexistence of God(s), nor do these good ideas require the minds of humans to give them reality by knowing them. Plato in his *Dialogues* (1892) found two basic beliefs relevant to morality:

- The doctrine of *teleology* in which everything in the universe has a proper function within a harmonious hierarchy of purposes. Thus, the ultimate of universal purposes have been explained in the nature of things. They are purposive rather than mechanistic. He emphasized the "why" of an event rather than the "how" as happiness. This indicates that a human's purpose is relevant to their proper functions. Their proper purposive values, like that of everything else in the universe, depend upon their excellence in fulfilling those proper functions. The moral purposes of individuals in realizing their objectives are determined by the effective functioning of the basic constituents of the types of their personalities. The morally virtuous person is one who is in rational, biological, and emotional balance, or in Platonic terms, one who is *wise, temperate, courageous*, and *just*. Bioscientists and researchers need to penetrate the nature through their relentless efforts in order to discover the truth.

- The doctrine of *Ideas or Forms,* which refers to a belief that general conceptions are not derived from experience but are logically prior to it. Each of us knows what honesty is. It is the truthful expression of an idea, reason, and/or motive. The idea of honesty is more real than experiencing truthful action. Plato culminated his account with the *Form*s or *Ideas* of the Good, the conception through which he united the principle of teleology and the theory of *Ideas* or *Forms* with morality. For example, a surgeon may claim that during a surgical operation finds that he/she needs to make a crucial decision by changing the routine surgical procedure and/or forms of surgery in order to avoid the death of a patient. He/she may claim that withholding these unusual procedural results in less overall harm or suffering for his/her patient without his/her consent. Thus, the surgeon may claim that his/her decision and action actually resulted in the patient suffering less harm than had he/she was obtained the patient's consent.

Aquinasian Moral Idealism: Saint Thomas Aquinas (1225-1274) is known as one of the theological moral theorists who have offered us a Christianized version of Aristotle's moral theory. He adds the concept of the beatific vision of God as humanity's final goal, a special doctrine of free will, and a theory of natural law as the reflective divine order. Aquinas (1945) believed that there is a twofold perfection of rational or intellectual nature: (1) natural happiness, and (2) supernatural happiness (God's image). Therefore, humans have two sources of truth rather than one:

- Those truths with human faculties provide us with virtues concerning our habitual choices of conduct. These choices are correct in outline but incomplete in details. Goodness involves choices, and choices include both appetitive and deliberative elements of moral conduct. A good character is constituted of habits and choices that are in accordance with appropriate principles. Identification of the "will" is the agency of good choices.

- The second types of truths are those truths that God reveals. He ascribed the source and authority of principles determining proper choices to the natural laws in which God makes them available to humans. These truths reveal God to be both creator of all good things and the determiner of their purposes in the state of existence. Nevertheless, each agent by its action intends an end.

As a result, Aquinas believed that the consequences of an individual's conduct are either foreseen or not. If they are foreseen, it is evident that they increase goodness or malice. But if the consequences are not foreseen, we must make a distinction. For if they follow from the nature of action, in the majority of cases, the consequences increase the goodness or malice of that action. On the other hand, if consequences follow by accident and are seldom, then they do not increase the goodness or malice of the act. For example, in the field of medicine, one can specify particular moral ideals that involve preventing unjustified violations of the professional moral rules. Insofar as a lack of proper understanding of morality leads to unjustified violations of the professional moral rules, providing a proper understanding of morality is also following a moral ideal.

Hobbesian Moral Idealism: Thomas Hobbes (1588-1679) is viewed as an idealistic materialist and as a highly pessimistic moralist. Hobbes's *Leviathan* (1839) presented a bleak picture of the innate qualities of human beings in the "state of nature." Hobbes, like us, lived in a time of extreme violence and exploitation of human rights. Consequently, Hobbes contended that fear of violent death is the primary motive that causes people to create a political state by constructing to surrender their natural rights and to submit to the absolute authority of a sovereign.

Hobbes believed that competition is viewed as a war of every human being or group against every other one. The notion of justice or injustice, fairness or unfairness, rightness or wrongness has no place. Where there is no moral rule, there is no moral power; where no moral law, no justice. At the same time, he believed that exploitive forces such as fraud and corruption are at war with virtues. Justice or injustice, fairness or unfairness, rightness or wrongness faculties are neither of the body, nor mind. They are comparative valuable consequences of conditions that insure there is no propriety, no dominion, but only that every human being gets what he/she can get, for so long as he/she can keep it.

While human beings are in war with natural conditions, they cannot be successful unless they establish a covenant of mutual trust among themselves. Therefore, before the notions of justice or injustice appear, there must be some coercive power to compel human beings to perform in accordance with their mutual trust covenants. What is such a covenant mutual trust? It is a moral power to ensure the good of the commonwealth. Where there is no moral good commonwealth, there is nothing just or unjust.

A *commonwealth* goodness is said to be instituted when a multitude of people do agree, and covenant, every one, with everyone, that particular individuals, or assemblies of individuals, shall be given by the major part the right to represent the entire group. With the establishment of the commonwealth goodness through the social contract, Hobbes tells us; the necessary and sufficient condition for morality is present.

Hobbes established the notion of civil authority and law as a foundation of morality. He argued that morality requires *social authority, and law as the foundation of morality.* Nevertheless, Hobbes rejected the individual's consciousness awareness as the main source of morality. Morality, then, is based upon law, the law of the absolute sovereignty of an individual, group, and/or nation. He assumed morality and legality proceed in the same path of perceptual reasoning, because morality is a pluralistic phenomenon that turns out to be the "dictation of reason" through absolute civil power.

Conclusions

The idealism moralists, like others, deal with certain basic beliefs in morality. They are very impressed with the thought that the universe is ultimately something mental or spiritual. They are uncompromising opponents to materialism. They believe that spiritual belief in goodness is the main cause for existence. They believe that the states and activities of the self, as we experience them inwardly through our mental vision, are the only realities that we can know directly and incontrovertibly. They believe that our moral vision becomes the world of appearances. They believe that a valid universal morality is apprehended by the mind as perfectly clear and self-evident intuition of good faith, good will, and good acts.

REALISTIC MORAL THEORY

The realistic moral theory is a more pragmatic, action-oriented view concerning morality. Moral realists hope to provide foundations for the moral guidance of mankind. The ideas of moral realists in the sphere of moral theory are varied and complex. A major problem for moral realists is how to cope with immoral actions and how they will be able to find remedies that are compliant with definitions and standards of moral virtues. In other words, idealistic absolute goodness should show how humans could achieve their moral objectives through intellectual wisdom and moral reasoning. In the realistic moral theory, we are trying to match our valuable practical behavior with our moral virtues.

A central difficulty of any moral theory is to do justice to both the absolute virtues and to the relative aspects of moral values. By an absolute goodness, we need to know the statistically mean one that is intrinsically and always good in human intellectual wisdom and reasoning. However, with an extrinsic judgmental valuable perception concerning goodness, we may come out with several degrees of relative goodness with different comparative value systems. Since morally good will is an absolute good, many of the good things of life are *relative, not absolute.* We need to consider valuable moral behavior through excellence, best, better, and good, or conversely vice, worst, worse, and bad. Within such a magnitude, we may in practice find morality not as an absolute phenomenon, but as a relative one when compared to higher and lower qualities. There are numberless values that are relatively higher than others. As Montague (1930: 44) indicates: "No amount of happiness enjoyed by pigs can be equal to the happiness of Socrates."

Principle Beliefs in Moral Relativism: How an individual's decisions and behaviors become good or bad depend on morality in a real pragmatic sense. Realism is old as existentialism, naturalism, and materialism. It deals with what "actually exists." This indicates that an individual desires the ability to deny his/her past and present nature of existence. He/she desires to become something different and better than that he/she was in the past, or he/she now is. He/she desires to do what he/she desires in a practical sense. He/she desires freedom to determine his/her destiny.

Realism's philosophical assumptions are based on common sense. Realists try to conceptualize moral convictions of humans in nature within conditional and situational circumstances. They try to find contingent practical solutions for human problems and conflicts. There are specific moral principles that realists have found in their beliefs. These principles are as follows:

- Humans possess natural convictions concerning the extrinsic existence of power. This indicates that they are part of a highly orchestrated system of universal ordination.
- Humans possess convictions regarding the existence of moral truths. Moral truths existed before we discovered them. They will exist after we pass away. For example, honesty has always been viewed by all generations as goodness. It will remain the same, in the moral sense in the future too.
- Humans possess convictions regarding the existence of spirituality in human nature. Attributes of moral virtues exist just as we know them, except for errors in our perceptions that are verifiable as mistakes. This indicates that life is a process of "trial and error."
- Humans possess convictions regarding conscientious awareness not only of external objects, forces, and derivative powers, but also of the causal and multiple linkages among themselves.
- Moral behavior and experiences are the touchstones of what is real, "seeing is believing."
- Such a knowable moral conviction shows us how material things, as external manifestations of nature, are perceived as interdependent linkages among all elements in the universe.
- We are living in the midst of external realities, which simply are what they are, or what they appear to be to our perceptions.
- Realism seeks to describe characters and their interrelated events as they really are without idealization, sentimentalization, and/or deception.

As we mentioned above, the term *moral realism* had to do with what actually exists; "seeing is believing." Immanuel Kant called this empirical knowledge as known science. Kant believed in empirical moral knowledge; the application of realistic patterns of goodness and happiness in daily human life. He believed science is based on observation and direct exposure to knowledge. Knowledge always comes after the evidence found in the process.

In contrast to the moral idealists that believe in good will as the basic foundation of moral judgment, moral realists believe that good will or intentions alone are not sufficient to reach the pinnacle of goodness. Good will should result in good deeds. In addition, the application of moral realism principles in human thought and behavior can result in a stabilized life.

- *Kantian Moral Realism*: Within the scope of real endeavor, we are examining Kant's views on morality that are based on "good-will as the means and ends of unconditionally good deeds." Immanuel Kant's (1724-1804) realistic morality is mainly set forth in his book *Fundamental Principles of Metaphysics of Morals* (1785). He sought a *priori* principles that prescribe universal laws of conduct. He found two objectives in morality:

- *Goodwill as Unconditionally Good*: Kant concluded that the only thing in the world that is good without limitation is the good will to do one's duty. There are no other "gifts of nature," such as intelligence, courage, and perseverance. These traits are desirable, but may be pernicious if the "will" which directs them is not good (Kant 1957: 539). He asked: What determines the nature of excellence? He answered this question in his own way: "The will is good when it is completely devoted to duty for the sake of duty."

- *Duty as Moral Imperative*: The "good-will" is not good unless it achieves excellent consequences. The "value" of good faith defines the nature of good will. For example, if a foolish person with his/her good faith commits a foolish act, such an act is not perceived as moral because the foolish consequence does not carry any moral value. This means that moral acts need to have moral values along with good-will in the agents' characters not only in means, but also in their ends. In the field of biosciences, if a biologist collects a series of vials of bacteria and suddenly, without thinking about his decision and actions, releases them into the environment in an inappropriate manner, such an action may cause serious harm or damages to people and their environments. Such an act is viewed as immoral. "Just causes" seek universal laws that are consistent or congruent with proper promissory conducts. Such a moral rule requires good faith in promises. To behave morally means to be able to properly *justify* self-conduct.

The formulation of categorical imperatives especially brings out the moral convictions held by realists in general that each individual has an intrinsic worth of consciousness in his/her conduct. We must not use all these worthy good faiths and good wills *merely* as means. We need to act within our community where each individual is at once ruler and subject. Kant (1898: 10) concluded that the only thing in the world that is good without limitation is the "good-will" to do one's intellectual duty. He believed that a moral person needed to be experienced with the universal principles of goodness.

Moral experience is the touchstone of what is real. There are different perceptions in morality. These perceptions raise fundamental questions such as:

- What is the common sense of existence?
- What is an individual's intellectual sense of existence?
- Does morality answer to a universal sense of understanding?

To answer to these questions we will explain the realistic views of Thomas Reid and John Locke.

***Reidian Moral Realism*:** Thomas Reid (1710-1796) was the champion of the realism of common sense. His views are set in his *Inquiry into the Human Mind on the Principles of Common Sense* (1764). He held that an individual has dependable and immediate intuitive convictions regarding the existence of the external world, of moral truths, and of the existence of the soul. He thought the universal conviction of human beings depended on moral truths. We have an immediate awareness, not only of external objects, but of the causal and other relations between them. There are at least two main ways of conceiving universal moralism:

- We may regard universal moral laws as a set of separate principles that govern *"forms"* in truth. Forms follow the natural ordination. These forms are *"mental"* in their empirical nature.
- The moral laws of nature do not govern natural processes, but only express specific *"knowable"* attributes to describe such processes. These laws are the essence of common sense, or as Kant called it, "science."

Reid believed that scientific empirical knowledge is based upon good choices and volitions in the human mind and actions. This is the surest moral decision and action. We can call a biotech employer a "real moralist" because we mean that he/she never loses sight of the bitter taste of "unprofessional consequences." The realistic moral bioscientists and biotechnologists who usually manage a medical laboratory or a biotech corporation achieve their moral objectives despite *"adverse"* circumstances. They never lie or deceive their stakeholders. These types of scientists and technologists believe that if there are realities that cannot be altered, then the realist scientists should alter themselves to suit those realities.

Lockeian Moral Realism: John Locke (1632-1704), whose moral theory influenced the American Founding Fathers, believed that every human is allowed to use what nature provides. Locke is known as a moral empiricist. People may make natural resources their own if they can use them and if others have as much, and as good, remaining for their use as well. The initial partition of the earth is a fact. Each person owns a portion of such partitions. The moral right of declaring ownership of natural resources is based on the fortunate condition of having been born in a country where resources exist.

Locke founded morality on religious authority, tempered with reasonableness. We are obligated to behave morally through God's commands. This is the ultimate sanction of morality. He believed that the truth in morality is not stabilized unless it is subject to periodic validation. There is abundant reasoning in nature that demonstrates their validity to unbiased reasons.

Locke's realistic ideas on morality are further set forth in his *Treatise on Government* (1690). His view regarding moral behavior of citizens in a country is that of a diffused relationship between religion and government. Locke conceived an original state of nature provided by God where humans are entitled to such rights as freedom, justice, and the ownership of property. But humans violate these God-bestowed rights by seeking their own selfish ends and by robbing and enslaving each other. Such intentions and acts are immoral.

Conclusions

Today, in a moral sense, we speak of human rights rather than natural rights. Human rights are rooted in law and protected by it. Natural rights are rooted in the sanctity of morality. In a just and moral society, legal rights are differentiated products of moral rights, and to a considerable degree they overlap with pragmatism. Legal rights perform a negative function by telling people what is *forbidden*. A positive morality tells people what is permissible and what they *should* do.

Realistic moral theory is a doctrine that perceives goodness as a real means and ends to be properly linked in their right path of intellectual wisdom. Both good faith and good will require not the will of God, nor the might of nature, nor the edicts of society to make them better than they are. Pragmatic real good faith and good-will demands of us that whichever of them is pragmatically relevant to a person's given good situation should be pursued. But demands are not commands. They should be congruent with the possibilities of achieving good consequences.

HEDONISTIC MORAL THEORY

There are two other moral theories whose principles we can apply as means and ends in examining our moral behavior. One is all *self-centric:* good behaviors endorse *hedonistic morality*; the view that "pleasure" is the only intrinsic goodness in life worth pursuing. Second is the *egoists'* belief that both intrinsic and extrinsic values are not simply pleasurable, which may differ in quality as well as quantity, but create *happiness*. This second view is called *eudaemonistic morality*. Since the basic value in terms of both assessments results in good ends, it is perceived as happiness, not pleasure. For clarity of meanings we describe pleasure through hedonistic moral theory and happiness through eudaemonistic moral theory as means and ends of morality (De George, 1995: 63).

The view that associates morality with self-interested decisions and actions believes that goodness is an intrinsic power can that manifest a pleasurable life as delightful life. The theory of morality that advocates a pleasurable life as the means and ends of goodness is known as *hedonism*, a name taken from the Greek meaning "pleasure." One question that surfaces in hedonistic moral objectives is: Is there some least common denominator in terms of which we can assess our perceptual goodness? The answer is yes. That is through the application of the moral theory of hedonism.

Principle Beliefs in Hedonistic Moral Theory

Hedonistic moral theory holds that basic human values should be oriented toward the promotion of pleasure and the avoidance of pain. According to this view, everything that people desire, wants, or needs could be reduced in one way or another to pleasure or pain. Pleasure means the absence of pain.

Pleasure, in its strictest sense, is the immediate accomplishment of delightful sensational, emotional, and physical ends. Pleasure is the powerful dynamic motive that urges individuals to respond positively to their good need-dispositions. The immediacy and vehemence of sensational and emotional delightfulness would probably be the main reason for stability of human life and the survival of the human species. Therefore, all people need to enjoy their lives and avoid suffering.

Pleasure is the avoidance of experiencing depravation from need-dispositions. Pleasure is a search for gratification to be experienced with the fulfillment of physical, sensational, and emotional consequences. Depravation is a kind of momentary suffering from the stabilized states of deficiencies. Also, depravation is, culturally, assumed to be an aversive state that may involve withholding desired psychological tendencies. For example, in both the Jewish and Moslem faiths, fasting, and in Buddhism and Hinduism, meditation, are considered conscious deprivation from such things as eating and drinking, in order to motivate people to appreciate and obtain fulfillment. The end-result is self-confidence and self-realization.

Recall that hedonistic morality encourages positive intentions and actions to prevent or relieve pains or harms. A general hedonistic morality is mentioned the general categories of harms and pains in the field of medical and health as in "relieve pain or prevent harm." Relief from pain is a desirable emotional and sensational end, but prevention of disabilities specifies particular harms to prevent malpractice. There is an idiom that states "no pain, no gain." Pleasure can be considered in two ways:

- As the end result of an action with a pleasurable memory
- At the beginning of an action with the "intention" of pursuing a life-lasting enjoyment

In analyzing these two processes, we acknowledge that the interpretation of pleasure is different from culture to culture. Some cultures conceive that pleasure, as the end-result, is the last in execution, for it is the last thing to happen. But in other cultures, the end is the first, not in the order of execution, but in the order of intention. For example, some people believe in financial depravation in the form of putting aside some income, saving for the necessity of their future needs, while in other cultures people perceive pleasure on the basis of the immediate action of spending their incomes to fulfill their immediate end-desires. This is the result of the complexity of human nature. There is no doubt that both types of cultures are striving for "goodness" one conceives pleasure in a long period of waiting (as with savings), while the other perceives it in a short period of time (as with spending). In fact, the sense of pleasure is a trajectory state of excessive sensational and emotional enjoyment which turns an individual's behavior from depravation and suffering to the climax of fulfillment and then gradually turns it back to the original state of depravation and deficiency again. This is considered the momentum of the survival of the human race. In viewing the hedonistic theory, we will review Spenserian views.

***Spenserian Hedonistic Moral Views*:** Herbert Spenser (1820-1903) was a hedonistic moralist who believed that *pleasure is the essence of the good*. Spenserian philosophy (1888) is a systematic thought, characterized by bringing various scientific thoughts into a systematic whole. To Spenser, pleasure has been defined as an individual's good experiences. Life approaches perfect goodness when it leads at once to present pleasure and remote pleasure. Spenser's hedonism also serves to define right and wrong decisions and actions. Conduct is right when it leads to pleasure for all. It is wrong when it entails avoidable pain and the depravation of pleasure.

Spenser believed that "egotism" must come before "altruism." Since egotism is a product of determination, then human beings are capable of searching for pleasure more than for pain. Society, therefore, exists in the service of its individual members. The pleasure of the group exists in terms of the pleasure of its individual members. Nevertheless, egoism and altruism are complementary. But as the moral status of a society evolves, it will see that altruism becomes a mandatory moral objective to be achieved.

Spenser's hedonistic moral hypothetical assumption is based on a belief in the necessity of finding a scientific basis for the distinction between pleasure and happiness and for the general guidance of conduct. Toward this end, he considered it necessary to examine the linkage between nature and human desires. Also, Spenser regarded moral conduct as good to the extent that it makes life longer, richer, and happier for the individual, for his/her children, and for the social group. He believed that hedonistic moral objectives are viewed as fulfillment in a society where there is durable peace and in which each individual achieves their desired objectives and aids others in achieving theirs.

Within the contextual boundaries of bioethics according to Spenserian hedonistic morality, stem cell engineering, transplantation of animal organs to human beings, gene engineering, and cloning are permissible because each technique provides more enjoyment for human beings. Spenserian hedonistic moralists believe that it is the moral commitment of bioscientists and biotechnologists to either prevent harm (aging) or relieve pain (death) from human beings. What is odd about hedonistic morality is that it provides scientific justifications to do everything to avoid pain and prevent harm to human beings, since in preventing harm or disability bioscientists and biotechnologists are morally obligated to humanity to strive to find new techniques to relieve pain and/or to prevent harm to humans.

Conclusions

We may take into our considerations any kind of conscientious judgment concerning our conduct that can be assessed by the end results of our self-conduct. Since a human being is a complex being, he/she possesses a vast range of intrinsic instinct, sensation, imagination, emotion, genetics, problem solving and innovation. He or she also possesses a sense of learning, memorization, and creation. He/she is a whole and unified being. He/she is searching for satisfaction within and beyond the self. This mandates him/her to accomplish pleasurable and delightful objectives and to avoid painful or dreadful consequences. For such reasons, he/she makes a priority of perceiving first pleasure in the self and then in others. This characteristic in a moral sense is called hedonistic morality. Therefore, hedonistic moral theory is based upon the principles that:

- Moral life is based on the mitigation of pain and the enhancement of pleasure first in the self and then in others.
- Everything that people desire, wants, or need could be reduced in one way or another to pleasure or pain, or to help or harm.

- Pleasure is an intrinsic process that can manifest and maintain a high egotistic status.
- Pleasure is the end result of self-satisfaction.
- Pleasure is an end in humans that manifests satisfaction.

To live well in terms of hedonistic moral philosophy is to live a life of pleasure. Hence, since the good life appears to consist of pleasurable activities and the good use of satisfaction, it seems to be very egoistical. Nevertheless, since the nature of human beings is to desire limitless pleasure, within such a contextual perception, they need to pursue goodness. In closing, pleasure is viewed first and foremost as a state of interior well being, even by those who perceive it as an extrinsic objective for accumulating wealth, power, and reputation because they enjoy the possession of the wealth, power, and reputation.

EUDAEMONISTIC MORAL THEORY

As we mentioned above, there are two approaches in being moral: (1) hedonistic and (2) eudaemonistic. We have explained that the hedonistic approach is based on pleasurable and delightful means and ends. The advantage of the hedonistic approach has been challenged by another group of moralists who claim that not all intrinsically valuable good faith and good-will can be used to convert pain into pleasure or to convert harm to benefit. Eudaemonistic morality is based on balancing pain and pleasure or harms and helps. They believe that life is based upon the unification or diffusion of pleasure and pain or harms and helps in a balanced unity of existence. Also, eudaemonistic moralists maintain that pleasure is not the one and only thing that is good in itself; hence, depending on the view that one adopts, it is just one of a number of things that are good in this sense. Such a process is the result of our sensations and emotions. Since both sensation and emotion are differentiated from our feelings, then they may or may not establish a rational basis for being moral. What is intrinsically valuable in our consciousness is not simply pleasure but happiness (De George, 1995: 63).

The most serious defect of pleasure is that pleasure does not satisfy the whole ego of an individual person, nor even the best part of that person. People can share their pleasures with others through sensational and emotional enjoyments. Pleasure would not seem to provide the sort of happiness suitable to all people. Since pleasure does not create long-range satisfaction for an individual or even the best intellectual values, what Aristotle called the *"moral virtue,"* it would not seem to provide happiness suitable to an *"intellectual virtue"* because it is short-lived. It may be intense, but it never lasts. The magnitude of pleasure is derived from its own restriction and at best, it is limited to certain levels of goodness. This suggests that a certain type of moral egoism is typical of those who are concerned with avoiding harm to the self rather than gaining benefits for the self.

We should remember that eudaemonistic egoism is a doctrine that maintains the sanctity of human rationality and directs us to seek only our own happiness through intellectual virtues. Egoism contends that an action is morally right if and only if it best promotes the individual's long-term goodness. Within the mechanistic boundaries of morality, we need to identify the difference between *selfishness* and *egoism*. *Selfishness* is the inherent nature of emotional and sensational pleasurable goodness, while rational *egoism* is the inherent nature of moral happiness in terms of intellectual virtue. Therefore, we need to identify what moral happiness is.

What Is Moral Happiness?

Eudaemonistic theorists believe that people use their best long-term advantages as the standard for measuring an action's rightness. If an action produces or is intended to produce a greater ratio of good to evil in the long run than any other alternatives, then that action is the right one to be performed or pursued. In such a case an individual should take that course of moral action to attain the state of happiness. Thus, we see how an eudaemonistic moral theorist perceives its means and ends on the basis of happiness.

We are now in a position to discuss what we mean by happiness. Within such a domain of inquiry, we need to face three distinctive questions:

- Can an individual attain moral happiness?
- Can an individual maintain moral happiness?
- Is such a moral happiness complete happiness for an individual's life-long process?

Again, let us recall what has been defined as moral happiness. Moral happiness is an ever-lasting process of having a good and clean life. All people agree that happiness is an ultimate end state of end when conscience awareness fulfills its proper mandates. In attempting to determine objectively what happiness consists of, we arrive in a state of "life with virtue." The state of life with virtue is known as living according to moral reasoning, extending and concluding it with intrinsic and extrinsic excellent results. We will analyze the original questions concerning happiness and then outline the doctrine of eudaemonistic moral theory.

Principle Beliefs in Eudaemonistic Moral Theory

Eudaemonistic moralists believe that morality is primarily an individual's convictions toward excellence in terms of intellectual virtue. If we perceive scientific endeavors as virtuous efforts that include science, understanding, wisdom, art, and prudence, then can we call them "knowledge." If our attention is focused on knowledge, then we need to define what we mean by knowledge, science, data, information, and alertness as intellectual virtuous awareness.

In today's free market economy, the basic organizational resource is no longer material capital, labor, or natural resources, but knowledge-wealth. Knowledge is not the same thing as scientific formulas, data, or information, although it uses all these phenomena. Knowledge manifests itself a step further, beyond scientific boundaries. It is a conclusion drawn from the application of scientific formulas and information data after it is linked to other known and unknown phenomena and compared to what is already known. Scientific formulas direct us not only to be knowledgeable about the functions of existence; they also direct us to know why something is true. This type of analysis is called syllogism.

Syllogism, as we defined before, is a conclusive argument in which two premises and a conclusion can be expressed either by demonstration or deduction. When we use scientific syllogistic formulas, we prove two domains of facts:

- The existence of logical truthfulness, demonstrated reasoning concerning a phenomenon, element, process, or the dynamics of a synthesized membership functional group.

- The possible deductive conclusion of a manifestation of premises that states why such formulas are true. For example, if a CEO of a biotech corporation is eligible to vote on the Board of Directors, that CEO is a member of the Board of Directors. Then the deductive result indicates that the board is a *codeterminative* one.

Science deals with human understanding concerning the discovery and formulation of the real world in which the inherent properties of space, matter, energy, and their interactions can be perfectly scrutinized and predicted. Science is a rational convention related to the generalization of the expected environmental norms, expectations, and values. It is nothing more than the search for understanding of the fundamental reasoning of the real world. Nevertheless, searching for discovery in the real world in practice is composed of ethical and unethical practices. Sometimes scientists ignore the rights of individuals or groups when they reveal the real world. A successful scientific innovation needs to apply innovations. The scientists' concern about innovativeness states that "excellence" needs a vision in order to be focused on the maximum prudence in achieving creative methods. This is the exact meaning of eudaemonistic moral practices. Such an eudaemonistic moral objective mandates that scientists question the answers of previous questions they wanted to answer, where the world of humanity is moving toward, and to which path of discovery they need to be directed. For example, in biotechnology and biobusiness industry, how should scientists pursue the notion of happiness for humanity through 'cloning human beings? Within such an important scientific endeavor, how can human dignity and integrity be guarded? What bioscientists and bioethicists need to consider is the collection of appropriate progenistic data through prodigical information systems in order to understand the consequences of cloning on the welfare of humanity.

Prognostic data are simple, absolute quantitative facts and figures that, in and of himself or herself, may be of little value or use. At this juncture, data is known as the raw facts, untouched by human minds. Nevertheless, we have more knowable data than we can tell. To be valuable and useful for humanity, data is processed into finished information by connecting parts with other data. Therefore, information is the end result of the functioning membership of prognostic data that have been linked with other data and converted into a workable and meaningful context for the identification of specific right or wrong usage of data.

From another prodigic point of view, technological breakthroughs are known as integrated innovative systems which access, through pragmatic processing of interlinked data, both deep and broad domains of know-why, know-what, know-how, know-who, know-where, know-who, and know-for cyberspace information systems in both corporations and industries as well as in modern societies.

By technological breakthroughs, we mean any consistent application of scientific discoveries about the natural world that is employed to achieve a purposive objective to modify the material world. Therefore, in a moral sense prodigic technology is purposive. It is applied to achieve both ethical and moral objectives. Technology differs from science. Science seeks knowledge while technology applies science for the manipulation of the natural world to achieve a goal (Marshal, 1999: 83). Within such a highly sophisticated cyberspace environment, cognivistic knowledge mapping, pragmatic operational designs of data gathering, and holistic processing of the interlinked distributive operational techniques can be potentially abusive systems.

Data processes and designed outputs can be easily misused by biotechnologies in order to inflate the biocorporation's performance. Therefore, within the context of the real business world, we can claim that development of a technological civilization may not be evidence of progress from an ethical and moral point of view. However, technological developments are facts reflected in humanity's physical and intellectual abilities to affect and shape the natural environment and direct it to their desirable objectives (Parhizgar and Lunce, 1994: 55).

Under the above circumstances, the question of whether bioinformation can be assumed to be equivalent to, or at least possessing all the intellectual values when compared to bioknowledge, may be seen as a matter of logical reasoning. While the common practice has been to use the terms bioknowledge and bioinformation interchangeably, a number of differences between the two phenomena have been distinguished. Marshal (1997: 92) has described knowledge as inside the human mind and information as the knowledge outside the mind. Nevertheless, information may become knowledge when introduced into one's mental model.

Knowledge always contains a human intellectual valuable factor. E-sites, books, and pictures, which contain nudity from the standpoint of biological sciences, can be moral, ethical, and legal as knowledgeable sources of discovery only when scholars, researchers, and bioscientists absorb their real values and put them to scientific use. However, nude pictures, images, and the E-sites in advertising can be immoral, unethical, and illegal (pornographic magazines, books, and Internet E-sites) if children and adults are viewing them as a source of sexual pleasurable medium. Within such an analysis, through a eudaemonistic moral approach, formation, illustration, and manifestation of nudity by bioscientists is moral because they are using it to discover the real valuable characteristics of human beings. However, pleasurable viewing by lay people is immoral.

Knowledge is perceived and applied to both means and ends. In its logical reasoning as a means, knowledge is information that can be used to secure valuable materials as abstracts for the purpose of the spiritual enhancement of the human mind. As an end, knowledge can be perceived as understanding logical reasoning or using it for the contemplation or reflection of human enrichment. Knowing can be perceived as the possession of knowledge, and learning as the process of the acquisition of knowledge. Training is viewed as the process of disseminating and contributing knowledge from a knowledgeable person to an interested intended audience in order for them to acquire wisdom. Knowledge languishes and fades if it is not cultivated by wisdom, intellectual virtue. Knowledge is not self-sustaining; it does not grow by itself. It has to be actively cultivated by scholars in order to remain updated.

Going back to our discussion concerning egoistic happiness, moralists have distinguished two kinds of egoism: personal and impersonal. Personal 'egoism holds that individuals should pursue their own best long-term goodness, but they do not say what others should do. Impersonal egoism holds that everyone should follow his/her best long-term goodness as a cultural value system. Egoism requires us to do whatever will best further our own interests and doing this sometimes requires us to advance the interests of others. An interesting aspect of eudaemonistic morality as they are expressed in different cultures, including professions, is that the prevention of harm often becomes the duty of individual bioscientists, biotechnologist, and biomedical practitioners, by virtue of their ethical and moral convictions. Several misconceptions haunt both versions of egoism:

One criticism is that hedonistic moralists believe that people do only what they like that they believe in "eat, drink, and be merry." Another misconception is that hedonism endorses self-interest and the view that since only pleasure is of intrinsic value; the only good in life worth pursuing is for self-pleasurable ends. This will promote selfishness. Selfishness corrupts human morality and turns people into savages. Therefore, by this reason eudaemonistic moralists believe in happiness not in pursuing pleasurable objectives. They believe that happiness is both intrinsic and extrinsic satisfaction. Eudaemonistic moral values spell out specific standards based upon the primacy of greatest value, which is known as liberty. Everyone should act to ensure greatest freedom of choices.

Jeremy Bentham's Eudaemonistic Morality: Within the domain of morality, Jeremy Bentham (1748-1832) is known as an eudaemonistic moralist who believed that morality is based on the principle that the objective of life is the promotion of the greatest "happiness" for all individual people. Also, Bentham (1823) is often thought of as the founder of utilitarianism ethics: "The school of philosophy that holds that the tendency of an act is mischievous when the consequences of it are mischievous; that is to say, either the certain consequences or probable." For our purposes within the boundaries of eudaemonistic morality, it is important to treat pleasure and happiness separately. Bentham's view on happiness is influenced by the principles of utility that specify "the greatest amount of happiness" is the purpose of life. In addition, he believed that the purpose of government is to foster the happiness of all individuals, and that the greatest happiness of the most people should be the goal of human existence.

Conclusions

Eudaemonistic moralists believe that there are multiple sources of happiness for individuals. People need to learn the right methods to choose the surest pathways in order to choose the best ones. They believe that the choice should be assessed by the greatest amount of prudence through intellectual virtue. Eudaemonistic moralists believe that standards are applied to both the processes and consequences of self-volition or decision, the principle that everyone should act to generate the greatest benefits for the largest portion of human life. Moral standards are applied to the intent of actions or decisions, the principle that everyone should act independently to ensure that others, given similar circumstances, for the purpose of happiness, would reach similar decisions.

Eudaemonistic theory holds that the basic values in terms of moral behavior are a calculation of goodness and badness in terms of moral judgment. Some maintain that *"happiness"* is the essence of the right kind of thoughts, habits or behaviors. Happiness is more a means than an end.

(Happiness) = (Means of Goodness) > (Ends of Badness)

(H) = (MG) > (EB)

and

(Happiness) = (Good Faith) + (Good Will)

$$(H) = (GF) + (GW)$$

Sometimes some people acquire wealth and power not really for their own sake but as a means of achieving something else and sometimes some people acquire wealth, power, pleasure, and reputation as an end. It should be noted that if the wealth and power have been accumulated for the sake of wealth and power, then the concentration of wealth and the exertion of excessive power could produce either pleasure or misery. The accumulation of wealth and power can be used for good or for evil. Therefore, it is perceived that happiness is an ultimate end when the satisfaction and fulfillment of all intellectual desires are met.

As previously stated, in attempting to determine objectively what happiness is, it is primarily, as Aristotle called it, intellectual virtues. Intellectual virtues shape an individual's life in accordance with the goodness of a holistic health of body and mind. There are two different ways to seek pleasure and happiness. The first is to search for feelings and experience practical values, and the second is to seek speculative cognitive knowledge in order to understand, either for the sake of simply knowing or for the sake of making decisions for conscientious actions. Nevertheless, if existence consists of both pleasure and happiness, decisions deserve specific attention:

- What do individuals conceive implicitly when they believe in goodness what does that say about pleasure and happiness?
- What can individuals learn from scientific values, which are the end results of scientific deliberations?

By fulfilling goodness, we mean an individual seeking satisfaction and happiness as the ultimate end. Therefore, eudaemonistic moralists believe that happiness is the life-long objective for a moral person.

AUTHENTIC MORAL THEORY

People have always searched beyond their ages, probing the real and the universal image for their origin and the prediction of their finality. The universal image of the origin of humans helps shed light on a variety of images in order to understand their nature and the entity in which they are living, perceiving, and proceeding. There are three major images concerning the nature of human beings: (1) unitarians, (2) binarians, and (3) trinitarians. Unitarians believe that the human is an independent agent beyond of the contextual premises of universe. Their spirits are subject to eternity. The Binarians believe that human nature is a composition of dual entity (e.g. matter and spirit; virtue and vice, good and bad; physical and metaphysical, etc.) within the context of the universal image. Their bodies are subject to defectiveness but their minds are subject to the evolutionary processes of development, spiritualism. The Trinitarians believe that human nature is a dependent agent within the context of *kinetic*, *kinesthetic*, and *telekinesis* derivative forces and power.

Kinetic forces and power exist on the surface of logic for the existence of human beings. Kinetic existence pays close attention to three domains of morality: (1) the positive imagery of the material need causes, (2) the realistic affinity of need quiddity causes, and (3) the positive conclusive need causes (Parhizgar, 2002: 124).

Kinesthetic forces and power represent the synthesis of *explicit* and *tacit* knowledge in the form of codified intelligence. It is the essence of sensational and rational movement within the brain. Explicit knowledge is a kind of intellectual wisdom that can be easily articulated and communicated. Tacit knowledge, in contrast, is knowledge that is not easily communicated or manipulated because it is deeply rooted in the very in-depth of experience. Tacit knowledge is more valuable and likely to lead to sustainable competitive advantages than explicit knowledge, because it is much harder for competitors to imitate.

Telekinesis forces and power represent intuitive knowledge as the cognitive production of spiritual motion in the body without the application of material forces the mind. It is a power long claimed by spiritualists within the domain of human existence. This is viewed as the real essence of morality.

Within the context of the above viewpoints, we must now pay attention to another moral theory that represents one rather extreme kind of psychosocial reaction to the traditional moral theories. This moral theory is known as the "authentic theory of morality." This is the morality which Freud (1949) called the super-religious moralism. It should be noted that in a real sense authentic morality could not be egotistic or even selfish, it should be altruistic.

The moral authentic theory is traced back to the views of Sigmund Freud (1856-1939). His ideas concerning the psychodynamic theory of personality involve unconscious motivation and the development of personality structure. Freud viewed personality as the interactive processes among three elements within a person: the *id*, the *ego*, and the *superego*. Freud pictured a continuing challenge between two antagonistic parts of the personality; the id and the superego, moderated by a third aspect of the self, the ego. He conceived of the primitive and unconscious part of personality (the unleashed, raw, institutional drive struggling for gratification and pleasure), as the storehouse of personality. The id is governed by the pleasure principle the unregulated search for gratification. The ego is the reality-based aspect of the self that arbitrates the conflict between id impulses and superego demands. It represents reality. It, rationally, attempts to keep the impulsive id and the conscience of the superego in check, and represents an individual's personal view of physical and social reality (the conscience that provides the norms that enable the ego to determine what is right and what is wrong). There is an ongoing conflict between id and superego. The ego serves as a compromiser creating a balance between the id and the superego. However, when id and superego pressures intensity in an individual's personality, it becomes more difficult for the ego to work out optimal compromises.

Authentic morality binds an individual with conscientious judgment. This means it is not a pattern of action or character trait, but it is compatible with being self-efficacious and unselfish in practice. For example, genetics holds a special foundational milestone in the mind of a bioscientist. Genetics can be shown by the perceptual role geneticists have to play as a group of geneticists or non-geneticists, an academic world in which widely different and divergent moral principles coexist. A moral geneticist looks for perceptual committed self-rule to respect the natural sanctity of each gene to be known and maintain it in harmony with other genes. Such a moral responsibility is rooted in the peaceful cohabitation of opposing philosophies to maintaining the survival balance among genes. Bioscientists must strive to induce genes to live without force, which can maintain the natural identity of each gene under the natural form of moral law, and with a sufficient synergistic quality of life. Non-geneticists follow the "amoral" rule of existence for the benefit of some genes to be preserved and others to be destroyed. According to the "amoral" philosophy of non-geneticists, bioscientists need to assess syllogistic judgment concerning the survival of the fittest genes and the demise of the sickest and weakest ones – the social Darwinism philosophy. In following these two paths of philosophical assumptions, both geneticists and non-geneticists choose different aspects and routes of survival with interlacing kinds of competencies and responsibilities for different objectives. It is trivial and misleading to claim that all geneticists have their most advanced bio-techno-scientific tools and techniques to analyze the real characteristics of each gene.

At the risk of being so absorbed in the idealistic notion of perfection in bioresearch, one can determine that the baseline of bioresearch should be focused on genetics because genetics can predict diseases much more that it can cure them. Therefore, genetic engineering (cloning) should be the main focal task of bio-techno-scientists in order to be innovative and advanced in basic research. Contrary to genetic engineering, genetic therapeutic research activities present the idea that genetics consists mainly of diagnostic and preventive activities. Its essential tool should be focused on the acquisition of bioinformation through "genetic counseling" in order to direct physicians as to how their patients are prepared with appropriate information to choose suitable techniques according to their genetic history.

Going back to the authentic philosophy of morality, we need to question by what measures and according to which evolutionary paths bio-techno-scientists should pursue their research. We need to answer this question ethically. We need to assess genetic engineering consequences according to their inherent natural characteristics with environmentally acquired conditions, or proteins. We need to know, first, what genetic diseases have evolved because each evolutionary mechanism of gene engineering or gene therapy can create contradictory consequences to natural selection. Within a super-religious moral judgment, a bio-techno-scientist should perceive his/her role to do things along with an altruistic judgment within the boundaries of modesty and consideration for others. This moral ground requires an individual to pursue honesty, integrity, and dignity in his/her judgments. He/she needs to avoid being egotistic, egoistic, narcissistic, and selfish. To deal with genetic enhancement, bio-techno-scientists should not interfere with the law of natural selection because they cannot predict the long-range synergistic prodigic consequences.

Principle Beliefs in Authentic Moral Theory

- Authentic moral theory is compatible with being self-effacing and unselfish in practice.
- An authentic moralist understands that goodness is not just the principle of judging as his/her own private maxim, but also, they must advance and/or advocate the notion of altruism to everyone else.
- An authentic moralist must be willing to see their principles of judgment actually adopted by other moralists who have the ability and intelligence to do so.
- An authentic moralist goes beyond his/her conscientiousness in the full sense of real understanding.
- An authentic moralist advocates the prudence as the whole foundation of judgment about their moral life.
- Since prudence is a virtue, the authentic moralists do have moral obligations to consider balancing their self and others' welfare in the time of judgment.

Conclusions

The principle of authentic moral theory is based upon the idea that the only factor relevant to whether the intentional, practical, and consequential result of a decision and/or an action is right or wrong is whether it is freely or authentically chosen by the person's superego, the conscience. The phrases: "Be true to yourself," "Be a judge for your own behavior," and "Do your own thing as your conscience commands you," suggest these sorts of view. If these phrases were interpreted as meaning that one should do that which brings about the super-conscience for oneself, then we would have an example not .of the eudaemonistic but of the restricted hedonistic theory of morality.

Valuable insights into an analysis of conscientious behavior may be obtained if we classify each of the individual faced with moral values within the three domains of superego, id, and ego. Such a classification within the self can solve moral conflicts within and beyond the self, when you are in Rome, do as your conscience commands you, not as the Romans do.

Authentic moral theory is about human nature; it claims that all moral values are ultimately differentiated from self-identity; humaneness. It claims to describe how people in fact ought to behave. Underneath such a theory is an altruistic judgment that binds humanity with goodness.

CHAPTER 4

ETHICAL THEORIES: RELATIVISM, DEONTOLOGICALISM, TELEOLOGICALISM, AND UTILITARIANISM*

CHAPTER OBJECTIVES

When you have read this chapter, you should be able to do the following:

- Know what syllogistic reasoning is.
- Know what we mean by Algebraic logic, Boolean logic, and Fuzzy logic.

* This chapter was adopted from Parhizgar, K. D. and Parhizgar, R. R. (2006). *Multicultural Business Ethics and Global Managerial Moral Reasoning*. Lanham, MD: University Press of America.

- Know what ethical theory is.
- Know what we mean by ultimate means and ends.
- Know what we mean by pleasant and pleasurable needs.
- Know what justness is.
- Know what fairness is.
- Know what righteousness is.
- To be familiar with ethical relativism, deontologicalism, teleologicalism, and utilitarianism theories.
- To be able to understand the arguments for understanding the principles of all ethical theories.
- Know different types of ethical theories.
- Know how to apply different types of ethical theories in managerial decision-making processes and actions in justifying bioresearch legitimacy.

PLAN OF THIS CHAPTER

There are different views on bioethics. Typically, ethical approaches are divided into two broad categories of philosophical reasoning: causal and consequential. Causal theories measure application of principles of ethics or correctness of any ethical act by the amount of good intention, decision, and action. Consequential theories, on the other hand, are unconcerned with intentions, decisions, and actions, but with the consequences of such a holistic process, and judge its ethicality, on the basis of the duty or obligation out of which the impulse to act arises. The usual approaches to analyzing foundational beliefs in bioethical theories are to present in greater detail the causal means or consequential ends, or the content of motives and practices of bioethics.

This chapter will present various approaches, along with the generally accepted strengths and weaknesses of each theory, within a multicultural context. It will summarize key concepts of each theory and the positions to be considered in order to enhance bio-techno-scientific research and avoid moral and ethical dilemmas. It also discusses impasses to which these theories give rise. This kind of discussion and analysis will provide appropriate knowledge for judging the validity of and grasping the significant reasoning for the application of each theory. It will be shown how ethical theories can build a foundation in progressive biological perceptions to examine the means and ends of human efforts.

Without some comprehensive understanding of ethical theories:

- How can we judge which theory is appropriate to be applied or followed in a given situation?
- What rationale is behind scientific decisions and actions?

- What guidelines are we using and applying to these different theories and approaches?
- What fundamental criteria for appraising bioethics are to be used in order to determine which theory is best for a given problem.
- What do we do if the application of different theories results in totally different means and ends?

To respond to these and other inquiries we will provide you with a theoretical basis for ethical beliefs from different cultural perspectives. In this chapter we will review four major ethical theories or approaches. These theories are: (1) relativism, (2) deontologicalism, (3) teleologicalism, and (4) utilitarianism.

INTRODUCTION

Since an individual's enriched moral and ethical conviction depends upon the daily cause-effect relationships of all good and bad factors, we need to begin by considering the first principle of ethics. The first principle of pragmatic bioethicality is related to good faith that can be originated in the realms of good-intention and good will. This principle manifests that not all individual actions or movement can be directed into a streamline of good-means or good-ends because some individuals do not know really "what good is." The meaning of good as we perceive it in ethics signifies everything that appears intellectually pleasant and worthy of appreciation. Therefore, we do not appreciate whatever we do because we are afraid of what we emotionally or sensationally desire. We do appreciate what we do because of what we intellectually ought to do.

In biochemistry, extracting something from an element and/or synthesizing natural elements in nature and/or artificial elements with natural elements can provide bioscientists appropriate opportunities to cure diseases or to cause diseases in an excessively inappropriate or unethical application of techniques, consumption, or usage. Nature has provided many elements with a universal philosophy of appropriate causes and effects. If human beings desire to accelerate good causes, the result will be good consequences. If human beings out of ignorance, greed, or an excessive desire for power, bad-will, bad-faith, and selfish end to accelerate wrong causes, the end result will be catastrophes. The best example is related to the Chernobyl atomic incident that contaminated the former Soviet Union's land and habitat, and caused the acceleration of cancerous cells among the inhabitants of the areas surrounding that plant.

Today, modern global citizens are no longer living within a socio-political euphoria that could easily be molded by the mind-manipulating false propaganda of global interest groups. In an extortionist economy, people have come to believe that the demand on the environment is more than that it can tolerate or deliver. Techno-scientific power failures have cultivated an image within the mind of humans that an avaricious appetite should have limits, to prevent selfishness and the rewarding of greed. Today global citizens are faced with an interesting paradox because the leading social-bioscientists and environmentalists have given warning to the ambitious political and greedy business leaders that cross alliances can cause adverse consequences in the real world. Multiethicalism encourages global citizens of this planet to avoid radicalism and "me-ism" which are destructive because they are contaminated with self-deception.

Apparently, politicians and business leaders have ignored the need for reevaluating the basic conceptual foundations of the industrial humans of the Renaissance of free research inquiry to serve humanity from which their value systems have emerged. Today, biosciences and biotechnologies are no longer homogeneously disciplined. To some, there is no doubt that biotechnology has violated the sacredness and sanctity of traditional biosciences. Biotechnology has moved traditional bioscientific values into "thinghoodism." In the time of the Industrial Revolution, scientists and technologists promised a better life style for human beings through the adequate accessibility of consumers to the rapid-response alertness of mass-production systems. Nevertheless, today we are witnessing how some mass-technologists have abandoned and/or diverted human welfarism ideology into gadgetry of "me-ism" and "thinghoodism.' We are witnessing how some bioscientists and biotechnologists have abandoned their ethical and moral professional causes to create mass-biogerms and mass-biochemical weapons such as anthrax, botulism, plague and ricin, small pox, tularemia, VHF, sulfur (the nerve agent Vx), tear gas, pepper spray, mustard gas, chlorine, serine, Hydrogen Cyanide, sodium hydroxide, white phosphorus, and cycloserine.

In arriving at a conclusive result concerning the cause and effect of a good action, we need to analyze both intentions and consequences. When we say that all of an individual's actions should be directed to some good, we need first to associate our intentions with good-will and second with good-faith. The meaning of good will in ethics is very broad. It signifies consequential results that appear desirable to us. Whatever is good, consequently, can be associated with whatever is desirable. This association is confirmed in our ordinary daily experiences. Judging a decision or action either by causality or consequentiality requires a very broad understanding of the ethical problems in the fields of bio-techno-sciences. Hosmer (1987: 12) has found five different views on the characteristics of ethical problems:

- Most ethical decisions have extended consequences.
- Most ethical decisions have multiple alternatives.
- Most ethical decisions have mixed ethical choices.
- Most ethical decisions have uncertain consequences.
- Most ethical decisions have personal implications.

On the basis of our discussion in Chapter 2, we assume that at this point the two views of morality and ethicality are two separated compartments of goodness in human behavior. One of these compartments is related to an individual's moral goodness and the other one is concerned with societal group goodness. As we mentioned before, morality is more focused on an individual's cardinal virtues, hence ethicality is related to a pluralistic societal cultivation of benevolent and altruistic life. We need to identify what is good and what is determined to be evil.

Finally, we have defined the meaning of good with desirable means and ends. The objection to such a definition raises an important difficulty, not about the nature of goodness as the first principle in ethics, but about interpretation and application of goodness to each individual as a desirable end. Therefore, since a desirable end is viewed as the result of the emotional, sensational, and rational means of an individual, seemingly all people cannot generalize it. In order to examine all related views within the contextual boundaries of ethics, we need to study different perceptions, positions, and directions of ethicists. We may now begin our review in the area of what is ethics.

WHAT ARE THEORETHICAL FOUNDATIONS OF EHICS?

In Chapter 2 of this text, we defined morality in terms of an individual's pursuit of self-intellectual interest and/or the search for self-egoism of goodness, but we have not seen what goodness is in terms of a collective socio-cultural value system. We need to search for such a definition through understanding the real meaning of ethicality.

Ethics involves the critical analysis of cultural values to determine the validity of their rightness in wrongness of human group behavior and their organization in terms of three major criteria: truthfulness, fairness, and justness. Ethics examines the relation of an individual to societal members and their groups, to nature, and to God through conscious awareness.

How individuals make an ethical decision is influenced by the way they perceive themselves in relation to goodness. Ethics is a purely theoretical treatment of moral virtues in terms of speculative and practical collective cultural value systems. In the speculative and practical knowledge of goodness, righteousness and worthiness, we are concerned with the cultural value systems in which they are operable, either in intending to do something or actually doing something in the realm of goodness. Although these two alternatives might seem to define what an ethical life should be, it is not the kind of intending or knowing goodness, but the complete practical execution of goodness through the collective behavior of a group of people.

Ethics is concerned with psychosocial intentions and actions and can deal with good deeds in a society. Ethicists have identified ethics with one or the other of these extremes. Some people have understood ethics as being speculative and demonstrating good thoughts and behavior (deontological), while others have tended to identify it as a complete practical good end-results (teleological).

In so far as the term morality is related to the definition of an individual's intellectual characteristics through his/her conscious awareness, ethics is the collective social conscious awareness of a group of people. Thus, morality is related to the individual virtue of excellence, and ethics is related to the society's fairness, justness, and worthiness, or goodness. Hence, as morality is the foundation of an ethical society it also relates to the existence of moral people who make the collective distinction between right and wrong judgments and good behavior from bad. Ethics generally requires people to behave in accordance with the valued norms and standards of goodness that they accept and to which they and the rest of society hold others.

Ethics, then, can be defined as a systematic collective attempt at social well-being in a society in order to make sense of our individual security and social peace in such a way as to determine the rules that ought to govern human social conduct, the values worth pursuing, and the characteristic traits deserving development in life.

THE ULTIMATE MEANS AND
ENDS OF BIOETHICS

In arriving at a final conclusion in an individual's daily moral bio-techno-scientific life, a bioscientist and/or a biotechnologist must analyze his/her activities within the end-result of goodness. The meaning of goodness is the attraction of our tendencies or desires positively for the efficient use of our energy toward more legitimate bio-techno-scientific productivity without side effects. Since the first principle of morals is the realization of the self-evidence of good faith, all moral desires needed to be decided by good will. The goodness that we strive for is whatever we do, because we perceive ourselves what we desire as goodness, and what we desire as goodness we appreciate in our desires as good-ends.

There is no doubt that everyone desires a *pleasurable* and/or *pleasant* life. The problem is what constitutes a pleasurable and/or pleasant life as two major components of goodness. People are the major operators for goodness and badness. Making legitimate profit and having money could be considered amoral goodness. A specific question arises: Is there any intrinsic value of goodness in a piece of paper called money? The answer is no. What is the value of that piece of paper? The answer is: the intrinsic and extrinsic money-power, value-power of that piece of paper that can be considered as *clean or dirty purchase money-power* with which we can buy our desirable and survival necessitated goods and services.

Dirty resources have been viewed as the result of conducting an illegitimate and unethical acquisition of bad things (e.g., buying and selling body parts for implantation, women's eggs, men's sperm). It is in some specific cases illegal activities such as selling and buying drugs, bodies, pornographic films and tools, gambling, and the like that are unethical, although in some communities they may be legal through licensing.

Clean resources are considered acquisitions of legitimate knowledge and techniques, bioscientific research and/or biotechnological innovativeness. What do we mean by legitimate bioscientific research and biotechnological innovativeness? If we believe bioscientific and biomedical efforts are legitimate professions, then we expect bio-techno-scientists and physicians must show some pragmatic valuable thoughts and behavior to profess. That is they cannot simply claim that they are highly specialized people who place their genuine abilities at the service of mankind, as if their professions themselves had no larger meaning of their own. We are expecting bio-techno-scientists to conduct research projects and manifest their expertise within the ability to maintain the sanctity and dignity of human beings. We are expecting them to have something to profess, with the intellectual deliberated ability to maintain a certain critical distance from the larger society (Churchill 1989: 30). By professionalism, we mean society has bestowed upon the professions special rights and duties. Ordinarily, these rights and duties are taken away from lay people. Indeed, the notion of professionalism in medicine, teaching and research, law, religion, and family society has provided a standing ground over civil society. As Callahan (1984: 348) indicated: "The Hippocratic tradition pictured medicine as a profession with its own internal goals and norms, providing the necessary and sufficient ingredients for a coherent medical ethic from within the culture of medicine itself." From this perspective, biomedical communities know at least some of their intrinsic professional duties entirely apart from more general extrinsic moral principles. They know they ought not to use their professional knowledge and skills, for example, as state executioners (via lethal injection), even though they have no principled objection to capital punishment. Moral meanings claim that bio-techno-scientists and practitioners discipline themselves to be committed to the physical and emotional life of human beings whose personhoods are " manifested on earth by living bodies" (Kass, 1989: 41).

COMPONENTS OF ETHICAL BEHAVIOR

Everyone is familiar, to some extent, with ethical behavior in relation to justness, fairness, and righteousness in decision-making processes and real action. Since ethical decisions and judgments are based on the cultural value systems in a society, there are certain ambiguities that are concealed in the signification of these cultural value systems. For example, in the biopharmaceutical industry, we speak of just causes (heavy investment in research and development: R&D), fair prices, and right profits. These meanings are closely related to each other. Nevertheless, they are not wholly the same. Let us begin, therefore, with the broadest meaning of ethics as a cultural value system. It contains justness, fairness, and righteousness.

What Is Justness?

The proper object of justness is right, that which is just. The proper Latin word for right is *jus,* and hence right is only another name for the just. From an ethical point of view, *justness* has had three clarifications:

- The first is that the source of justness is natural law. Natural law is a generalized principle for an individual's action, inclining his/her feelings toward what is goodness in nature.
- The second point is related to his/her extrinsic cultural reasoning as it is related to econo-political and sociocultural value systems for a happy life. These value systems are called civil rights in relation to and their consequential effects upon the end-results of goodness.
- The third point is related to an individual's intrinsic cognitive conception concerning human rights, as pleasurable or pleasant or life experiences, or both.

An individual's main concern is about happiness in terms of the consequences of the common goodness. It is based upon individual liberty as the pleasant means and ends of rational decisions and actions in upholding justice. Individual liberty is the most important pleasant moral order. Therefore, in a moral sense, we can say that we are free to do; we have a right to do. In the fields of bio-techno-scientific research and practices, bio-techno-scientists need to consider all the above rights at the time of ethical decision-making processes and actions. In effect, in bioethics there must be a harmonized valuable system to integrate bio-techno-scientific professional rights and duties and the civil rights of citizens. Such a harmony mandates the bioethicists command for the application of general ethical norms into the practice. The compartmentalization of human dignity and integrity with professional rights and duties will integrate moral virtues and ethical values as wholeness in society, justice.

What Is Fairness?

We divide ethical fairness, in regard to holistic sensational, emotional, and rational judgments, into three main deals of prudence. The term *prudence* is defined to be free from bias and dishonesty. Prudence needs to have the following meanings:

- Prudence is a careful, unbiased consideration that comes from the special relation between duties and obligations, impartiality.
- Prudence is viewed as those obligations that come from particular causes for right or wrong actions, straightforwardness.
- Prudence is viewed as those obligations that come from the particular rationalized means of actions, legitimacy.

A bio-techno-scientist needs to make a fair judgment on the basis of impartiality, straightforwardness, and legitimacy.

What Is Righteousness?

The term of righteousness means that what everybody does should be suitable to what is or that judgment should be in conformity with facts, standards or principles of reasoning. From an ethical point of view any decision or judgment could be weakened or deviated from the right course of action by too little or too much. An obvious instance is found in our daily attachment to special habits, tendencies, or extravagancies such as workaholism, alcoholism, sexism and others. A bio-techno-scientist needs to reason rightly at the time of conducting research, expressing scientific judgments, and suggesting decisions according to the speculative order of knowledge. The right reason is true knowledge of bioethical principles.

The biosophy of righteousness addresses the promotional aspects of Life Ethics. Life Ethics is related to an understanding of the wisdom of life, as distinct from the objective study of life; biology. Life Ethics will be familiar to those who are familiar with theosophy, which claims that everything in the universe possesses a special insight into the divine nature and thus humans need to respect them. As distinct from theology, biosophy is a complimentary field of human inquiry that grounds theosophy in all aspects of life. In Asian cultures, theosophy is viewed as a doctrine based largely on Brahmanic and Buddhistic ideas. It motivates us to live in accordance with a creed of commitment to wisdom to pursue ethics in all aspects of life. It calls us to action whenever there is justice and humaneness is required to assist other sentiment beings through biosophical wisdom.

IMPORTANCE OF FACTUAL BIOETHICAL KNOWLEDGE

It is very puzzling when we analyze moral conscience and ethical judgments concerning what an individual should do in a certain situation. What one needs is not really any ethical instruction, but simply either more factual knowledge or a greater conceptual clarity of the nature of means and ends. Certainly, a large part of the debate about what to do concerning a bioethical issue arises because we are ignorant of much of what bears on those problems. In the field of bioethics, much of our difficulty about this field is related to its important issues concerning life and death. Some people believe that there are intrinsic norms and values in bioethics and those bio-techno-scientists should observe them. They believe bioethics is the essence of universal sanctity and bio-techno-scientists should not disregard it. This doesn't mean that they should not conduct their research in order to discover new things. These bioethicists believe in creation and a universal cause of goodness.

Others believe that bioethics is a branch of politics or that it is a sub-field of political philosophy. They believe that the intrinsic norms of bioethics are not simply derived from a universal morality, but that it is an integration of universal morality within the context of a community in which there is an agreement not just on a few general principles but also on the meaning of an innovative and progressive good life. Therefore, continued efforts for a liberal political tradition must be inevitable. This group of bioethicists believe that if the community as a whole needs to formulate their ethical views on a substantive vision of what is good for human beings, we should accept bioethics as being not static, but dynamic. It needs innovativeness in assessing moral virtues, ethical values, and political doctrines in order to constitute proper bioethical visions. These bioethicists believe in evolution. We stress these points because we think that ethical principles cannot overstress the importance of factual knowledge and conceptual clarity for the solution of moral and ethical social problems. To understand an ethical life and/or society, we need to review different views on theories of ethics.

THEORIES OF ETHICS

There is two core assumptions of ethical perceptions: (1) the atomistic universal of moral laws (intellect, wisdom, and knowledge) and (2) the relativistic ethical systems (familial, organizational, and national). Nevertheless, through our intellectual cognizance of value systems, the most fundamental agent is the universal self. All people are subject to a universal equitability, regardless of the separation of contextual value systems and the compartmentalization of sociocultural and politico-economical classes of people in which they exist. Perhaps the most significant reasoning for such a declaration in ethics is related to the isomorphic nature of human beings. Human beings are not different in nature; however, their characteristics and behaviors are different based upon their genetic and societal learning characteristics in a microanalysis. The second core assumption is attributed to the atomistic self. Personal behavior is rooted in personal traits and value judgments. It is the starting point of our intellect and wisdom and it is a part of our ontological makeup as human beings. In the realm of our ethical reasoning and moral decisions and/or intentions, there is no consultation with other agents, we consult nothing outside of ourselves, and we consult with our consciences. However, in ethical decisions and actions we follow the cultural value systems. Thus, the manifestation of ethical intellect and wisdom is the deliberation of thoughts and actions extracted from our immediate intellectual cultural environment.

In spite of the implications and chained value systems of both morality and ethics, there are two major approaches in the realm of value systems: either (1) that *objective* moral values are the universal beliefs of humanity, or (2) *subjective* ethical values are the products of societal valued cultures in the form of cultural choices.

When we speak of ethics, we refer to our cultural value systems concerning collective judgments of right and wrong and good and bad thoughts and behavior. However, in multinational cultures, there are different perçeptions concerning what is right or wrong and good or bad. This variation comes from the personal gains and lifestyles of individuals. In a more moderately sized text like this, however, we must confine ourselves to working out fairly general theories about what is right. Two major dimensions can achieve a fair judgment of what are right and wrong decisions and actions: (1) consequential end-results, and (2) causal reasoning. In fact, the best way for us to proceed in working out such an endeavor with a reasonable breath is to review some of the main theories of ethics that have been proposed: (1) relativism, (2) deontologicalism, (3) teleologicalism, and (4) utilitarianism.

THEORY OF ETHICAL RELATIVISM

There is a basic question concerning ethics: what is ethical in relation to absolutism or relativistic logic? That question raises another question: are there objective universal principles of the human race upon which one can construct an ethical system of cultural valuable beliefs, religious faith, and political ideology that would be applicable to all groups in all cultures at all times? The answer is no. The negative answer is not related to different ethical values, faiths, and beliefs that exist among nations. It is related to all experiences that we confirm as facts in our behavior. There is no doubt that there are certain common phenomena in all societies that are the same. What are these commonalities? They are those in which people do have faiths, beliefs, and values. To what degree is the matter of relative? If all ethical beliefs in all societies are equally valid, then there is no variety of moral judgments concerning individual thoughts and behavior. We believe in one faith. Then, there is one faith in all cultures, so that all people believe and behave in the same manner. Such a presumption is far from reality. There is no doubt that all people should be socially responsible for their acts. All people should work together in order to make their lives happy. The question is to what degree? With minimum, or medium, or maximum sacrifices? This creates different judgments in different societies. Such a fact establishes ethical relativism.

Ethical relativism is not a fact, but a theory that attempts to account for this fact. This theory arises from a failure to distinguish universal moral rules, and particular moral judgments, from moral principles. It involves a failure to distinguish the invariant moral principles from the variable conditions that, in accordance with these universal principles, require a variety of different rules and practices. Through ethical practices and principles we assume that ethical behavior may be relative. It does not follow universal principles around the world. Yet ethical relativism theory supposes that it does with different interpretations and applications of reasoning. It should be obvious that ethical principles do not require any uniformity of practice in different cultures, for they do not require any uniformity of practices in different circumstances.

Some people maintain that ethicality just does not boil down to religious faiths. Others have argued that the doctrine of ethical relativism indicates that right and wrong are only a function of what a particular society takes to be right and wrong. Thus, for the ethical relativists there is no absolute ethical standard. It is dependent upon religious and/or cultural contextual faith and beliefs. There is no universal criterion of right and wrong by which to judge other than that of particular societies (Shaw, 1996: 11).

Principles of Ethical Relativism Theory

Since some ethicists believe that ethics is largely a matter of perspective on what is worth doing and not worth doing, what is worth of knowing and not worth of knowing (e.g., sex education), and what is worth wanting and having, and what is not worth wanting and having, therefore, the objective of good living and a good life is different from culture to culture. Some cultures believe in depravation for an appreciation of a pleasurable life, others believe in preparation and enhancement as the pleasurable fullness of life. Because of such diverse views on ethics, some ethicists believe that ethicality is a matter of relativism. There are some ethical principles concerning ethical relativism as follows:

- For the ethical relativists there are no absolute ethical standards.
- Multicultural diversity value systems are the main causes of ethical relativism theory.
- Because of multicultural differences among nations what is right in one cultural context of circumstances may not be right in another one.
- Right and wrong thoughts and behavior are viewed only as a function of what a particular society takes to be right and wrong.
- The only ethical standard for judging an action is the ethical system of the society in which the act occurs.
- Ethical relativism depends on religious and/or cultural contexts, not on criteria for right and wrong by which to judge other than that of particular societies.
- Ethical relativism holds that no universal standards or rules can be used to guide or appraise an ethical decision or action.

Arguments

Ethical relativism theory holds that since people are different in terms of their religious faiths, cultural value systems, and econo-political ideologies, naturally their ethical standards for judging their decisions and actions will be different too. The only societal group interests, political ideologies, and cultural value systems that are relevant for judging the ethical status of their societies are their own. Throughout history, what one group of people assumed to be right, fair, or just, many others believed to be wrong or evil?

The logic of ethical relativism extends to cumulative religious-cultural perceptions on goodness. Religious faiths and cultural beliefs require people to follow the rule of the society. It argues that "when in Rome, do as the Romans do." Religious-cultural relativists would argue that bioethics should implement the ethical value systems of each nation. In addition, ethical relativists claim that when any two individuals or two cultures hold different ethical views of a sociocultural value system, both can be right on the basis of circumstances of time, place, and their own people's beliefs.

Different ethical views are products of religious faiths, cultural beliefs, and political ideologies. Thus, a mode or trend of behavior can be right for one person or one society, and the same action, taken in the same way, may be wrong for another person or society, and yet the two persons or societies are equally correct. In a monolithic religious society, laboratory bioscientists and biotechnologists working on recombination DNA technology or in the area of human genetics have been subjected to broad scrutiny out of concern about playing God, while in a non-monolithic religious nation, as in Western civilizations, bioethics is concerned about biohazards. Moreno (1995: 47) indicated:

> A serious threat to an understanding of consensus in bioethics as Platonism is relativism... It would be irresponsible not to acknowledge that the historic emergence of the field is closely associated with the horrific abuses of concentration camp inmates during the Holocaust, and with the scandalous treatment of vulnerable subject populations in Tuskegee and at Willowbrook. Surely many regard those experiences as powerful warnings about the hazards of doing ethics without net....

For example, some members of our society believe that abortion is immoral and unethical because it is viewed as murder and it is a sinful action. Others who are pro-choice believe that abortion is morally and ethically permissible because it is purely related to a woman's choice and desire to have or not have a child. The differences are rooted in their religious faiths, econo-political ideological beliefs, and sociocultural value systems. These differences are examples of transcultural, multicultural, and intracultural relativism.

Different Types of Ethical Relativism

Many people dispute that some judgments should be based upon the basis of their personal rational reasoning. In other cultures an action or judgment may be right for one person or society, and the same action or judgment, taken in the same manner, may be wrong for another person or society. What exactly is meant by these claims? Frankena (1973: 109) stated:

> We must distinguish at least three forms of ethical relativism. First, there is what may be called *descriptive relativism*. When careful, it does not say merely that ethical judgments of different people and societies are different... Second, there is *meta-ethical relativism*, which is the view we must consider. It holds that, in the case of basic ethical judgments, there is no objectivity valid, rational way of justifying one against another; consequently, two conflicting basic judgments may be equally valid. The third form is *normative relativism*. While descriptive relativism makes an anthropological or sociological assertion and meta-ethical relativism a meta-ethical one, this form of relativism puts forward a normative relativism a meta-ethical one,... of relativism puts forward a normative principle: what is right or good for one individual or society is not right or good for another.

Therefore, ethical relativism theory has some unpleasant implications. First, sometimes it may ignore universal humanitarian value systems. Second, ethical relativists believe that ethical development and progress exist. Thus, we cannot say that our codes of ethics today will be viable for tomorrow; because we will have changes; our society will be changed, and consequently, our codes of ethics ought to be changed too.

Conclusion

Since ethics deals with theories of justice and injustice, the meanings of fairness and unfairness, worthiness and unworthiness, rightness and wrongness depend on operative judgments in certain situations. While reviewing the historical cultural value systems around the world, no attempt is made to pass judgments on the basis of superiority or inferiority of these various ethical reasoning. Therefore, ethical relativists hold that the matter of ethics is a conditionally operative one in different parts of the world or in different institutions. Consequently, this type of reasoning is neutral because it does not advocate one set of ethical values over another. It depends on specific circumstances.

DEONTOLOGICAL ETHICAL THEORY

Deontological theory is a moral based ethics. It is not based upon a casting vote system like in politics, for or against moral principles relating to human conduct, with respect to the rightness or wrongness of certain decisions and actions and to the goodness and badness of the motives and ends of such actions. It is based upon a consensus of valuable agreements as to what fundamental principles of goodness or badness are. *Deontos* in Greek means obligations or duties. The foundation of deontological ethical theory is based on reasoning about the basis of duties or obligations to the self and others. Deontologicalists believe in the standardization of prevailing moral principles.

To be unethical in bio-techno-scientific research is to bring evil into the world of humanity. By evil we mean that which is defined as morally wrong, immoral, harmful, and injurious to the self and others. It is unfortunate that some bio-techno-scientists have sold their spirit to the devil and contributed their intellectual abilities to produce biological germs and biochemical weapons to conduct mass killings of other human beings. Those who claim that in the animal kingdom predators must be evil because they harm and kill other animals for food, commit what Fox (2001: 12) called this term the *zoomorphic fallacy*. Unlike humans, it is the natural instinct of animals to be amoral, because they have no intellectual choice. Yet, natural predation is used to justify bio-techno-scientific research for the advancement of biosciences and biotechnologies on the one hand, and to argue that nature is flawed on the other.

Which bioethical perspectives or frameworks can most helpfully illuminate and direct bio-techno-scientific ethics? For many centuries a principles-oriented perspective has caused the field of ethics to fall within the savage world of the *zoomorphic* fallacy. In general terms, deontologicalists reject having different alternative choices in the interpretation of specified rational reasoning for moral and ethical decisions and actions if just causes are clearly known for all parties.

Deontologicalists believe that application of different principles in similar cases for moral and ethical judgments can cause mixed outcomes (double standards). As an ethical belief, harming the self and others is immoral and unethical. They insist that an individual must always avoid harming the self and others, whereas teleologicalists assume that harming the self and/or others will sometimes be necessary to proceed towards a consequential goodness. Teleologicalists in the field of bioethics believe that in the kingdom of nature humans are viewed as the "cream of the crop" of the nature. They should have alternative choices to use animals for biological experiments. If they don't use them, biosciences and biotechnologies are never able to improve and advance human happiness.

Deontologicalists believe in bioethics on the preferential arguments of the good over the right as a starting point in bioresearch. Conversely, teleologicalists appeal to the assessments of the priority of the right over the good. Deontological ethical theory is known as causal or nonconsequential ethics. Many ethicists have argued that the moral goodness of a decision and an action is determined by its means, not solely by its ends. They believe that if the means of a decision and an action are good, then the ends will be good. If they are bad, the ends will be wrong. Ethicists who adopted this approach are therefore called deontologicalists or causalists. They believe that a good act is one that initiates and applies good principles, to direct it in the right direction, and to conclude it with the right ends.

Philosopher Joseph Butler (1692-1752), (1949: 45) who is known as one of the proponents of deontological ethics stated:

> Any plain honest man, before he engages in any course of action, asks
> himself, is this I am going about right, or is it wrong? ... I do not in the
> least doubt but that this question would be answered agreeably to truth and
> virtue, by almost any fair man in almost any circumstance [without any
> general rule].

In addition, in Butler's philosophical reasoning he holds that the ground for
morality is conscience. In his ethical deontological theory, conscientiousness is
conceived as a reflective or rational faculty that discerns the moral
characteristics of actions. Consequently, he is not a defender of the popular
votes theory in a society concerning the rightness or wrongness of conduct. His
conception of ethics is closer to the view in which conscience is understood as a
term for mere reasoning approval or disapproval due to psychological and social
conditioning. For him, the judgments of conscience are not based on sensational
or emotional feelings, but on moral reasoning.

Principles of Deontological Ethical Theory

There are certain fundamental ethical means and ends for the application of
the deontological theory of ethics. These principles are as follows:

- Deontologicalists believe that an ethical individual should be sincere in
  his/her faith and reasonableness in judgments.
- Deontological ethical theory is known as a causal or nonconsequential
  ethics.
- Deontologists argue that the moral rightness of a decision and an action
  is determined by the good means, not solely by their good ends.
- Deontologicalists contend that more than the likely consequences of an
  action determines right and wrong decisions and actions.
- Deontological theory of ethics maintains that we must act on the basis
  of truthful principles of morality regardless of what the consequential
  results will emerge.
- Deontologicalists view ethics as manifestation of causal reasoning for
  the truthfulness, righteousness, and goodness of decisions and
  judgments.
- Deontologicalsts believe in three characteristics that are considered to
  be usually associated with good judgments. First, ethical judgment
  about the righteousness or wrongness of an action is held to be
  universally applicable. Second, being truthful and honest can be
  logically derived from the basic principles of all ethical systems. Third,
  mutual understanding concerning rules or principles that govern
  decisions and actions should be observed by all involved parties.
- Much of deontological theory is also termed universalism. The first
  duty of universalism is to treat the self and others as means and not as
  ends. Other people should be seen as valuable means in themselves,

worthy of dignity and respect, and not as impersonal means to achieve our own ends.

Arguments

Deontologicalists contend that more than the likelihood of consequences of actions determines right and wrong actions. They do not necessarily deny that consequences are morally significant, but they believe that other factors, including intentions with good faith and goodwill, are also relevant to the ethical decision-making processes and actions. They hold that there are some principles for distinguishing right judgments and/or actions from wrong. For example, we have in some sense become favorably predisposed to the idea of human cloning. We have become accustomed to new practices in human reproduction: not just *in vitro* fertilization, but also embryo manipulation, embryo donation, surrogate pregnancy, and pre-implantation genetic diagnosis. In addition, we are oriented towards eugenic animal biotechnology, which has yielded transgenetic animals and a burgeoning science of genetic engineering, and could soon easily be transferable to humans, cloning. Even more, we are oriented towards changes in the broader multiculturalism that now makes it vastly more difficult to express a common cause solely in terms of national cultural beliefs concerning a perfect understanding of natural sexuality, procreation, nascent life, family, and the meaning of fatherhood, motherhood and the links between the generations. The only thing that we are not concerned about ethical and moral issues in cloning is humans without sexual desires, and the confounding of normal kin relations who are the mothers and fathers: the egg donor, the surrogates who carry and deliver the babies, or the one who paid for it? Isn't it a new form of monogamous marriage?

Deontologicalists believe in some ethical and moral foundations concerning the principle of the cohesive one pair-family system, monogamy. They are against polygamous marriages, those males and females who are living together in civil communal setting of free sexual practices and/or open marriages, and those having children who have acquired either three or more fathers through bio-techno-scientific gene engineering; form of unnatural selection. How is biotechnology redesigning humanity? This is a fundamental controversial issue in the field of bioethics. The problem with unnatural selection is that you are treating the human person as an object to be manufactured for your purposes. Also, humans will be subject to the marketability trends as commodities to be bought and/or sold; slavery. Thus, ignoring ethical and moral values of human beings to materialism status within unknown natural environmental conditions is viewed as the result of such a perception.

The deontological theory of ethics maintains that we must act on the basis of truthful principles of morality regardless of their consequential results. We must judge ethical issues in our society regardless of a group's interests or the majority and minority votes of people. We need to look at what really promotes the greatest goodness for oneself and the world of humanity and not the greatest goodness for the greatest number of people.

There are two deontological philosophers whose views are related to the obligatory principles of right, ought, and dutiful responsibilities. These philosophers are George Edward Moore (1873-1958) and William David Ross (1877-1971).

Deontological Views of George Edward Moore

Moore (1948: vii) stated in his *Principa Ethica*:

> It appears to me that Ethics, as in all other philosophical studies, the difficulties and disagreements of which its history is full, are mainly due to a very simple cause: namely to the attempt to answer questions, without first discovering precisely *what* question it is which you desire to answer. I do not know how far this source of error would be done away, if philosophers would *try* to discover what question they were asking, before they set about to answer it; for the work of analysis and discussion is often very difficult: we may often fail to make the necessary discovery, even though we make a definite attempt to do so. But I am inclined to think that in many cases, a resolute attempt would be sufficient to ensure success; so that, if only this attempt were made, many of the most glaring difficulties and disagreements in philosophy would disappear.

In addition, Moore found, upon his debatable analysis: what is intrinsically good? That, is, what is good unconditionally and invariably? He found that the question is in fact two questions, namely: (1) how is good to be defined? and (2) what things are good? Moore (1922: 273) insisted: "We must analyze the former before we address ourselves to the latter." He concluded that *good* is *indefinable*, but the term *good* refers to a property of things. He explained that the term *good* refers to a quality that is analogous in some ways to sensory qualities. The principle objective of goodness consists in its being intrinsic, that is, it is unchanging and absolute. When anything possesses it, it would be necessary, under all circumstances, to possess it in exactly the same manner. In sum, Moore determined that the ethical characteristics of human perception and behavior depend upon either self-evidence or external-evidence.

Deontological Views of William David Ross

Deontological views of William David Ross resemble that of Moore in terms of intrinsic goodness to being defined as the quality of things. There is a decisive difference between them concerning the concept of obligation. In Moore's views the concept of obligation indicates rights, oughts, responsibilities, and duties that are linked to maximizing intrinsic goodness. In Ross's views there is no such linkage. Ross contends that rightness is a distinct and identifiable characteristic of an act and is generally independent of whatever good may result from their occurrence. In Ross's arguments for ethical intuitionalism, he insisted that the difference between what he termed *prima facie* (first appearance at the first glance), and *actual* duties make all difference. Ross perceived such an act that has the characteristic of generating ethical claims as prima facie duty. Therefore, deontological ethicists believe that our prima facie duties do not arise in prearranged harmony of ranked priority and/or nor do they occur singly. Nevertheless, some *prima facie* duties have a greater claim on us than others. As Ross (1930: 41) insisted, in his book *The Right and the Good*: "A great deal of stringency belongs to the duties of 'perfect obligation' the duties of keeping our promises, of repairing wrongs we have done, and of returning the equivalent of services we have received." Thus, there are circumstances in which beneficence takes precedence over all other considerations. Ross's deontological views on obligations conclude:

- All other ethical theories fail to recognize the complex relations involved in circumstance of obligations.
- The basic concept of prima facie includes a catalogue of many types of duty:
    - o Some duties rest on previous acts of ourselves: implicit promises and the duty of fidelity.
    - o Some rest on previous acts of others: duties of gratitude.
    - o Some rest on the fact or responsibility of a distribution of pleasure or pleasant: duties of justice.
    - o Some rest on the mere fact that there are other beings in the world whose condition we can make better in respect to goodness: duties of beneficence.
    - o Some rest on the fact that we can improve our own condition in respect to goodness or intelligence: duties of self-improvement.
    - o It is a mistake to regard every dutiful act as being for one and the same reason. We need to make a distinction between prima facie and actual duty.

Deontologicalists believe in specific conditional characteristics that are usually considered to be usually associated with good judgments. First, ethical judgments about the righteousness or wrongness of an action are held to be universally applicable. Through the conscious intellectual cognizance of an individual, if an action is right for an individual, it should also be right for anyone else in the same manner. If it is wrong for everybody, it is also wrong for anyone else on similar occasions. They hold that general ethical principles can be applied on the basis of particular similar cases and may then be useful in determining what should be done on later occasions. However, it cannot be allowed that a causal principal rule may ever supersede a well-taken particular judgment as to what should be done.

Different Types of Deontological Ethical theory

Deontological ethics emphasizes decisions rather than intuitions. This, also, is the view of most existentialist philosophers. Existentialists, led by the famed Jean-Paul Sartre (1905-1980), believed that standards of conduct cannot be rationally justified and no actions are inherently right or wrong. This view finds its roots in the notion that humans are only what we will ourselves to be. Sartre's famous interpretation of existence describes existence before essence. Sartre (1947: 27) stated:

> If existence really does precede essence, there are no explaining things away by reference to a fixed and given human nature. In other words, there is no determinism, man is free, and man is freedom... So in the bright realm of values, we have no excuse behind us, or justification before us. We are alone, with no existence.

Thus, existentialism holds that what people are, is a function of the choices they make, not that the choices they make are a function of what they are. Each of us is free, with no rules to turn to for guidance. Just as we all choose our own nature, so must we choose our own ethical percepts? Therefore, each person may reach his/her own choice about ethical principles. In or less extreme form, there are two types of deontologicalism: (1) rule deontologicalism, and (2) act deontologicalism.

Rule Deontologicalism: In choosing and judging on every ethical issue according to rule deontologicalism, one is at least able to first establish mechanical principles and structured reasoning rules. This suggests that in similar ethical circumstances applying the rules and principles is a viable foundation for the treatment of self and others similarly. Usually, rule deontologicalism holds that the expected ethical principles and rules consist of a number of rather specific criteria, like those of telling the truth or keeping promises, so as to always act in a certain kind of manner.

Rule deontologicalism holds that the standard of right and wrong consists of one or more rules. We ought to tell the truth. It cannot be right for treating some people in a manner and to treat others differently while both types of people have similar characteristics, and/or because merely on the ground that they are two different individuals. For example, genetic engineering is viewed as a fundamental scientific reality for improving medical diagnoses and therapeutics and to develop vaccines against specific epidemiological diseases (e.g., small pox, tuberculosis, plague, etc.). Genetic engineering can also provide safe immunecontraceptives to enhance the quality of life.

Act Deontologicalism: Act deontologicalism holds that ethical behavior must follow ethical rules. The main point about act deontologicalism is that it does offer us anticipated intellectual standards concerning the recognition of right or wrong intentions and decisions in particular circumstances. It spells out specific ethical judgments for similar cases that are basic and general rules. These are to be derived from similar cases, not the other way around. Rule deontologicalism provides people with actual pragmatic standards to be followed. In the case that there are no ethical rules then we need to act on the basis of the rule of thumb, the moral conscience.

Conclusions

In sum, deontological views of ethics are concerned with causal reasoning for the truthfulness, righteousness, and goodness of decisions and judgments as follows:

- They are not concerned about applicability of consequential results in pre-judgments about right or wrong actions. These ethicists focus their attention on the right causes regardless of consequences. This theory is concerned with perceptual values in bio-techno-scientific activities. For example, bioethicists assess ethical and moral values concerning the selling of human organs and limbs by those individuals who are financially desperate. Another example is related to the assessment of socio-cultural values and religious faiths concerning *in vitro* fertilization (IVF) and embryo transfer. Deontological bioethicists believe that while IVF is ideal for many people, it is unethical and immoral because IVF has an ambiguous status in terms of the well functioning of the somatic sexual capability of a pair of human beings. The prime socio-cultural and religious issue of IVF is about matrimonial parental rights (husband and wife) and offspring harms. From another dimension, some people believe that IVF is not necessary surrogacy; it uses the sperm and egg of the natural (unmarried) individuals, implanted into the wife's body of a couple. Many deontological bioethicists argue that due to parental rights the entrenched marital interests of reproductive biotechnology decreases the autonomy and almost exclusive natural rights of the surrogate mother. Deontologicalists argue that reproduction through surrogate motherhood violates societal normative rights of family cohesiveness and ideals that degrades the moral integrity of marriage. They believe that surrogacy exploits women's dignity through the power of money. For example, in the Islamic faith through following *Koran*, the offspring of a son in law and his mother-in-law (even through surrogate pregnancy) or between a woman and her father-in-law is prohibited, because the offspring will be viewed as illegitimate children. The major reason is that parents should have a desire to have children not primarily for the sake of their desire to have children, but for the sake of having children on the basis of children's rights. Therefore, deontologicalists argue that IVF is not morally permissible on the grounds that there is no matrimonial marriage between a surrogate mother and the husband of another wife. IVF is viewed as a biomarriage, a modern type of biopolygamy.

- Ethics is a cultural value judgment and overrides other considerations. We are ethically bound to do that which we sometimes may not want to do. Again for example, deontological bioethicists believe that IVF is morally illicit because the process produces embryos that are not transferred back into the womb. Kass (1985: 102) argued that the early embryo at the blastocyst stage is only potentially a human being. It may be allowed to die, but because it is nevertheless potentially human it must be treated with respect, which means, concurrently, that as long as the deaths of preimplantation embryos are not significantly more than those that occur naturally in procreation it is permissible to let them die, though not to conduct experiments on them.

- Ethical judgments should properly direct the individual's behavior towards morally right actions, and moral blame can properly accompany acting immorally. As a deontological bioethicist Kass (1985: 72) opposes IVF on the grounds that it is dehumanizing. He stated:

  Human procreation is not simply an activity of our natural wills. Men and women are embodied as well as calculating creations... [Human procreation] is a more complete human activity precisely because it engages us bodily, erotically, and even spiritually, as well as rationally... Before we embark on new modes of reproduction, we should consider the meaning of the union of sex, love, and procreation, and the meaning and consequences of its cleavage.

Therefore, while morality is considered a personal goodness of an individual, ethics is the collective intellectual goodness of a cultural value system of a group of people.

Since moral theories provide us with freedom of choice based upon conscious judgments, they indicate that all moral convictions seem to vary from person to person. The most serious objection, perhaps, is the fact that the ethical rules of a society may be good or bad, moral or immoral, right or wrong, just or unjust, fair or unfair, and enhancing or impoverishing of human life. Through moral rules, we have agreed on one ground or another that the moral standards have offered us with alternative choices. In general, these choices have been of two sorts: (1) deontological and (2) teleological. We already have analyzed the deontological ethical theory, now we will turn to the teleological analysis in the next pages.

TELEOLOGICAL ETHICAL THEORY

Telos in Greek means goals or results. As defined by the Roman Stoic philosopher Epicurus (336-264 B.C.) (1866), ethics deals with those things to be sought and those things to be avoided, with ways of life and with the *telos*. *Telos* is the chief aim or end in life. It measures the outcome or result of a course of decisions and actions in human activities. In sum, deontological bioethicists are futurists who concentrate on side effects of bio-techno-scientific research outcomes and their impacts on future generations. Of course, future generations are not present to claim their rights, but the present generation ethically and morally should extend to them the right to live. Perhaps the notion of reciprocity is the consequential problem, and we can simply extend a reciprocal right to exist to the future generations on the same grounds as we do for infants, namely because they are our progeny.

Ethically and morally, we are obligated to ensure that our progeny will have no grounds for complaint about the conditions of their existence, somatically and ecologically. The bio-techno-scientific gene enhancement, gene engineering, and human and animal cloning may end with good or bad conditions. Then, it is possible that future generations would praise or condemn us for enhancing them or depriving them of a natural life span. In this regard McKenny (1997: 54) indicated:

> One might think of the gratitude future persons might have toward us for programming the equivalent of Nozickian pleasure machine into the brain or germ line after we had finally identified the appropriate neurotransmitters or genes and developed the techniques, assuming they would still be capable of gratitude.

Teleological ethicists hold that the position of moral grounds and the ethical worth of humans are solely related to the consequences of their behavior. This means, if a decision and an action are right, then their results should be right too, and if decisions and actions were right but the outcomes were wrong, then such a discourse can not be ethically right.

Teleological ethicists are unconcerned with intentions, decisions, and actions, but they are extremely sensitive to the consequences of such a holistic process. They judge the ethicality of the actions on the basis of the duty or obligation out of which the impulse to act arises. In sum, teleological ethicists hold that the rightness or wrongness of an ethical issue is determined by the results that these processes produce.

Principles of Teleological Ethical Theory

Teleological theory indicates that the basic or ultimate criterion or standard of what is ethically right, wrong, obligatory, etc., are the ethical and unethical norms that are brought into being by decision makers and operators with their final end-results. The final appeal, directly or indirectly, must be focused upon the comparative amount of good produced, or rather to the comparative balance of good over evil produced. The ethical and moral duties of bioscientists, biotechnologists, and bioinformationalists are unconditional for mankind to exist and survive. This mandate stands above both selves and future human beings. It is therefore, not their rights or wishes, but their humane duty to decide and act responsibly, and their duty to be truly human. Bio-techno-scientific thoughts and practices should maintain the sanctity of their duty over their commitments to their duty. They should not mix it with politics, because in politics involves win-lose outcomes. This indicates that bio-techno-scientific practices should not be in the hands of politicians, so as not to jeopardize the future of human race. Jonas, 1984: 43) clearly expressed his opinion voice: "No condition of future descendants of humankind should be permitted to arise which contradicts the reason why the existence of mankind is mandatory at all." Thus, an act is right for a biologist, biotechnologist, and bioinformationalist if it meets the following criteria:

- They produce some good results for all humans. In such valuable ethical version of the ontological principle, the idea of humanity makes the existence of humanness an imperative.
- The end-result is based on the extension of social responsibility to discover legitimate opportunities through the use of resources in order to the increase quality of life. It is ethical if biologist, biochemist, biophysicist, and biotechnologist continue an action as long as he/she stays within the rule of humaneness.
- It does not corrupt the public image and ruthlessly eliminate honest thoughts and actions.
- The elementary canons of face-to-face bioresearchers' civility (honesty, good-faith, good-will, and good-ends) are observed.
- Anti-fraud, anti-deception, anti-force, anti-corruption, and anti-pollution are valued in the course of any and all contractual agreements between society and the biopharmaceutical industry.
- Open and free competitions on win-win based (not win for biotech and biopharmaceutical corporations and lose for people) strategies between buyers and sellers, through profit optimization strategy, are promoted.
- The biopharmaceutical and biotechnological corporations' social responsibilities are legally known not only as artificial persons, but also have social conscience to provide effective and harmless products, avoid pollution, and respect human rights.

Arguments

The usual approach to analyzing foundational beliefs in ethical theories is to present greater detail on causal means or consequential ends or the content of motives and practices of ethics. The teleological approach in bioethics places complete emphasis upon the bases of the practical measurable consequences of decision-making processes and actions, not the intent and/or decisions of an action by bioscientists, biotechnologists, bioinformationalists, and biomedical practitioners. According to teleological ethical theory, all researchers and biopharmaceutical business ventures should be concerned about the question of: (1) what sort of consequences is relevant to determining right and wrong actions? and (2) what consequences are they seeking for whom? Let us look at this latter question first. Suppose for a moment that we have agreed that a scientist's objective is to seek a secure life-long employment. Then the question arises: whose objectives are legitimate or illegitimate that determine whether the scientist's activity is ethically right or wrong? Two basically different kinds of answers may be given to this question:

- Mutual professional interests for all stakeholder parties in an organization
- Benefits for the personal interest of the scientist and organization and/or benefits for mankind

The teleologicalists would hold that every stakeholder's interest is relevant to others according to the ethical principles. In contrast to this is the other kind of consequences, which might be called restricted interests, which would be unethical. The teleological ethicalists hold that every stakeholder's profit is relevant to humanity's goodness for the present or future generations.

Teleological ethical theory assesses the general public opinion concerning ethical and unethical businesses, including biopharmaceutical and biotechnological ventures, through the results of the Gallup Poll, which surveys the public's opinions of the ethics of major corporations in the United States. Survey data from the fall 2000 Gallup Poll on Honest/Ethics in the Professions reveals that the honesty of American executives is thought to be high by only 22 percent of those surveyed. Over the past decade, this percentage has fluctuated between a low of 17 percent in 1996 and a high of 22 percent in 2000. It will be interesting to see the data after the collapse of three corporations: Geron, ImClon, Enron, and Word.com (Carroll and Buchholtz, 2003: 167). The above survey result of the Gallop Poll is not surprising, because as we mentioned before, the American business system functions on the basis of amorality, expressing a portion of truth, not the whole. Nevertheless, the survey reveals the troubling fact that a majority of consumers have lost faith in the integrity of businesspeople, and expect businesses to observe ethics.

From the standpoint of ethicists a specific question will arise: how can the magnitude of the bioethical problems be more detectable today that they were once before? To answer this question, one must assess the consequences of both descriptive bioethics and prescriptive bioethics through the value judgments people have made about the practice or behavior of bioscientists, biophysicists, biochemists, biotechologists, bioinformationals, and biomedical practitioners. For this we need to know what we mean by consequential bioethics.

Teleological bioethics assesses the consequences of bioresearchers as they have been observed and evaluated. This theory does not rely on what they are saying but of what they are doing. For example, the mission statement of Johnson and Johnson Company <http://www.jni.com/who_is_jnj/cr_usa.html> addresses its corporate beliefs about its principles of responsibility to:

> The doctors, nurses, and patients, to parents and all others who use our products and services ... to our employees, the men and women who work with us... to the communities in which we live and work and to the world community as well.

In practice, by evaluating Johnson and Johnson's operation, we have found that there is a discrepancy between what they believe and how they operate. Johnson and Johnson is under investigation by the Securities Exchange Commission for possible book cooking of profits in order to keep the value of its stocks very high. *The Multinational Monitor* (1996) reported that approximately 17 percent of the corporate executives who attended the White House Conference on Corporate Citizenship in May 1996 were CEOs of corporations with criminal records, corporations that have been convicted of everything from price-fixing to pollution, from procurement fraud to obstruction of justice. Among them was Johnson and Johnson's CEO Ralph Larsen. In January 1995, Johnson and Johnson's Ortho Pharmaceutical Corp. unit pled guilty to ten counts of obstruction of justice and destruction of documents in connection with a federal probe of the company's marketing of an anti-acne cream. This indicates how some corporations violate their started mission for the sake of greed.

Conclusions

Teleological ethical theory focuses on the result of what a biopharmaceutical or biotech corporation has done in practice. In sum, teleological bioethics relies on what we see, and what we believe. In other words, how do we get from what is to what ought to be? Or what makes a bio-techno-scientific issue ethically right is the good that is produced by the outcomes of intentions, decisions, and actions, not the sole nature of the declared bioresearch mission. The teleological bioethical approach appraises the net consequences of decisions and actions, not the individual's or group's intentions.

Teleological bioethicists do not hold that intentional, decisional, and operational processes possess intrinsic values in and of themselves, but all processes must be evaluated in terms of their consequential virtues and vices, or the good and bad consequences that they produce. The teleological bioethicists hold that rules have to be followed not because of acknowledged obligations but because of the fear of punishment for breaking those rules. They are concerned with avoiding harm to the self rather than gaining benefits for the self. These bioethicists believe that since cultural values vary from culture to culture, then it is relevant to judge a bioethical value system based on their outcomes in relationship to the cultural and religious standards.

The origin of a bioethical action, its efficiency, not its final cause, is based on choice, and that choice is a desire to rationalize its ends. Ethically, the primary bioethical act of a good choice and a good will is bio-techno-scientific devotion. Devotion is promptness to do whatever pertains to the manifestation of a good end via a good choice. An act of devotion is the most important end of the behavior of intellectual virtues. This is why good and right choices cannot exist either without wisdom and intellect or without a purified emotional state of harmony between mind and body, bioscientists and biosciences, and bioinstitutions and people. Good decisions and actions cannot exist without a combination of biointellect and moral character. Intellect and wisdom themselves, however, move nothing, but only the wisdom and intellect which aim at an end through the human sensational and emotional body dynamics provide practical movement through the synergistic combination of the personal and social embodiments of cultural value systems. In sum, teleological bioethical theorists reject the absolute universal ethical commitments because they believe that there are exceptional circumstances that can turn a good action to bad or vice versa.

UTILITARIAN ETHICAL THEORY

In analyzing different logical arguments concerning ethical theories, we already have reviewed three theories: relativism, deontologicalism, and teleologicalism. Now we are turning to another ethical theory known as utilitarianism. Utilitarian ethics is more oriented towards politics. This means that if we want to understand and ratify an ethical principle, we need to turn to a political voting system in order to acquire a majority votes for the approval of that principle (e.g., anti-abortion law, anti-cloning law, etc.).

Speaking briefly, relativism theorists focus on a variety of principles that indicate that there is no absolute ethical standard for having a happy life. Having a happy life depends on variable perceptions within multicultural value systems. Multiculturalism identifies a variety of reasons to believe in diversity among nations. This indicates that what is right in one cultural context may not be right in another (e.g., the issue of abortion, or the transplantation of a pig's heart artery valve into human's heart in Moslem countries). From another perspective, the teleological ethical theorists focus upon the net consequences of ethical means and ends. They believe that bioethics needs to be concerned only with the net profit for specific interest groups. Utilitarian bioethics is concerned with the utility of bio-techno-scientific innovativeness for the benefit of majority of people.

In a comparison of analytical ethical theories, deontologicalists and utilitarians vehemently disagree on pursuing goodness in biosciences and biotechnologies. The major disagreements are often about how best to justify means and ends. The deontologicalists focus upon application of ethical principles during decision-making processes and actions. Deontologicalists believe in the standardization of prevailing moral principles not to search for degradation, debasement, and dehumanization of biosciences and biotechnologies. For example, if you believe in honesty, you will believe in human dignity and human liberty. According to deontological theory of bioethics, bio-techno-scientific activities should be pursued not as an end for the benefit of small interest groups, but it should be pursued for the virtue of wisdom, by an independent minded quest for the sake of knowledge for the promotion of public health.

Challenges to the use of animals to benefit humans are not new. Their origins can be traced back several centuries through religious cultural beliefs. The European utilitarian bioethics concerning goodness for animals' traces back to the Cartesian-utilitarian debate presented by the French philosopher Descartes. He defended the use of animals in experiments by insisting that the animals respond to stimuli in only one-way: "According to the arrangement of their organs." He stated that animals lack the ability to reason and think and are, therefore, similar to a machine. Humans, on the other hand, can think, talk, and respond to stimuli in various ways. These differences, Descartes argued, make animals inferior to humans and justify their use as a machine, including them as subjects in experimental research projects (Leob et al., 1989: 2719).

Principles of Utilitarian Ethical Theory

Philosopher Jeremy Bentham was motivated by the idea that the *Public Good* ought to be the object of the legislator, *general social utility* ought to be the foundation of reasoning. McCollum (1998: A28) stated:

> Bentham is often thought of as the founder of utilitarianism. The school of philosophy that holds that the purpose of government is to foster the happiness of the individual, and that the greatest happiness of the most people should be the goal of human existence.

To implement this social and political ideal, people need to measure pleasure and pain. In this way good and bad acts can be evaluated in terms of such factors as intensity, duration, and extent. Bentham (1838: 16) composed the following verse to aid the student in remembering the criteria of utilitarian measurement:

> *Intense, long, certain, speedy, fruitful, pure --*
> *Such marks in pleasures and pains endure.*
> *Such pleasures seek, the private be thy end:*
> *If it were public, wide let them extend.*
> *Such pains avoid, whichever be thy view:*
> *If pains must come, let them extend to few.*

Utilitarianism ethicists such as Jeremy Bentham (1838) and John Stuart Mill (1806-1873), (1897) tried to work out an algebraic assessment in assessing pleasure and pain by using nine principles as follows:

- *Intensity* means vehement thoughts and feelings towards extreme degrees of pleasure and avoidance of pain (but not the disappearance of pain).
- *Duration* means continuance in time for having a pleasurable time.
- *Certainty* means having confidence and assurance without doubt concerning the whole assessment of pleasure and pain. Such a course of judgment can establish further truthful and indisputable bases for goodness.
- *Propinquity* means appreciation of the nearness or proximity of pleasurable experiences for experiencing continuous goodness.
- *Fecundity* means the quality of producing a great number of pleasurable experiences and minimizing the greatest number of painful ones.
- *Purity* means the condition of being free of evil and the freedom from extraneous matter or quality of pleasure that can enhance our spirit.
- *Extent* means the space or degree to which pleasurable acts are continued.

Another utilitarianism ethicist, John Stuart Mill, added two more dimensions to the assessment of pleasure and pain as follows:

- *Quality* means the extreme usefulness and utility of a pleasurable judgment with respect to excellence.
- *Quantity* means the identification of an infinitely great amount of pleasurable judgments or actions in accordance with a· set of consistent define rules.

Therefore, utilitarian ethicists hold that what is ethically right or wrong is ultimately to be wholly and quantitatively judged by looking to see what promotes the greatest general balance of good over evil.

UTILITARIAN BIOETHICS

A utilitarian approach in bioethics can be extremely helpful in thinking through an ethical dilemma. In sum, bioethical utilitarianists believe, in the following principles:

- The greatest number of virtuous values over vices (enhancement of human somatic nature such as gene engineering and gene therapeutic).
- The greatest balance of pleasure over pain (eugenic biotechno-scientific activities).
- The greatest good for the greatest number of the population (irradiation of somatic infectious diseases through incubation of viruses, germs, and microbes).
- The greatest profits over costs (promotion of biopharmaceutical and biotech corporations).
- The greatest benefits for the greatest number of employees (advancement for bioscientific education and development of biotechnogical innovativeness, stem cell research and cloning).
- Whatever satisfies the principle of utility also satisfies the requirements of justice. Since justice is built into the principle of utility managing the preferential medical and health research projects according to the demand and supply in the marketplace (e. g., fatal diseases such as cancer and AIDS).
- The greatest net amount of happiness over misery (life-time research and innovativeness against aging; reheorology).
- Actions affect people to different degrees in different circumstances (opening a new academic branch of medical practices in pharmacology to assess physicians' prescribed drugs, the practice of pharmaceutical prognosis in parallel with physicians' practices).
- To maximize happiness not immediately but in the long run (the conversion of medical practices to the prevention of diseases).
- The most certain likelihood of happiness for the greatest number of people (nationwide universal health and medical care policy).
- No personal or societal bio-techno-scientific issue will remain unsolved, because in practice, utilitarianism provides some formulating and testing judgments (creation of a bioinformation

system to tackle the nationwide health and medical problems and issues).

- Utilitarianism provides an objective and attractive way of resolving conflicts of self-interest (universal health and medical care insurance for each citizen/resident).
- Utilitarianism concerns itself with the total happiness produced over miserable means and consequences (the conversion of commercial health and medical services into professionalism).
- Utilitarianism searches to sacrifice minority happiness for majority happiness (conversion of public policies into altruistic biomedicine).

ANALYSIS OF AMERICAN UTILITARIAN BIOETHICS PHILOSOPHY

In addition, we use the word utilitarian for situations when the value of something is proportional to how useful it is to humans. White Jr. (1967: 1203) predicted that Americans would regard nature in utilitarian terms; due to the Judeo-Christian belief dictated in Genesis that humanity should have mastery over nature. Americans believe that the Creator intended that humans use nature. American utilitarian bioethicists believe that nature does not stand apart from humans. Nature should serve humans, and if humans see that what they are doing is ultimately against their best interests, then they obviously have to correct it or clean it up. Therefore, what the preceding suggests is that perhaps we should recognize two basic principles of obligation: (1) principles of utility and (2) principles of justice.

Principles of Utility

The literature in bioethics in the last thirty years or so has identified several ethical principles, often but not always the same ones. For example, the American National Commission for the Protection of Human Subjects of Biomedical and Behavioral Research (1978) justified its recommendations for policies by appealing to three major principles: (1) respect for persons, (2) respect for beneficence, which includes what some have called nonmalfeasance, and 3) respect for justice. Within the domain of bioethics, Childress (1994: 75) expressed his utilitarian principles as follows:

> Whatever the principles in biomedical ethics are called, they represent the following sorts of general moral considerations:
>
> - Obligation for respecting the wishes of competent persons (respect for persons or autonomy).

- Obligations not to harm others, including not killing them or treating them cruelly (nonmalfeasance).
- Obligations to benefit others (beneficence).
- Obligation to produce a net balance of benefits over harms (utility).
- Obligation to distribute benefits and harms fairly (justice).
- Obligations to keep promise and contracts (fidelity).
- Obligations of truthfulness.
- Obligations to disclose information.
- Obligations to respect privacy and protect confidential information (confidentiality).

Principles of Utilitarian Justice

Utilitarian bioethical theorists believe that all other ethical theories such as relativism, deontologicalism, and teleologicalism, do not take the promotion of good biosciences seriously enough. Utilitarian bioethicists believe in the *pareto-principles*. They argue that if a social state of affairs "X" ought to be regarded as socially preferable to a state "Y" at least one of the parties' concerns is better off, and none is worse off. Consequently, a state of affairs is optimal if it cannot be changed in such a way that at least one party would gain more and the other party would lose less (Koller, 2002: 10). For example within the perspective of utilitarian bioethics concerning the rights and duties of humans and animals in bio-techno-scientific research, Moros (1996: 319) stated:

> Even if the case against the strong and weak positions on animal rights were convincing (I hold it is not), the utilitarian could maintain that "rights talk" fails to capture what is morally significant about our treatment of animals. If we grant that animals can experience pain in biotechno-scientific experimental research projects, utilitarianism can maintain that our duty to minimize pain applies to animals as well as humans.

To quote philosopher Jeremy Bentham (1970): "The question is not 'Can animals talk?' but 'Can they suffer?'" Also, utilitarianism eliminates the problem of a possible conflict of basic ethical principles. They ask: "What could be more plausible than the right to promote the general good for the greatest number of people?" They answer this question by a reasoning: "The major point is that an act may be made right or wrong by the facts surrounding it, rather than the amount of good or evil it produces. This indicates that an act is not only either moral or immoral; it may be amoral. This argument opens new doors to the field of bioethics, where a biologist's job in a competitive ·biotech marketplace is not to reveal all secrets to the public. Nevertheless, this does not mean that he/she should lie or deceive people. But he/she may act amorally to disclose a portion of the truth, not the whole. This is the exact meaning of utilitarianism bioethical justice.

Arguments

The utilitarianism that is the essence of the thoughts of Jeremy Bentham is derived from the word *utility*. Utility value denotes that things are good because of their usefulness for some purpose. Hosmer (1987: 98) states:

> Such a perception has come from the eighteenth-century meaning that referred to the degree of usefulness of a household object or a domestic animal; that is, a horse could be said to have a utility for plowing beyond the cost of its upkeep. *Utility* has this same meaning, and this same derivation, in microeconomic theory. It measures our degree of performance for a given good or service relative to price.

Therefore, utilities in reality should be assessed according to a cost/benefit analysis for both parties, and have to be computed equitably for everyone. This means that in the field of bioethics, the biologists' satisfaction cannot be considered to be more important in some way that the human subjects' satisfactions. What is more important than the interests of both parties is the decisional-rule that should then be followed in order to produce the greatest net benefit for society.

Utilitarianism holds that an act is right if, and only if, it produces the greatest net benefit for society over any other act possible under any circumstances, social justice. Utilitarianism differs from the economic concept of cost/benefit analysis in the field of economics in that the distribution of the costs and benefits has to be included as well. That is, these are net benefits to society, and each individual within the society has to be considered equitably (not equally) in the decision-making processes and operations, and also needs to be treated equitably (not equally) in the distribution of goodness.

Utilitarianism holds that the sole standard of right, wrong, and obligation is an observation of the principle of utility. It dictates quite strictly that the ethical means and ends to be sought in all courses of transactions should be based upon the greatest possible balance of good over evil or the least possible balance of evil over good as a whole. The utilitarianism of bioethics lies in its promise to provide for the humane, tough-minded biologists away of resolving complex moral problems and disagreements by rational pragmatic means. With such a perception, another question appears: How, within the context of bioethics, can we include the least evil? The answer is that whatever the good and the bad are, they are capable of being measured and balanced against each other in some quantitative way or at least in an algebraic perceptual assessment.

Application of Utilitarianism in the Field of Bioethics

There are two major views to be analyzed when utilitarian bioethical objectives are considered: (1) obligations and (2) values. These two views assess: Are means more important than ends in biotechno-scientific research projects and innovativeness or vice versa? First, utilitarianism holds that when we are faced with two dissimilar facts concerning the utility of a decision and/or an action, or in other words, trying to see which decision and/or action is likely to produce the greatest balance of good over evil, then that decision and/or action will be ethical. This kind of judgment is called *pragmatic act utilitarianism*

Conclusions

Application of the utilitarian ethical theory remains particularly important in the fields of biomedicine, biology, biochemistry, and biophysics for a variety of reasons. First, utilitarian thinking underlies much of the bio-techno-scientific research activities and innovativeness on the basis of risk assessments, to gain or to lose. Second, the balance of cost/benefit assessments in biopharmaceutical and biotechnological practices may very badly hurt a minority group. Consequently, there is always the possibility of justifying benefits for the greatest majority of population by imposing sacrifices or penalties on minorities. Such a preferential decision and action may not violate the civil rights or the human rights of minorities, but it will violate their natural rights. Another difficulty with utilitarian bioethics is that the rights of a minority group can easily be sacrificed for the benefit of the majority. For example, if biopharmaceutical research were designed on the basis of color, race, ethnicity, religion, and economic classes of majority and minority groups of people, then there would be serious problems in drug development and/or testing. The side effects would violate humans' natural rights (e.g., the Tuskegee syphilis study, the Jewish Chronic Disease study in Brooklyn, New York, the Willowbrook State School for the Retarded experiments etc.).

Through the utilitarian philosophy of social goodness, *economic-class*, ruling-*class,* and *lay-class* are three major terms that make ethical issues contentious. These concepts immediately put *money-power* and *elite-power* on guard. The idea of economically well-endowed and privileged classes of people may dominate the ruling-class and/or the lay-class and may go against the ethical grain of a society. Then, through application of the utilitarian principles of the greatest good for the greatest number, we may face difficulty. To avoid such a difficulty it is necessary to establish and maintain constitutional checks and balances against the ruling or power-elite class.

In addition to the above problems, it is often difficult to obtain the information required to evaluate all of the cost/benefit assessments for all individuals who may be directly or indirectly affected and/or injured by an action or decision. Then our judgments may not be right or wrong. Within the context of utilitarian cost-benefit analysis and the greatest profits for the greatest number, we will be exposed to variety of judgments such as: excellent, best, better, good, right, proper, suitable, beneficial, improper, inappropriate, bad, worse, worst, and vice. According to the bioethics of utilitarianism, biotechno-scientists should keep the following guidelines in mind when they are handling cases of conflicting ideals, causes, processes, and effects (see Figure 4.3):

- When two or more ideals conflict, honor the best ones.
- When two or more causes conflict, choose the right one.
- When two or more rival processes conflict, choose the proper one.
- When two or more effects conflict, choose the suitable one.
- When two or more obligations conflict with consequences, honor the more beneficial one.

Nevertheless, the selection of one of the above attributes would make our judgments more difficult.

As a decision maker, a biologist needs to be knowledgeable about all direct and indirect attributions related to bioethical issues. Some biologists who are not attuned to ethical and moral problems and make some mistakes may claim that they did not know about consequences of their mistakes. It would sound innocent to present the claims that I didn't intend that to happen, or I honestly didn't consider that alternative, or I just didn't know. Such claims are not acceptable within the context of utilitarian cost/benefit assessments. In the *Republic*, Plato claimed that ignorance is an aspect of evil since it is the opposite of being a (Plato: *Apology, Crito, Republic I-II: 343)*. Using Plato's line of thoughts, the right to act ethically implies a responsibility not to speak and/or act from ignorance.

CHAPTER 5

BIOETHICAL PROFESSIONALISM, PARAPROFESSIONALISM, OCCUPATIONALISM, AND VOCATIONALISM

CHAPTER OBJECTIVES

When you read this chapter you should be able to do the following:

- Develop conceptual knowledge concerning what a profession is.
- Distinguish differences between a profession and a paraprofession.
- Distinguish differences between a profession and an occupation.

- Distinguish differences among professional codes of ethics, occupational codes of conduct, and vocational code of behavior.
- Define what the special rights, duties, entitlements, privileges, and autonomy of a professional person are.
- Understand why society has allowed professionals more autonomy and self-management than paraprofessionals and occupationals.
- Be able to argue in favor of or against allowing a profession to govern itself.
- Develop a sense of logic for understanding under what conditions self-governance by a profession is justifiable.
- Know why professional codes of ethics are justifiable for professionals' autonomy to perform their duties.
- Be familiar with characteristics and procedures codes of ethics should have in a profession.
- Argue that an occupational and/or a paraprofessional person should not have the same rights and duties as professionals in a democratic society have.
- Be able to make distinctions among the different themes and objectives of professional academies, associations, and organizations.
- Know the limits of moral, ethical, and legal ordinations among professions.
- Be familiar with members of a profession on the issue of collective bargaining power.
- Know what the difference is between restricted professionalism and extended professionalism.
- Understand the logic behind the differences among registered, licensed, and certified paraprofessionals.
- Know what different types of management philosophy are concerning moral, ethical, legal, and amoral behavior and conduct.
- Be familiar with prohibitions and injunctions against advertising by professional members with regard to justification in the professional codes of ethics.
- Analyze different moral and ethical commitments through professionalization of a group of experts.
- Be familiar with professional experts and their moral and ethical commitments in relation to different governmental agencies.
- Know the relationship between professional employees and employers.
- Know what the ethical, moral, and legal boundaries are between experts and their organizations.
- Know how to recognize business organizations as professional entities.
- Know how amoral behavior differs from moral behavior.

PLAN OF THIS CHAPTER

This chapter begins with an *ism*. In the English language, *ism* is used as a suffix that illustrates a holistic meaning concerning a chain of integrated and interrelated thoughts and beliefs towards a desirable end. It can manifest a quite specific train of thought through which the meaning of the word can be fixed. Changes in deliberated traditional thoughts within a compounded collectivistic words can manifest a sense of emotional content, often reflect changes in opinions and ideals about aesthetic and virtuous meanings of the world in which they stand for. The best examples for such a connotation are the meanings of principlism concerning *professionalism, paraprofessionalism, occupationalism, and vocationalism*. These suffix *isms* represent neologistic thoughts concerning opinions and beliefs in bioethics.

There are several moral, ethical, and legal issues concerning decision-making processes and operations in bio-techno-scientific activities. Accordingly, there are several obligations concerning moral commitments, professional-group ethical convictions, and societal legal mandates. In addition, there are several attributes such as trust, loyalty, and rationalism among people in society. As we defined in chapter one, *moralism* is related to a conscious awareness on the part of an individual to pursue right things; *ethicalism* is defined as excellent cultural behavioral values that fit into customs and traditions. Ethicalism is referred to as a societal benchmark or instrumental assessment of a society as a whole for the guidance of good social behavior for individuals and groups.

We hear constantly of professional bioethics: bioscientific ethics, biotechnological ethics, bioresearch ethics, biopharmaceutical ethics, bioinformational ethics, and biomedical ethics. Are these professional bioethical attributions making up their own specific schools of thoughts? Are they each distinctive? The answer is "no." Our view of professional bioethics is roughly analogous to our practical convictions about certain ethical rules and principles. Our plan in this chapter is to provide you with a neologistic ethical framework and the conceptual tools to sufficiently allow you to behave morally and ethically in your operations. We shall devote primary attention to the following questions:

- Is professionalism bound with ethics?
- Is occupationalism bound with professionalism?
- Are there any other terms than professionalism and occupationalism such as paraprofessionalism and vocationalism in the scientific community?

We may begin by recognizing a broad moral and ethical distinction among the ideas of professionalism, occupationalism, and paraprofessionalism. We have seen that biomedical practices have ethical convictions and legal mandates not to harm, abuse, misuse, neglect, or defraud the patients. These ethical convictions and legal mandates fall primarily on those who treat, diagnose, prognosis, and provide physical therapy to patients. In this chapter, we are going to examine what responsibilities biologists, biotechnologists, bioengineers, biopharmacists, and bioinformationalists have. What duties they have and how bioacademic institutions, private research centers, biotech corporations, and biopharmaceutical companies and their employees can be accountable to the public?

INTRODUCTION

People have different ideas and perceptions concerning the kind of world in which they want to live in. Some strive to build their own personal power through manipulation, domination, and greed, while others feel fear, sadness, empathy, anger, depravation, and injustice. Some are very materialistically oriented, while others are spiritual. Some are very prudent, conservative, and value only their own personal lives and benefits, while others sacrifice their lives for the happiness of others. Nevertheless, such visions must be realistic and pragmatic. For those people who are highly materialistically oriented, their visions are based upon a cost-benefit analysis and/or gains-losses. For those people who are spiritually oriented, their visions are based on humanistic concerns. Accordingly, we recognize two major groups of people: (1) altruistic, and (2) egoistic. Altruistic people are very generous in their mind-set and egoistic people are very stingy and greedy. You need to evaluate your own personality according to these characteristics. Those groups of people who are altruistic scientists are called professionals.

SCIENTIFIC IDEOLOGY OF HUMAN SURVIVAL

Biosciences and biotechnologies are promising to eliminate all practical degenerative diseases of the human race. They are promising to enhance human life through mitigation of suffering and increasing happiness. Moral principles, ethical beliefs, and legal doctrines describe scientific foundations of a bioethical system: ideals, bids, requirements, encouragements, consents, and injunctions. They define, describe, and prescribe a rule-based ethics. So in the Twenty First bionic century, people consider well care as the most important value in their lives. They demand that physicians to offer them prolonged lives. As people perceive a longer life as being consciously alive, the more valuable life is. For the purposes of well-care and prolonged life, people will survive by borrowing body parts, through transplantation of another's body organs and/or with reproductive neo-organs laced with neo-vessels and an inorganic implant from self-provided stem cell cloning parts. There remain some questions as follow:

- Who will these people be?
- With what courage and compassion do they proceed with their lives?
- How will bionic issues such as causes, signs, symptoms, courses, diagnosis, prognoses, and treatments be redefined?
- What would be the known validity of discoveries of physiology, pathology, bacteriology, and quantitative medical and health data and methods to be rewritten?
- How will clinical competency by physicians and/or by nanorobots be viewed as mastery of life sciences?
- How can nanorobots appreciate personal and social needs of the patient?
- What will happen to humanistic qualities, sympathy, and the empathetic healing power of physicians, bioscientists, and biotechnologists toward patient's suffering?
- Who will be responsible for penetrating the past, discovering the present, and guiding the future toward better or worse scenarios of life?
- Should we strive for the mastery of scientific medicine to discover the mystery of life?

The only response to the above concerns that we have found is the indication that human beings, through application of bioscientific discoveries and biotechnological innovativeness, can mitigate their sufferings. Within this context, human beings are consciously and deliberately changing themselves. They are operative agents of themselves to open science and technology to self-manipulation in every dimension of physiological, psychological, and societal life. Nevertheless, bioethicists are worried that the gene pool will become polluted and could create epidemic contamination of blood banks, sperm-banks, and synthesized eggs and engineered genes, together with the new techniques of reproduction processes. The end result can be complicated by controlling human breeding systems, which can lead humanity to a totalitarian form of Social Darwinism manipulation: "the survival of the fittest and the demise of the sickest and/or the weakest."

THE HEALTH AND MEDICAL TECHNOLOGY

Biomedical, biotechnological, and biopharmaceutical corporations are involved in research and development, through manipulation of biotechnological prodigy in order to prolong the well-care life-system of human beings. Technological prodigy facilitates researchers in the development and application of their know-how knowledge in practice, in order to accurately realize the significance of their research findings and biotechnological breakthroughs. Biomedical technological prodigy evolves from the scientific pragmatic construction of extraordinary synergistic scientific techniques, tools, and processes according to the size, amount, extent, and degree of manipulative functional power of the intended prodigy. Technologically, through application of highly sophisticated integrated software and hardware a physician looks inclusively at the syndrome, trauma, disfigurement, defect, and abnormality of a patient's medical disorders. In the application of medical and biotechnological methods and tools, there is a controversial bioethical issue for physicians that indicate physicians and bioscientists such as pathologists, entomologists, ecologists, microbiologists, and pharmacologists moral and ethical duties in the labs. Those diffusive moral and ethical duties should be centered on the integration of the well care and sick care of their patients. This raises a question: Is there a different temperament required to integrate well care and sick care at the same time? This question raises several controversial implications regarding moral and ethical obligations of physicians to their patients. The biomedical code of ethics and the bioethics of professional obligations of bioscientists and biotechnologists may differ from each other concerning diagnosis, treatment, and prognosis of patients. Bioscientists such as pathologists, microbiologists, and radiologists look for applications of innovative methods for detecting abnormality of cause and effect of symptoms, syndromes, and disorders of genes, proteins and cells. Pharmacologists look for matching consequential results of the physician's prescribed drugs and the experienced validity of the physician's judgment in diagnostic and treatment, and the discovery of their side effects. A physician looks towards receiving the scientific laboratory results of a patient's examination in order to make his/her final decision how to diagnose and treat patients' maladies.

A bioethicist looks for the preservation of human dignity and integrity in the well care and the sick care of patients. The end-result of all of the above is that scientists and practitioners manifest their ethical and moral obligations to their professions and to their clients as patients.

THE RISK OF UNCERTAINTY

Biomedical technological research activities are based on trial and error. Trials promise good news and consequences, and errors manifest mistakes and catastrophes in bioresearch experiments. We group the bioethical obligations of scientists, scholars, and researchers into three major headings. The first can be called their obligations to each individual client not to physically or psychologically harm the patient. The second group of moral obligations is related to the general public concerning the safety of those who live with patients and their future genetic offspring. The third group of moral obligation is to not pollute the gene pools, including sperm and ovarian tissue banks and/or the cell-transgenic (ovarian tissues) mutation.

Guterman (2001: A19) indicates that men can father children well into old age, but women go through menopause and lose their fertility. Men can save sperm in a sperm bank, and put off reproducing indefinitely. But eggs don't freeze well, so women's choice may be limited. Instead fertility clinics use ovarian tissues to be frozen and then transplant them back into women's body. Research underway may erase those inequities. Scientists have found a new technique for providing women the option of removing their ovarian tissues and transplanting strips of them back into their bodies, where they regain their functions by producing the monthly hormone cycle and mature egg cells. This early research technique raises the prospect that young, healthy women could bank some of their ovarian tissues for future use, perhaps delaying or even eliminating menopause. Kutluk Okay (2001: A19) at Cornell University's Weill Medical College found new techniques to freeze immature eggs, but has had difficulty ripening them in the lab, as the procedure it results in the boiling of water in the cell, so that all the structures are damaged. In addition, they found that mature eggs are so large (at a tenth of a millimeter, the largest human cell) that damaging ice crystals form within the cells when scientists try to freeze them. Although researchers are working to improve the egg-freezing techniques, the first human born from a frozen egg is now four years old; the success rate is still low. These and other biomedical research experiments raise different bioethical questions. How can bioscientists and bioresearchers observe the professional codes of bioethics in their experiment? In order to respond to this question, we are analyzing the inherent natures of professionalism.

WHAT IS PROFESSIONALISM?

We may begin our discussion by recognizing a broad distinction between ideas of professionalism, paraprofessionalism, and occupationalism. Since such a debate is arguable, certain types of activities reflect a certain vacillation among professional, paraprofessional, and occupational concepts. In this section we will first describe all the relevant ethical and moral characteristics of professionalism, and then in the following sections we will define and analyze the other three terms, paraprofessionalism, occupationalism, and vocationalism.

Professional biomedical practitioners should love to exercise a benevolent power over patients. They need to avoid self-centeredness and narcissism in their medical research and practices. Professionalism means to enhance the professionals' mind with updated technical and pragmatic knowledge and skills. It is a relentless lifetime effort to enhance the proper treatment of patients in acute care medicine. Respect in looking at and paying attention to clients' interests on the part of professionals involves maintaining a distance from ego gratification.

Physicians exert their power expertise through their desire to fulfill their humane mission. Through acquisition of the patients' voluntary consent they diagnose, treat, and prognoses their patients. They may exert their power of expertise by at first causing pain to patients, but eventually such unpleasant actions will help patients by curing their sicknesses or injuries. They never abandon their patients to ignorance, confusion, powerlessness, helplessness, or hopelessness.

The notion of professionalism does seem to involve more impersonally regulated concepts; it often has been structured in terms of serving beyond the self. Everyday we hear the terms of profession, professional, and professionalism. At one level, we describe a member of a profession as related to a group of experts who are committed to certain ethical rules and regulations through observing a pluralistic professional "codes of ethics." These professional codes of ethics require a member of a profession to observe them in addition to the legally mandated rules. Edgar Schein (1966: 3-11) sketched out the basic elements in conceiving the concept of professionalism as follows:

> A professional is someone who knows better what is good for his client than the client himself does... If we accept this definition of professionalism... we may speculate that it is the vulnerability of the client that has necessitated the development of moral and ethical codes surrounding the relationship. The client must be protected from exploitation in a situation in which he is unable to protect himself because he lacks the relevant knowledge to do so... If [a biologist] is... a professional, who is his client? Who needs protection against the possible misuse of these skills?

In an economic term, professionalism is more oriented towards elitism. This means more power should be given to those who have developed their intelligence rather than those who have not.

The historical process of professionalization merged an appeal to the self-interest of the members with an emphasis on the common good. Social goodness could only be achievable on the basis of a strong internal professional organization and self-imposed standards of associates' behavior (DuBose, Hamel and O'Connell, 1994: 102). Although all ethical concepts of professionalism, paraprofessionalism, and occupationalism refer to human social goodness, there are significant differences, as well as interesting emphases among them. Colleges and universities train individuals for the practice of professions that require systematically studied knowledge for their practice and which are necessary for the well being of society as a whole. Such professions include medicine, law, higher education, engineering, architecture, and the administration of private and public institutions. Also, it should be noted that colleges and universities are not the same as a vocational school or a polytechnic institution.

It is common for the incumbents of a profession to regard themselves as people whose services are given to others in a way that leaves room for their personal selfishness. The idea of professionalism does seem to be more impersonally regulated and has often been viewed as client-centered in the precise separation of selfishness from altruistic perceptions. In a philosophical term, professionals have been supposed to enter their professions for love rather than money. In practice, professionals have been paid more than other occupations.

Professionals are perceived as practitioners of a specific scientific branch of knowledge and practitioners of a pragmatic profession who voluntarily set values and standards for the integrity of their own professions. They possess all possible pluralistic competencies to practice their jobs and morally, ethically, and legally are accountable for their success or failure. This perception enshrines a range of virtues more than a set of scientific skills. This means that professionals practice their skills with very high levels of virtuous standards.

Professionalism is known as a concept and practice that resents the bureaucratic objectives of a group of people who are loyal to their specializations. This notion conduces the level of performances more to avoid the self-serving interests than to meet the needs of others. Professionalism avoids dehumanization of a group of people whose intentions and practices serve people rather than the making of a profit. Within the practice of professionalism philosophy, clients easily perceive the integrity of practitioners who are judged to be "on their side." Professionalism avoids hypocrisy and professionals are authentic in dealing morally and ethically with their clients.

If we accept that biologists' moral convictions should be devoted towards the discovery of somatic mysteries, then they should be bound with moral rules. One view of professional bioethics is roughly analogous to the altruistic desire to pursue an intellectual search for achieving goodness for humanity. Professional bioethics should not be seen as a unique and distinctive discipline or as a different kind of ethics. Morality and ethicality are the basic and universal system of professionalism that can apply their principles in all human activities within different contexts, but only accomplish the same common purposes, humanely. Although the disciplinary characteristics of all professions depend upon circumstances, concepts, relationships, and actions, all follow the same altruistic intentions. Professional ethics requires experts to avoid the evil act. All professional individuals would agree on what the goods are insofar as they are against the evils. Furthermore, no committed moral and ethical professionals would avoid goodness unless they understand their selfishness to enjoy illegitimate end results in order to satisfy their personal greed, pleasure, and passion. In order to elaborate on the issues of professionalism, we need first to analyze different dimensions and issues in biomedical practice concerning maladies.

THE MYSTERY OF MALADY

Within the contextual boundary of having a healthy and happy life, medical professionals and health care paraprofessionals are looking for precision in their patients' life-balance. Since human beings are exposed to many diseases, they can feel and understand the end-result of diseases, handicaps, defects, illnesses, sicknesses, disorders, abnormalities, injuries, lesions, and their effects on their daily lives. Maladies can cause an individual to be aware of pain or disorder through the presence of abnormal symptoms. Sometimes, symptoms are apparent through an understanding of the stages of development, while others could be internally developed without awareness of a patient. Some abnormalities are inherently related to genetic disorders and some are the results of the daily-generated abnormal proteins. In fact, many people have symptoms but do not yet feel the original causes. For clarity of use, the term *malady* can refer to all causes, processes, and effects of abnormal symptoms. Gert *et al.,* (1997: 98) define a malady as something that is wrong with an individual who is in pain, disabled, or is dying. Therefore, in such a cultural value system, happiness, which is the essence of well being, is not regarded as an objective of health and medical care systems.

The common starting point in well care is the agreement that happiness is possible for human beings; otherwise there would be no opinion on what this happiness is. Happiness consists of something that satisfies an individual as a human being. Happiness is not pleasure. To live well as a human being is to live a life of purpose. Hence, an individual's good life is achievement of a happy life; it is interpreted as a pain-free. Happiness is first and foremost a state of intrinsic genetic and somatic harmonious functional structuring. Nevertheless, human nature is an intimate union of intellectual, sensitive, emotional, and somatic life. It seems logical to conclude that an individual can be really happy so long as he/she continues to live safely.

Maladies vary in terms of the intensity of the harm being suffered, from relatively minor to extensive pain and suffering. Maladies are highly integrated, interdependent, and correlated within the mechanical structuring of a patient's physical and mental body. The American Medical Association's Standard Nomenclature of Diseases and Operations has broken down the range of medical conditions into the following categories:

- Disease due to genetic and parental influence, (e.g., a gamma glubolinemia, Down syndrome, etc.)
- Disease or infection due to a lower plant or animal parasite, (e.g. Cholera, malaria, etc.)
- Disease or infections due to a higher plant or animal parasite, (e.g., Athlete's foot, fleas or lice, etc.)
- Diseases due to intoxication, (e.g., Arsenic, Cyanide, etc.)
- Diseases due to trauma or physical agent, (e.g., scars, stab wounds, etc.)
- Diseases secondary to circulatory disturbance, (e.g., coronary occlusion, gangrene)
- Diseases secondary to disturbance of the integration of psychic control, (e.g., macular paralysis or spasm, seasickness, etc.)
- Diseases due to or consisting of a static mechanical abnormality, (e.g., dental malocclusion, gallstones, etc.)
- Diseases due to disorder of metabolism, growth, or nutrition (e.g., malnutrition and obesity, vitamin deficiency, etc.)

- Diseases due to unknown or uncertain cause with the structural reaction manifest, (e.g., atherosclerosis, liver cirrhosis, etc.)
- Diseases due to unknown or uncertain cause with the functional reaction alone manifest, (e.g. epilepsy, migraine, etc.)

BIOSCIENTIFIC COMMON CRITERIA FOR PROFESSIONALSIM

Carr (2000: 23) and De George (1995: 468) indicate that the idea of a profession should serve specific commonly altruistic criteria of professionalism as follows:

- Professionals should provide important public services beyond their self-interests.
- Professionals should be involved theoretically as well as practically in-grounded expertise.
- Professionals should have a distinct ethical dimension that calls for expression in the code practical ethics.
- Professionals should require structural organizational regulations and practices for the purposes of recruitment and discipline in their fields.
- Professionals require a higher degree of autonomy in their decision-making processes and actions than do others independent judgments for effective practice.
- Professionals should impose upon themselves pluralistic "codes of ethics" and live up to them.
- The specific demands for "careful consideration" in a profession should protect the welfare of society. Such careful consideration should protect the public interest, the rights of clients, and the duties of professionals within the domain of their expertise.
- The monolithic document of the "professional codes of ethics" for each profession should be assumed as the bedrock foundation for judgments in the process of legal actions.
- Professionals should not only fulfill their expert roles to share their knowledge and experiences with colleagues and peers, but they also should exercise their individual moral obligations without fear.
- Professionals should relentlessly strive for the restructuring of their professional mechanical performance according to the legitimate environmental forces if they pluralistically need to reform their "professional codes of ethics."
- Professionals are sometimes faced with moral and ethical problems and issues, because of conflicts of interest and conflicts between one's professional ethical obligations and the demand of civilian bureaucratic

authorities. They should wisely resent and express their truthful professional opinions as experts.

- Within the domain of their judgments, professionals first are viewed as moral agents, ethically responsible second, and legally accountable third. To decide to be a member of a profession is to choose greater, not lesser personal moral commitments, professional ethical convictions, and legal expertise in decision-making processes and actions.

- Professionals have been allowed, permitted by a general rule of societal trust to govern themselves by their autonomous collective "professional codes of ethics." They need to implement these codes without prejudice and/or favoritism.

- Professionalism depends in large part on the quality of personal deliberations and reflection upon novel problems. In critical situations, they need to make extraordinary decisions and actions to solve problems with good faith and good will.

- Any profession is governed by "professional codes of ethics," which reflect clearly the obligations and responsibilities of their expertise by recurrence to the rights of clients. They need to be faithful to their clients.

Different Types of Professionalism

There are two types of professionalism: (1) restricted professionalism, and (2) extended professionalism. Although the distinction between the two is usually observed in the interests of arguing in favor of the latter over the former, both notions of professionalism appear to be within the holistic context of professionalism.

Restricted Professionalism: Restricted professionalism is defined as the notion of procedural specialization competence, mechanical operational skills, and contractually bound commitments to the principles of a profession. These notions are more along with the lines of exchanging expertise than the notion of acquisition of legal intellectual knowledge property (e.g., patents or copyrights). The responsibilities of restricted professionalism are inclusively defined in terms of procedural cooperation among professionals, and more directed toward accountability or conformity to the relationships among peers.

In restricted professionalism the bench bioresearchers study and test the nature of suspicious symptoms and tissues by running viable routine procedures in order to detect abnormal somatic cells and their dysfunctional consequences. For example, pathologists who examine cancerous cells of patients and/or conduct a routine procedure in forensic research to assess and identify the DNA of criminals or severely burned victims are subject to professional guidelines, the counsel of their own personal moral dignity (conscience), and their' ethical integrity (professional codes of ethics) in their workplace. Therefore, restricted professionals follow the protocols of clinical researchers and are subject to guidelines and to oversight by their professional associations and organizations. These professionals are as vigilant in guarding against personal inclination in relations with patients as they are about maintaining a professional level of competence in diagnosis, prognoses, and therapy.

Restricted professionals are not allowed to conduct non-routine procedures in order to detect abnormal genes and/or abnormal dysfunctional proteins. Laboratories need to follow the attending physicians' orders to conduct their routine testing systems. They are not allowed to conduct more research on received sampling tissues. Therefore, laboratory professionals and paraprofessionals do not have the liberty of conducting their research in much depth in detecting non-routine symptoms. They are focusing on the sick care rather than the well care of patients.

Professionally, to speak of the value of a person's well care and sick care is very ambiguous. Many people make daily decisions that implicitly or explicitly place different values on their lives. Though often not consciously considered, the values of well care and sick care are involved in decisions that many people make everyday. Nevertheless, many decisions appear to value peoples lives inconsistently.

Extended Professionalism: Each profession or each domain of expertise has its own logic, understanding, practices, and dilemmas that call for a specific fashioning of their various "codes of ethics" and "codes of conduct" to deal with particularities and extended extraneous information regarding its activities. Among these extraneous informational domains, obtaining intimate information from human subjects is crucial for generalizing of the effectiveness of new bioresearch projects. Generally, people do not want their intimate information about themselves to be revealed. Disclosure of obtained intimate information outside of a profession can cause social pain and psychological suffering for human subjects. Traditionally, it has been understood and expected that biotechno scientists and biomedical practitioners would not violate and/or breach confidentiality.

An extended professional view aspires precisely and specifically to the relentless acquisition of knowledge and innovative procedures through the practice of a dynamic profession. It is related to maintaining continuous independent judgments rather than merely being obedient to the bureaucratic professional authorities. For example, in forensic expert testimony and/or in the court-witness hearing, the matter of telling the truth is crucial. The general moral and ethical rule is "do not deceive."

Another example of biomedical particularization of extended professionalism is the cause-effect processes of laboratory bioscientists and bioresearchers working on recombination DNA technology or in the area of human eugenic reengineering assuming products stem cell which have been subjected to a broad public scrutiny out of concern about "biohazards" in the first case and "playing God" in the latter case (Moreno, 1995: 4). It is vital to practice medicine within the boundary of natural selection. Directing the decisions of doctors concerning diagnosis, treatments, prognosis, and therapy is a matter of professional policy and practice rather than an administrative or financial one. In addition, within the domain of the health and medical care system, the notion of extended professionalism is related to the level of superiority in knowledge acquisition and seniority in professional pragmatic services.

Notoriously, however, the recent general erosion of professional autonomy in the field of medicine in relationship to the health insurance industry has shifted from professionalism to occupationalism. Professionalism has been marked by a more centrally prescribed de-professionalization or de-skilling of restricted professionalism through governmental and/or insurance superiority over physician autonomy. One effect of such a restricted professionalism can be seen in the popularity of HMOs, in which the medical and health industry is focusing more upon managerial, particularly economic-administrative aspects of the quality care system.

WHAT WE MEAN BY VALUING HUMAN LIFE?

Professionally, there are three ways of valuing human life: (1) personal value, (2) social value, and (3) total value. The *personal value* of a life is its value to the person whose life it is. The *social value of life* is its value to other people. The *total value* is then the sum of its personal and social values, its value to everyone (Bayles, 1987: 265).

In the field of medicine, many discussions about sick-care, well care, and total quality care are confusing. There are different life values among people. Some are quantitative values, others are qualitative values, and the rest are total values; both qualitative and quantitative. These distinctions are important in a professional and paraprofessional health and medical care system. Therefore, the need for a clear analysis of sick care, well care, and total quality care, as well as the scope and limits of these phenomena, is a major focal point for bioethics.

Within the contextual boundaries of restricted professional bioethical sick care and well care phenomena; controversy may be of many factorial types. We will now try to provide you with a general analysis of the processes of the above issues in order to be able to respond to the following questions:

- What is sick care?
- What is well care?
- What is total quality care?
- Are these culturally value judgments?
- Are these professionally scientific judgments?
- Are these econo-politically judgments?
- Are these actual physiological or psychological judgments?

- What is a disease?
- To what extent do these definitions determine the scope of the restricted clinical professional responsibilities of physicians and health and medical care institutions?

WHAT IS SICK-CARE?

When people talk about sick care, they are concerned with total care. Patients presume that they get what they need from their physicians, when they need it. Today, the health and medical care systems function according to the business mentality of either insurance companies or their economic conditions. Patients get health and medical care according to their medical package plan deals. Patients should be aware of the fact that when they get sick, they have different alternatives for seeking diagnosis, treatment, and prognosis of their sickness. For example, when they get a cold, they do not go to doctors to get medication because it may be expensive and time consuming. They go to the drug store and buy their medicine over the counter. When women are pregnant, they buy a pregnancy self-test set, in order to be sure that they are pregnant. When an elderly woman gets to specific age, she goes to her physician or to a clinic to be advised as to what types of vitamins or hormones she needs for good bone density. In a general term, the sick care business is a manner in which it is provided, the way in which it is financed, and the type of patients they will be serving professionally or occupationally. Therefore, sick care is a kind of medical service that is generally provided by professional and paraprofessional experts to specific patients, not to the public as mass-care.

There are two distinctive sick-care systems: (1) simple sick-care, and (2) complex sick care. The simple sick-care system does not need hospitalization. It is an uncomplicated health problem. The complex sick care system requires comprehensive diagnosis, treatments, prognostic, and in some occasions therapeutic care. People usually develop some specific illness that requires treatment in a hospital. The sick care system is more complex, more expensive, and more elaborated. For some patients and some illnesses, long-term, supportive, rehabilitative, and recovery care systems may be necessary.

WHAT IS WELL CARE?

The World Health Organization's (WHO) famous definition spells out the means and ends of *well care* as: "Health is a state of complete physical, mental, and social well being and not merely the absence of disease or infirmity" (Caplan, Englehardt Jr., and McCartney, 1981: 83). Within the scope of such a broad definition, the classification of an individual's health and medical conditions varies from person-to-person and culture-to-culture. Some include pregnancy, drug addiction, abortion, alcoholism, emotional temperament, psychological disorders, familial problems, women's aging, and psychopathic as medical disorders, while others do not. These issues identify the differences between well care and sick care perceptions.

The term *Sick care* is about prevention of deteriorating cells, tissues, organic functional disorders, somatoform tissue disorders, and the improving, recovering, healing, and curing of human maladies. The *well care system* is concerned with enhancing human life toward the full realization of both physical and mental development and growth. Therefore, each nation according to their cultural, legal, bioethical, biomoral, professional, and religious systems. defines different perceptions of well care and sick care systems.

WHAT IS THE TOTAL QUALITY CARE?

Based on a review of the literature, researchers have found different factors as the main microanalysis and macro-influential philosophical and operational functions in the health and medical care industry. Sick care focuses on micro relational values among patients; family members, physicians, health and medical care centers, and financial sponsors (e.g., insurance companies, social medicine, private medicine, and free medicine). Well care function focuses on the macro-issues of the quality of human life. Nevertheless, the total quality care (TQC) focuses on both sick care and well care within the contextual boundary of a highly effective econo-political policy, without defect or deception. The total reliability of today's health care efficiency and effectiveness depends on the availability of effective and efficient medical technology. The total quality care (TQC) system comprises the major issues concerning:

- Scarcity of medical and health care resources
- Availability of physicians and medical technology
- Accessibility of patients to health care facilities
- Durability of prescriptive chain relationships of professionals
- Qualitative efficacy of prescribed drugs and medications
- Flexibility of health care policies and plans to fit sick care, well care, and total-quality-care systems
- Suitability of treatments to illnesses and sicknesses
- Profitability of healthcare insurance companies and their professional relationships with physicians, hospitals, clinics, health centers, and above all their clients (patients)
- Cost-benefit analysis of the health care facilities
- Malpractice premiums for physicians and paraprofessionals
- Comprehensive compensatory insurance policies for abnormal institutional events, emergency incidents, and negligence
- Consistency in diagnostic decisions regarding treatments and prognostic outcomes

- Matching health care effectiveness with health care efficiency (effectiveness equals doing the right things; efficiency equals doing the right things correctly)
- Accuracy in medical and health care procedures
- Carefulness in writing and distributing of prescribed drugs and medication administration
- Professional and humanitarian nursing care
- Prudence in trial and error practices in medical and health care research experiments
- Assessments of the side effects of treatments and medications by synthetic drugs, laser surgical instruments, radiation therapy, or herbal medicine
- Follow up treatments and prognoses of diseases and illnesses
- Assessments of progressive prognostic treatments

HEALTH AND BIOMEDICAL CARE INSTITUTIONS

One difficulty in writing about the health industry is that the idea of health institutions such as biotech and biopharmaceutical companies, bioscientific research centers, hospitals, clinics, insurance companies, and physician offices brings different things to people's minds. What people usually think of when they think of a medical and health care institution is the architectural structure owned by professional practitioners and investors. When people get sick they visit physicians in health and medical care institutions, as they say, by which they mean they visit attending physicians either in hospitals, clinics, and/or in their offices. Nevertheless, nobody, not even physicians, nurses, or staff has ever seen investors. The health care institutions are actualized, concretized only in a set of legal papers. Whatever is tangible about a health and medical care institution is on these papers, its charter of corporation, its by-laws, its mission, its responsibility, and the titles to its properties.

Patients in hospitals can't tell much about who owns and runs these institutions for any purpose. Patients are like laymen, in a biological metaphor, do not know about molecules, atoms, and sub-atomic particles, or about principles of mechanics. Their knowledge has to do largely with principles of cost-benefit analysis in terms of recovering from illnesses, taxes, and prices of rooms, laboratory, x-rays, pharmaceutical costs, and physicians' fees for services. Patients know far more about tax exemptions than about the atomic structure of their own somatic cells. They do not know which groups of providers are known as professionals, paraprofessionals, and/or occupationals. They rely only on the expertise and codes of medical ethics observed by their attending physicians.

Among the social activities of well care and sick care endeavors, the rise and the size of bioscientific discoveries have increased pressure on biologists and biotechnologists to integrate occupational and know-how knowledge to search for the discovery of more bioscientific truths. Critical to the new conception is the notion that a bioresearcher should be concerned with finding new truths and that he or she should adopt the attitude that knowledge (or, rather, what we think we know) is speculative, contingent, and subject to revision in the light of new evidence. The professional obligations of physicians, bioscientists, bioresearchers, and bioethicists are not only relevant to what is known to be true, but also they are obligated to those that were known, based on evidence and subject to alteration in the light of evidence. This causes the creation of a new motive for inquiry and scholarship among academicians within the context of conflicting ideas, in a context in which they might be encouraged to actively participate in the development of new knowledge.

DIFFERENCES BETWEEN CODES OF BIOETHICS AND CODES OF BIOCONDUCT

The argument for making a distinction between a profession and an occupation in a moral, ethical, and legal sense is based on two claims: (1) codes of bioethics and (2) codes of bioconduct. We discussed above in a general way in some organizations (e.g., a hospital, a law firm, a laboratory, a plant, etc.) that there might be three groups of employees working together: (1) professionals, (2) paraprofessionals, and (3) occupationals. Within the field of bioethics their own area of expertise regulates each group. Professional experts are highly educated and skillful and serve their clients beyond their personal interests. They are altruistic people. Paraprofessionals are trained to help professionals perform their duties. Occupational experts are trained to safeguard their personal interest by serving others via safeguarding their institutional interest. In terms of moral, ethical, and legal boundaries each group possesses specific disciplinary codes of behavior. In a general term, all three groups must comply with the law and in addition, professionals must observe codes of bioethics.

WHAT ARE PROFESSIONAL CODES OF BIOETHICS?

What is a code of professional bioethics? The Hippocratic oath, generally recognized as the earliest expression of such a code in relation to medical practice, seems to be a simple principle to the effect that the physicians' first concern should be for the well being of their patients above any personal interest or profit. Within the domain of professional bioethics, professionals must always treat people as *ends* not as *means*. Kant's distinction of the morally grounded categorical imperative from the hypothetical imperatives of instrumental agency seems tailor-made to distinguish the endeavors of professionals from those of occupations such as trades-people or sales-persons. Professionals are required to possess, in addition to specific theoretical expertise and technical skills, a range of distinctive personal moral virtues, cultural values, and legal knowledge to elevate the interest and needs of their clients above their self-interest.

Within the contextual boundary of a code of professional bioethics there are three main attributions: (1) basic human needs, (2) civil needs, and (3) quiddity needs. Basic human needs extend through the essential needs for survival. Civic needs, such as medical and health care needs, judiciary and justice-service needs, and educational opportunity needs are the prime societal needs in a society for achieving peace and harmony. As Parhizgar (2002: 126) stated:

> The professional codes of ethics require the quiddity needs to be considered as matters common to all concepts of the existence of a person. In Latin and Arabic languages, the term *quiddity* means: 'what is it?' This concept in English-speaking cultures is closely related to the holistic essence of humanity. It is said, morally and ethically, that basic human needs are viewed as natural needs, the right to live; civil needs are viewed as liberty and freedom in intellectual expressions within the establishment of structural justice systems, how to live? and quiddity needs are related to the holistic essence of humanity, what is good to live? Basic needs are known as *natural rights*. Civil needs are apt to be known as welfare rights. The quiddity needs are known as human rights. Quiddity needs, holistic needs, demand freedom from diseases, injustice, and ignorance.

Therefore, a professional code of bioethics spells out what constitutes appropriate education, adequate experiential skills, genuine justice, and sufficient careful consideration in a profession.

The professional codes of bioethics require not only the acquisition of appropriate theoretical knowledge (e.g., scientific, evidential, observational, deductive, tacit, technological, legal, and ethical) they also require competencies and experiences in practicing knowledge. The professional codes of bioethics must sufficiently include enough matters of normative, evaluative, and behavioral criteria rather than solely bioscientific or theoretical reflections of problem solving. The professional codes of bioethics must focus on the pursuit of what is true and good rather than upon the discovery of what seems to be good or true. For example, in biotechnology, biosciences, and the biopharmaceutical industries, experiments in human cloning seem to be a rational method for changing defected genes and the replacement of degenerated cells of the human species. Such an attribution is apparently evidential because bioscientists, biotechnologists, biopharmacologists, and biochemists pursue their professional research on the normative or evaluative experiments as the good and truthful evidential reasoning for changing the natural path of evolution to a desirable artificial one. Since all present bioresearch activities emphasize the domain of "trial and error," researchers are not sure about the strategic prodigical consequences of cloning in the human species. Therefore, they first need to know what are good and truthful ethical and moral consequences of their experiments, and then they begin their experiments with careful consideration. Such a recommendation provides a clear guideline for establishing a code of bioethics in these professions.

Professional codes of bioethics should have the following characteristics:

- A profession should be regulated by pluralistic self-rule of professional members. This means that all members are entitled to freely express their moral, ethical, and specialized concerns through collective debates, hearings, and testimonies. The inclusion of ideal codes of bioethics is not necessarily inappropriate.
- Authoritative societal representatives provide appropriate room for professional bioethical autonomy and accountability for the performance of their services. The government will not interfere in the regular practices of professionals, unless it finds a serious harm has been rendered to the social fabric. Professionals must make expected professional moral norms, ethical behavior, and technical procedures publicly available to patients before providing them with any type of services.
- Professional codes of bioethics should provide both providers and clients with appropriate rights and duties.
- Professional codes of bioethics should not be self-serving for the individual objectives of professionals. Codes should be initiated in consideration of the interests of the profession and the total interests of society as whole.
- Professional codes of bioethics prohibit professionals for competing with peers and colleagues by spreading false rumors.
- Professional codes of bioethics should prevent false advertisement and promotion by a professional person. It must prevent negative comments by peers against colleagues in a profession.
- Professional advertisement (e.g., biopharmaceutical, biochemical, and biotechnological) should be designed as honest pieces of information not for the promotion of their businesses but for public awareness concerning the availability of their public services.
- Professional codes of bioethics should provide sufficient room for professional institutions to regulate immoral, unethical, and illegal practices by professionals.
- Professional codes of bioethics should provide society with appropriate procedural channels to enforce punishment for unprofessional actions and those who have broken the codes of ethics. In return, society must appropriately provide special channels for controlling illegal activities of professional members.

Professional Causal and Consequential Responsibilities

Some responsibilities are moral and ethical, some are legal, some are moral, ethical, and legal, and some are amoral. We need to identify in what sense we are responsible and accountable. Sometimes, we are causally responsible or consequentially responsible in our moral judgments. Causal responsibilities are ingredients in moral, ethical, and legal deliberations. This means that an individual is responsible for specific courses of decisions and actions. Consequential responsibilities are ingredients of sole conscientious judgments and behaviors. This notion indicates that the individual's judgment and/or actions are based on their being knowingly and willingly deliberated.

There are degrees of knowledge and degrees of deliberation in moral and ethical judgments. Such a variety of responsibility and accountability is based on conditional and situational factors. The conditions that diminish moral and ethical responsibilities are known as excusable conditions. For example, a pathologist may not be responsible for informing an attending physician in a hospital and/or an outpatient immediately after detecting a cancerous cell, either because of not having the address and telephone number of the attending physician, a patient, or both, because of the sloppiness of medical records. This condition provides room for the lessening of professional negligence. This condition is viewed as a managerial responsibility rather than a professional responsibility. Those conditions that preclude or diminish the exculpatory responsibilities of judgments and actions fall into one of the three following categories:

- Those conditions that preclude the possibility of action are excusable. This means that to be morally and ethically obligatory, an action must be possible.
- Those conditions that preclude or diminish the required knowledge are excusable. Bioscientists and biotechnologists are morally and ethically responsible to be highly skilled and specialized within the domain of their expertise. The excusable responsibilities could be lessened when one of the conditions is absent. With respect to knowledge, there are two excusing conditions: (1) *excusable ignorance* and (2) *invincible ignorance*. Excusable ignorance is related to an insufficiency of knowledge. Invincible ignorance is related to unpredictable consequences of our judgments or actions. Professionals are responsible for the immediate and obvious consequences of their judgments and actions. Nevertheless, both excusable and invincible ignorance are failures due to the lack of sufficient knowledge.
- Those conditions that preclude or diminish the required freedom are excusable. A bioscientist or pilot may be excused by the lack of freedom in independent judgments. They need to follow standard procedures in their performances. This means excusable conditions may

be viewed as the result of four conditional factors: (1) the absence of alternatives, (2) the lack of control over courses of actions, (3) external coercive forces, and (4) internal coercion (De George, 1995: 115).

WHAT IS PARAPROFESSIONALISM?

The words *paraprofession* and *ancillary* refer to the engagement of specific training and pragmatic skillful activities for a group of academicians and scientific skillful practitioners in which individuals regularly devote their daily activities to assist professionals in order to acquire a living income. Most paraprofessional groups aspire to the "rule bioethics" (e.g., physician aids, nurses, paralegal, lab technicians, etc.). There are a number of component parts to the definition of paraprofessionals as follows:

- Paraprofessionals need to acquire formal theoretical education, practical skills, technical training, and qualifying examination in order to be certified and serve in their career areas (e.g., Registered Nurses – RNs).
- Paraprofessionals are required to be certified as having specific qualifications reflecting community sanctions or approvals (e.g., Certified Teachers, Certified Occupational Therapists, Licensed Appraisers, Certified Custom Brokers, etc.),
- Paraprofessionals are required to acquire licenses through skill tests in order to be allowed to independently practice their jobs in specific communities (e.g., Midwives, Licensed Psychologists, etc.).
- Paraprofessionals need to have specified qualifications in order to be a member of local, regional, or national associations (e.g., American Nursing Association, American Dietician Association, American Physical Therapist Association, etc.).
- Paraprofessionals are required to observe certain "codes of conduct."
- Paraprofessionals are required to follow certain legal mandates (Greenwood, 1962: 206).

Different Types of Paraprofessionals

As modern society becomes more complex, it requires greater specialized knowledge and practical skills. We may recognize differences among paramedical, paralegal, and paraeducational people with a variety of ideas and mandated patterns of responsibilities and accountabilities. Within the contextual boundary of a broad distinction between paraprofessionals and occupationals, we may find a certain vacillation between these concepts. Genealogically, there are significant and illuminating tensions as well as interesting differences of emphasis between paraprofessional and occupational people. It is common for the incumbents of the so-called paraprofessions to give their career lives to the service of others in a way that leaves relatively little room for personal gain (e.g., firefighters, police officers, soldiers, emergency crews of medical helicopter pilots, co-pilots, and nurses). Wilson and Neuhauser, (1976: 52) indicate that there are three major groups of paraprofessionals: (1) registered, (2) certified, and (3) licensed paraprofessionals.

Registered Paraprofessionals: Registration is a legal process by which qualified individuals are included on a listed roster maintained by governmental or non-governmental agencies. Registration in some cases allows individuals to carry recognizable designated titles after their names. This group of people needs to have sufficient experience and knowledge in sensitive lines of professional activities. Nevertheless, members of this group of people are not required to have a maximum theoretical educational expertise in their own fields. They are more practical. For example, a cytotechnologist registered by the Board of Registry of the American Society of Clinical Pathologists may use the designation title of CT (ASCP).

Certified Paraprofessionals: Certification is a process by which a non-governmental agency and/or a scientific association grant recognition to an individual who has met certain predetermined qualifications specified by that agency or association. A *diploma* is one form of authorized certification by a recognized agency or individual that has been issued for a qualified person to perform specific skillful job.

Licensed Paraprofessionals: A licensed paraprofessional degree is the process by which a qualified governmental agency grants permission to people meeting predetermined qualifications to engage in a given occupation and/or use a particular title.

DIFFERENCES BETWEEN PROFESSIONALISM AND PARAPROFESSIONALISM

As modern society becomes more complex, it requires more greatly specialized knowledgeable experts. Most highly specialized groups in the field of medicine and health care systems aspire to be considered professionals. We may recognize a variety of different ideas and innovations among medical and health occupations. Within the contextual boundary of a broad distinction between *occupation* and *profession,* we may find a certain vacillation between these concepts. Genealogically, there are significant and illuminating tensions as well as interesting differences of emphasis between occupational and professional conceptions. It is common for the incumbents of so-called occupational researchers in the field of biosciences, rightly or wrongly, to give their lives to the services of others in a way that leaves relatively little room for their personal gain. Identically, this idea of a significant continuity between bioscientific occupational researchers' personal and occupational concerns and interests has probably been one reason why traditional occupations (e.g., biologists, biochemists, biophysicists etc.) have been less financially rewarded than other professions such as physicians and lawyers. Maybe one of the moral reasoning for such a discrepancy is the fear that raising the salaries of bioscientists and bioresearchers would attract the wrong kind of people, those of mercenary inclinations, into the occupations. There can be little doubt that teaching and researching in the field of biosciences has often been regarded as an occupation, that it has also been regarded as the kind of profession which people enter for love rather than money, and that it has also frequently been woefully underpaid.

In any medical and health organization there are two types of employees: (1) professional experts and (2) auxiliary staff. Professional experts perform their duties beyond their personal interest, while paraprofessionals perform their duties on the basis of receiving economic incentives. As we have analyzed professional codes of ethics, we will analyze "occupational codes of conduct" in the following pages along with the notion of occupationalism.

WHAT IS OCCUPATIONISM?

We may begin our discussions by recognizing a broad distinction among professionalism, paraprofessionalism, and occupationalism. These ideas carry different definitions, power, authority, responsibility, and accountability in society. Although all of the above terminologies refer to specific ranges of activities, there are significant and illuminating differences among them. Occupationalism is viewed as a societal bureaucratic ordering (legal) system concerning the values, contributions, effectiveness, and efficiency of all types of jobs and jobholders in society. It mainly focuses on the distribution of wealth and resources among citizens according to the econo-political doctrine of a nation.

Occupations and occupational incumbents attempt to convince the public, legislators, and community authorities that they are deserving of high respect, prestige, privilege, and special treatments in society because of two major reasons: (1) they claim that they begin to generate their own esoteric and useful knowledge including branches of scientific expertise, skilful pragmatic know how methodological doing things, and both possession of experiential and experimental valuable data, (2) on the basis of acquisition of knowledge and rendering services to their clients, they believe that like professionals (e.g., physicians and lawyers) should be entitled to regulate their own conduct from within the occupation, rather than solely being imposed by authoritative funding agencies. These people believe that ethical values and moral convictions are created for outside public consumption, so that an occupation can gain a monopoly, and have little impact within the group. Some ethicists like Douglas (1978: 13) takes strong issue with this view and sees occupational ethics as "a deceit and a snare," a means by which the establishment within an occupation can control and hide its activity from the public and thereby create a monopoly. Furthermore, he argues that even if the occupation takes its self-policing seriously, it could be used as a club to control deviance of the more creative nonestablishment members whose new ideas are vital, particularly for young people.

Through a lens of occupationalism, bio-techno-scientific experts, especially in the field of biomedicine, perceive patients as objects, albeit scientific objects, exhibiting certain pathological features. Bio-techno-scientists who are disposed toward dominating pathological objects and demonstrating their technical expertise may become competent medical diagnosticians and prognosticians, but they lack the professional qualities required for performing services beyond self-interest. They may lose the notion of moral commitment and love of patients and become cold and aloof.

A cold and impersonal behavior makes bio-techno-scientists inattentive to the broader dimensions of patients' lives. Such bio-techno-scientists may multiply diagnostic tests and therapeutic interventions for their own economic benefit. Even though these bio-techno-scientists' specific decisions and clinical operations might not violate a particular "code of conduct" (legally), they may not serve a patient's best financial interest. Consequently, the preference of such a perception and action will endorse first the interest of bio-techno-scientists first and patients second. They may undermine "core medical and professional value systems and professional codes of ethics." Such a deviant outgrowth makes the difference between professionalism and occupationalism.

The consequence of bio-techno-scientists' engagement in a type of self-interest is the narrowing of their scientific perspectives and their reliance solely on biotechnology and failure to generate proof of pathology. Not all bio-techno-scientists are medical doctors. They may obtain their doctoral degrees in a graduate school. They were never under the "oath" of the medical profession. Therefore, they assume their roles as occupationals rather than professionals. Professional medical practitioners never abandon a patient. But bio-techno-scientific experts may abandon patients; if they find that bio-medical techniques are ineffective. Nevertheless, medical doctors who are under the medical oath never abandon their patients to the last moment of the patients' lives as long as the patients refer back to them.

An occupation is a kind of vocation in which people perform specific jobs for receiving economic incentives as incomes, wages, salaries, commissions, and fees for services. It is common for the incumbents of so-called vocations to regard themselves as occupationals.

Whereas professionalism seems to be viewed as loyalty to the notion of "expertise codes of ethics," occupationalism is viewed more as having loyalty to the "civil codes of conduct." The "expertise codes of ethics" mean that physicians' professional commitment is to provide diagnosis, treatment, and prognosis to all types of people within the boundary of humanity without any discriminating policy such as race, religion, color, ethnicity, political ideology, nationality, and wealth. The "civil codes of conduct" mean that jobholders must act within the legal boundaries of their power and authority. For example, peacekeeping officers' (e.g., a police, constable, or state trooper) responsibilities require them to perform their duties according to their geographical areas of "jurisdiction and /or services."

Occupationalism is enshrined with legal standards and requires a specific set of skillful training programs. Occupationals may not be professionals, because they do not require the same equivalent qualifications of professional expertise. The main objective for an occupation is the pursuit of self-interest. From this perspective, if university professors, lawyers, or physicians convert their jobs from professionalism to occupationalism through self-interest, their clients will suffer from such self-interest. Then they will not be trusted to serve people.

Another dimension of occupationalism is related to the priority of the notion of economic self-means and ends. From this perspective, occupationalism's priority is to first fulfill self-interest and second to serve others. As we indicated before, the notion of professionalism is a personal attachment to a kind of job expertise that requires avoidance of preferential personal welfare and/or self-interest. It is a fact that all occupations in society are no more than that they get paid for what they do, "fee for services." Within this sense of understanding in an occupation, specifically in the fields of biosciences, biopharmaceuticals, and biotechnologies, we may find that some people can fairly compare their responsibilities with the quality of their performance to satisfy their employers' interests.

One consequence of regarding human social activity as an occupation rather than as a profession is that it changes the idea of significant continuity between selfish and altruistic values and concerns in terms of moral commitments and ethical convictions. The notion of occupationalism is focused on the nature of the division of labor, the economic value of work. Although much recent emphasis has been put upon the economic status of paid work, "fees for services," and has therefore, sought to stress the broader econo-political values of work, the urgent need for total quality care systems has been neglected. Thus, it is common for the incumbents of a so-called occupation to regard themselves as people whose services are totally dominated by financial rewards.

Occupationals are known as having a "cultural custodian" view of performing their jobs in return for receiving a specific financial reward. One reason for including such a financial view among different types of occupations is that a certain anti-professionalism stance has been found within the organizational bureaucratic mandates. Thompson (1961: 170) states:

> The bureaucratic culture makes certain demands upon clients as well as upon organizational employees. There are people in our society who have not been able to adjust to these demands. To some people bureaucracy is a curse. They see no good in it whatsoever, but view the demands of the modern organization, and is not simply a reaction to bureau pathology. Its source will be found within the critic himself, not within the organization. It is, in fact, a kind of social disease, which we propose to call bureausis.

What Are Occupational Codes of Conduct?

The arguments in favor of the following issues concerning codes of conduct are based on two claims. The first is that the know-how knowledge and skills that members of an occupation have mastered have usefulness for the economic welfare of a society. The second is that members of an occupation are expected to observe the legal standards for themselves that society expects of them. Codes of conduct in an occupation do not exhaust the issues of ethics. Ethical codes of conduct are general behavioral and procedural rules for both professions and occupations. They specify particular legal prohibitions and ideals, each of which can be evaluated from moral and ethical points of view. For instance, bioethical issues in biosciences and biotechnology often gain media attention as the result of advances in cloning. These issues raise moral, ethical, and legal legitimacy not only for those in research centers but also for those in society in regard to their religious faith. The ethics of organ transplants, the use of fetal tissues, the various genetic engineering, and stem-cell cloning press issues in socio-cultural and econo-political endeavors. Therefore, bioscientists and biotechnologists are not under oath like physicians to observe codes of ethics. What are they expected to observe are the codes of conduct.

The "codes of conduct" consist partly of ordinary ethical rules, partly of rules of etiquette, and partly of rules of professional conduct (Dawnie, 1974). Bio-techno-scientific research is not considered a merely scientific enterprise that can be ethically evaluated from some exogenous standpoint.

Occupational "codes of conduct" spell out the rules among a group of people that are expected to have behavioral standards, for effectively communicating those standards to all people. A study by the Ethics Resource Center in 1990 revealed the following topics in the codes of conduct:

- Conflict of interest
- Receiving gifts, gratuities, entertainment
- Protecting institutional proprietary information
- Giving gifts, gratuities, entertainment
- Discrimination
- Sexual harassment
- Kickbacks
- General conduct
- Employee theft
- Proper use of institutional assets including patents, copyrights, and job shops

Schwartz (2001: 247) indicated that there are eight themes through which jobholders perceive "codes of conduct," as follows:

- As *a rulebook,* the code acts to clarify what behavior is expected of employees.

- As a *signpost*, the code can lead employees to consult other individuals or institutional policies to determine the appropriateness of behavior.
- As a *mirror*, the code provides employees with a chance to confirm whether their behavior is acceptable to the institution.
- As a *magnifying glass*, the code suggests a note of caution to be more careful or engage in greater reflection before acting.
- As a *shield*, the code acts in a manner that allows employees to better challenge and resist unethical requests.
- As a *smoke detector*, the code leads employees to try to convince others and warn them of their inappropriate behavior.
- As a *fire alarm*, the code leads employees to contact the appropriate authority and report violations.
- As a *club*, the potential enforcement of the code causes employees to comply with the code's provision.

The point is that whereas the professional "codes of ethics" are self-sustainable, the occupational expected conducts are authoritative tailor-made rules. In professional codes of ethics, professionals are known as guardians of their professions, while from occupational custodian view. This means that job occupants are viewed as guardians of their institutions. In addition, within the philosophy of professionalism, professionals strive for precisely how to be *neutral* and observe a clear line between professional obligations and institutional loyalty and occupationals try to safeguard their institutional interest.

Whereas professionalism seems to be viewed as loyalty to the notion of independent commitments to "expertise rules and principles," occupationalism is viewed more towards the notion of being loyal to the "civil policy." Expertise policy is a set of shared values flowing from the part of an individual's intellectual self-disciplinary perceptions of professional membership; professionalism. The civil policy is viewed as top-down desired conceptions of elite groups of power-holders concerning societal ordination of citizens in a society, occupationalism.

DIFFERENT VIEWS CONCERNING PROFESSIONS AND OCCUPATIONS

The distinction between an occupation and a profession is a notion that clearly outlines what the general and specific characteristics of these two phenomena are. That distinction clearly makes a difference between private or personal and public or professional opinion. In a profession, there are specific pluralistic rules and regulations, in addition to knowledge and skills, in terms of professional self-imposed disciplines namely, the "codes of ethics, COE," while in occupations there are specific qualifications and expected behaviors which are prescribed and imposed by the elite groups of authorities, in which they are defined as the organizational "codes of conduct, COC." The point is that whereas the professional codes of ethics are viewed as self-sustained sanctions against self-interest, the occupational expected codes of conduct are authoritatively tailored-rules made by elite societal authorities.

In professional codes of ethics, professionals are known as guardians of their conscience commitments for respecting their peers and their work integrity, while in the occupational custodial view, the codes of conduct are viewed as guardians of their own self-interest and their institutions. In addition, within the philosophy of professionalism, professionals strive for "cooperative" enhancement of their tasks, while in occupations occupationals compete with each other in order to win the market edge. Professionals share their findings from experimental research towards more accomplishments, while occupationals keep their achievements secret in order to maintain their competitive superiority. In addition, within the philosophy of professionalism, professionals strive for precisely how to be neutral and observe a clear line between professional obligations and institutional loyalty, while in occupationalism there is no clear line to separate organizational loyalty from professional commitments.

Professionalism is viewed as having commitments to the cause of altruism and the promulgation of the scientific partisan doctrine. Professionals believe and act according to the sincerity of their expertise and pragmatic values. Professionals strive to achieve pragmatic scientific outcomes to be measured by good-intention, good will, good operations, and good consequences. Whereas professionalism seems to be viewed us having loyalty to the notion of "expertise policy," occupational people strive to have loyalty to the "civil policy." To explain these differences, we may assume the role of a physician in wartime. According to "expertise policy," a physician's professional responsibility is to cure injured people – both friends and foes. If that physician changes his/her ideology to occupationalism, then he/she has to cure only friendly soldiers not foes, because he/she was hired and paid by friends, not by foes.

Expertise rules are professional sets of shared humanistic values that pursue the goodness of humanity. Professionals put aside their self-interest and/or prejudice in order to serve humanity. The "civil rules" are viewed as top-down ideological political desires concerning the elite interest groups of power-holders in a society. For example, the role of biopharmaceutical companies in the international marketplace is to follow their home political ideology, capitalistic, socialistic, communistic, or nationalistic. Each political ideology applies specific strategy to fulfill such an ideology.

WHAT IS VOCATIONALISM?

Parks (1993: 217) indicated:

> The word vocation connotes the *relation* of self and the world. To have a
> vocation is to have more than a position, a job, a role, or even a career that

one arbitrarily chooses on the basis of personal reference or inclination because one is forced to answer the perennial questions posed to the self: What are you going to do when you grow up? How are you going to earn a living or otherwise secure livelihood?

The word *vocation* is rooted in the Latin, *Vocare*, to all, it connotes a sense of being beckoned or invited, and it requires a response. Vocation is a profoundly ethical question; embedded in the issue of vocation is a question of the good: What is good for myself in relation to world? Thus, the question of vocation conveys a sense of financial attachment of being called to relationship and to an interdependence that possesses a financial magnitude within the context of earnings.

Vocationalism depends on relationships between an individual and a technical task to be done such as plumbing, carpentering, and trading. Vocationalism conveys a pragmatic commitment to solve the problems of others rather than self-fulfillment. A vocation is a profoundly ethical question of the good: What is good for myself and for my customers and/or clients? Any response to this question affects primarily both the self and others and their relationships. Since the notion of occupationalism is more focused on self-fulfillment such as my job, my position, my pay, the ethical question of vocationalism can be neither posed nor answered by the self-alone. Parks (1993: 217) states: "Vocation conveys a sense of being called to a relationship and to an interdependence that is larger than self." Therefore, vocationalism is a vehicle for social mobility through pragmatic problem solving. Within such an endeavor of thinking, society needs a group of people to be involved in vocations and trades.

Vocationalism is the notion of the development of the necessary skills and docility to be successful employees within a capitalistic framework system. It channels working-class people into working-class jobs. Indeed, it seems to be a fairly common sociological view that such distinctions reflect differences of social or class status. Within such a magnitude of ethical deliberation there are two types of arguments concerning vocationalism: (1) ethical functionalism, and (2) ethical instrumentalism.

What Is Ethical Functionalism of Vocationalism?

Ethical functionalists tend to come to the defense of vocationalism by describing several vital "social necessities." Social ethics mandates some people in society to serve pragmatic problem solving by training middle-level workers, and to preserve the notion of excellence. Vocationalism provides a facility to democratize vocational options and maintain lower prices for services rendered to the community. Vocationalism will serve society in all different types of needs. This means that when a kitchen is flooded because of a burst water pipe, it is likely to be more urgent that there is a plumber than that there is a doctor or lawyer in the vicinity. Therefore, it is not necessary to ask a mechanical engineer to come and fix it and charge the homeowner at excessive rates. Because of social necessities, there should be another group of workers with a lower cost to fulfill this social task.

Ethical functionalism is a matter for normative or evaluative, rather than scientific or theoretical reflection, focused on the pursuit of what is *good* rather than upon discovery of what is *true*. Evaluative or normative ethics is considered by through evidential patterns of social necessities; goodness.

What Is Ethical Instrumentalism of Vocationalism?

Ethical instrumentalists tend to come to the defense of vocationalism by describing several vital *"civil necessities."* There are three major reasons for having vocationalism as an instrument in balancing civil needs:

1. Vocationalism provides those workers who have developed the necessary pragmatic skills and docility to be successful as small business owners. These opportunities allow society to enjoy lower costs for having immediate services by small businesses and avoiding bureaucratic red tape processes and/or expensive sophisticated technological systems.
2. Vocationalism is used as an instrument to serve professionalism in order to avoid class confusion in a capitalistic society.
3. Vocationalism maintains class equitability reward systems by channeling *"working-class people into working-class jobs."* This facilitates changing the trends of the labor market from unemployment to employment. Also, this converts scientific aspects of problem solving to technical, territorial societal ideology.

It is important to provide grounds for distinguishing professionalism and paraprofessionalism from vocationalism in areas such as trades, manufacturing industries, and mercantile enterprises. It is important to emphasize here that this sense is focused upon the idea that enterprises such as medicine, law, and education are implicated in questions and considerations of a particular ethical and moral character which are not to the forefront of, for instance, plumbing, joinery, auto repair, wholesale or retail sales, and hairdressing. Any community possesses numerous vocations, although we are not able to analyze the ethical and moral issues of each in this text.

What Are Vocational Codes of Behavior?

Vocational codes of behavior are just another type of culture in which an individual should behave within the context of societal rules. Each vocation or each domain of life earning has specific practices, understandings, and dilemmas that call for a specific fashioning of the various societal commitments to deal with the particularities of its pragmatic activities. Vocational codes of conduct are highly related to contractual bindings between buyers and sellers in execution or management of the content of a contract. The very nature of the practice of a vocation is viewed as an act of guidance to behave (oneself); just to do expected his/her job.

ACADEMIA, ASSOCIATIONS, ORGANIZATIONS, AND UNIONS

The primary determination for establishing an academy, an association, an organization, or a union is related to know how society expects its members to fairly and justly relate and behave to each other and towards their customers or clients. According to social ordinations professionals, paraprofessionals, occupationals, and vocationals form either pluralistic or collectivistic gatherings that are known as academia, associations, organizations, and unions. In a democratic society these institutions strive to create an enhanced social system in the areas of their expertise, practices, concerns, and benefits in order to establish a societal balance system to protect their rights and duties.

The primary objective of members of academic institutions is to promote scientific knowledge by a group of academicians. Academia's mission is to promote the doctrine of scientific free expression of ideas without interference from institutions, or social and governmental authorities. Academies are viewed as scientific forums for discussions, analysis, and dissemination of scientific knowledge concerning societal issues and problems (e.g., The Institute of Medicine, IOM, the National Academy of Sciences, NAS, Hastings Center, the Kennedy Institute of Ethics, RAND). Also, the primary mission of academia is to establish a system of collective scientific understanding for scientists, researchers, and practitioners to enhance and promote theoretical and practical knowledge discovery by conducting annual conferences for sharing their discoveries, innovations, and inventions of new methods and procedures with their peers and colleagues.

Professional associations also tend to establish a self-ruled professional policing system concerning the behavior and practices of their members. In addition, professional associations tend to establish and enforce their "professional codes of ethics," in addition to their legal occupational obligations (e.g., National Advisory Board on Ethics in Reproduction, American Medical Association, American Academy of Pediatrics, American College of Physicians, American Association of University Professors, and American Bar Association).

Societies are those ethical, moral, legal, and social entities that strive to maintain the highest disciplinary standards of personal conduct of their members in society. Societies emphasize codes of conduct. Affiliated members of a society strive to enhance their humanitarian and philanthropic awareness by raising voices against injustice, unfairness, and wrong doings of authorities or organizations. Societies try to improve public understanding of organizational roles in public and private and their power, authorities, responsibilities, and accountabilities (e.g. American Thoracic Society, Society for Civil Rights, Society for Advancement of Management, Cancer Society, National Abortion Rights Action League, the National Right to Life Committee, the AIDS Coalition to Unleash Power, ACT-UP, etc.).

Organizations in the field of business are known as those entities which are committed to specific causes and effects such as commercial, trade, exchange materials, goods, and services either as buyers or sellers. The best example of such organizations are known as "trusts," "monopolies," "cartels," and consumer organizations e.g., Health Maintenance Organizations, HMOs, such as Group Health of Puget Sound, Harvard Community Health Plan, etc.) Domestically and internationally, these organizations play very important functional roles in the marketplace.

The illicit activities of organized criminals for receiving continuous profit are one of the ladders of social mobility for some political and financial authorities in all nations. Indeed it is not too much to say that the whole question of organized crime in the international market cannot be understood unless one appreciates: (1) the distinctive role of organized gambling as a function of mass-consumption economy, (2) the specific role various demographic movements around the world have in creating marginal businesses and crime, and (3) the relationship of criminals with some societal authorities to the changing character of national and international machines (Bell, 1960). Nevertheless, we should indicate that not all uncharted domestic or international organizations are criminals. Some have specific business causes for organizing their collective power while others organize their power to protect their rights (e.g., International Labor Organizations – ILO).

International organizations include some oil cartels such as OPEC, the Organization of Petroleum Exporting Countries (Algeria, Gabon, Indonesia, Iran, Iraq, Kuwait, Libya, Nigeria, Qatar, Saudi Arabia, United Arab Emirates, and Venezuela). The members of OPEC control prices of energy by establishing oil production quotas in the international marketplace. These organizations may not be directly harmful to their own countries and others. They possess an uncontrollable financial power to influence moral and ethical issues for good or evil. Ralph Nader (2000: 3) indicates:

> Over the past twenty years, big business has increasingly dominated our political economy. This control by corporate government over our political government is creating a widening 'democracy gap'... The unconstrained behavior of big business is subordinating our democracy to the control of a corporate plutocracy that knows few self-imposed limits to the spread of its power to all sectors of our society.

There are two other types of organizations: (1) unions and (2) employee organizations. Both types of organizations join employees of public and private organizations. A union is a formal and legal association of workers that promotes the employment rights and duties of its members through collective decisions and actions. Unions' primary concerns are related to wages, benefits, incentives, work rules, sanitation, safety, and the security of employees. The status of unions varies among countries, depending on the culture and the laws that define employer-employee and/or union-management relationships. Employees in different nations are represented by many different kinds of unions such as craft unions, industrial unions, and federations. A craft union is a type of collective bargaining system in which members do one type of work, often using specialized technical or vocational skills and training (e.g., the International Association of Bridge, Structural and Ornamental Iron Workers). An *industrialized* union includes many workers working in the same industry or company, regardless of jobs held (e.g., United Food and Commercial Workers, The United Auto Workers). The federations are groups of autonomous national and international unions. This type of union is the most complex organization in which individual unions work together and present a more unified front to the public, legislators, and members (e.g., American Federation of State, County, and Municipal Employees and American Federation of Labor and Congress of Industrial Organizations- AFL-CIO).

Employee organizations in contrast are said to have a greater concern for the occupational aspects of employment, including the quality of public services and of the people performing it. Employees of state and local governments serve in a variety of capacities. Among public employees are police, firefighters, sanitation workers, nurses, health aids, clerks, prison guards, utility workers, and others. This is a substantial range of occupations that demonstrates the wide range of matters with which public employees are concerned.

CHAPTER 6

PARADIGM OF BIOSOPHY, BIOPHILIA, AND BIOKNOWLEDGE

CHAPTER OBJECTIVES

When you have read this chapter you should be able to do the following:

- Analyze and further explore the factors that inhibit bio-techno-scientific responsiveness to ethical changes in our contemporary society.
- Know whether ethics is adequate as science or as a holistic knowledge.
- Analyze different types of biosophy and their relationship to biosciences, biotechnology, and biomedical practices.

- Identify crucial societal factors that influence the biopharmaceutical industry over the long term.
- Identify both dimensions of material and non-material cultures in relationship to the importance of ethical values in evaluating, financing, and accumulating wealth through bioscience, biotechnology, and bioinformation.
- Describe why bioethics must be related to practical bioscience.
- Know the meaning of practical ethics.
- Know how ethics is both a process and an end product of bioresearch.
- Know not only what type of bioresearch is right but also precisely why it is right.
- Know how an individual who is intellectually well informed in regard to doing good and evil can be characterized as an ethical bioresearcher.

PLAN OF THIS CHAPTER

Bioscientific formulas, biotechnological breakthroughs, and knowledge-based bioinformation systems are essential component parts of critical thinking. These phenomena help us to examine human wisdom so that we can act, as we believe, as free from natural errors as possible. Natural errors or abnormalities occur in nature when a product deviates greatly from structured standards, pre-designed rules, and expected types of formation. Abnormality is a malformation and prodigious monstrosity. Abnormality is usually characterized as circumstances that deviate from physiological or psycho-social ideals regarding the proper levels of natural functions, freedom from pain and suffering, and the achievement of expected human form and grace (Engelhardt, Jr., 1996:189). Thus, abnormality is defined as irregularity within a particular context of natural expectations.

Biosciences medicalize reality. They create pragmatic methodologies to eliminate deviated natural malformations. They translate sets of normality into scientific formulas in their own terms. They deal with abnormalities in the ways in which the natural world of experience takes place. The difficulties human beings have are then appreciated as medical abnormalities, deformities, disabilities, diseases, illnesses, and sicknesses, rather than as innocent vexations, normal pains, or possession by the devil. These phenomena are beyond the immediate control of the individuals afflicted, and they are presumed to have scientific bases in physiological, anatomical, or psychosocial causal matrices.

Within the contextual boundaries of the ordered natural system there are some errors that make normal human life impossible. Humans, through their limited intellectual deliberations, assume that all natural errors can be corrected by seeking the establishment of a final and absolute coherence in the enumeration of the finite instances of the error. Specifically, most bioscientists are rather of the opinion that the order that biosciences find in nature has only a statistical probability, not an absolute rigor. According to this principle, bioknowledge can only *tend* to be congruent, and does not attain the absolute congruence to be found in a purely rational system like geometry. Nevertheless, an absolutely truthful congruence assumes the existence of an absolute mind or reason where all facts are known and are seen to be in perfect congruence. Therefore, we should accept that in bioscientific deliberations, bio-techno-scientists and biomedical practitioners try to find congruence to be identical with *truth*, while in reality congruence is identical with their *thoughts*. This makes it difficult to prove that all bio-techno-scientific breakthroughs are not error free.

This chapter examines the evolution of bioscientific advancements, biotechnological developments, bioinformational prodigies, biopharmaceutical strategies, biomedical practices, and their holistic integrative affects in relation to synergistic bioknowledge and biomedical practice systems. It discusses how bioknowledge can provide moral, ethical, and legal strategic advantages through examination of the ways they affect bioorganizational operations, vertical and horizontal organizational structural design, and interorganizational relationships among individuals, institutions, industries, human generations, and environmental conditions.

Human beings need to know how to change the environment in order to enhance their existence. One of today's most prominent views concerning biosciences and biotechnology indicates the historical record of total views concerning the tension between traditional and innovative values. Generations of bioscientists, biotechnologists, and bioethicists work to develop both theoretical and experimental concerns, or a *paradigm of bioknowledge,* which has two primary characteristics: (1) a spirit that attracts adherents from competing rational modes of scientific activities and (2) an open-ended phenomenon that reveals new moral and ethical problems for bio-techno-scientists and bioresearchers to consider. We call this holistic paradigm biosophy. The term of *biosophy* is related to an intellectual activity based on multidimensional perspectives that guides us to consider how natural selection and innovative solutions should work together to achieve progressive objectives.

Within the paradigm of the *biosophical* conception of natural selection, the evolutionary Darwinist vision of the tree of life, Freud's notion of the unconsciousness instinct, Dalton's views of the atom as tiny solar system, and James's view on the change and growth of personality, human beings need to be creative in order to be the masters of their own domain and to enhance the embodiment of their existence. Thus, in this chapter we shall seek to know:

- What is a paradigm?
- What is a paradigm of bioknowledge?
- What is a paradigm of bioethics in bioacademic circles and bioresearch centers?

Furthermore, this chapter examines the biosophical revolutionaries of bioscientific advancements, biotechnological developments, bioinformational prodigies, biopharmaceutical strategies and their attributes in relation to bioethics. Therefore, first we should know what biosophy of the natural world and bioknowledge is, second what a paradigm is, third what a paradigm of bioknowledge is, and fourth what a paradigm of bioethics is.

INTRODUCTION

Just as there are errors in nature and there are also errors in the paradigm of bioknowledge, and thus it seems strange to speak of erroneous thought as being identical with reality. Bioscientists and biotechnologists are trying to understand the effectiveness of the efforts that influence their actions. They first inquire into the ways in which new ideas emerge. Then they integrate historical records of research findings with their ideas in order to eliminate the tension between scientific tradition and techno-scientific innovation. Such a multidimensional research work is called a *paradigm* of biosciences. A paradigm of biosciences has four primary characteristics:

- The breadth to reexamine traditional bioscientific findings that have established branches of integrated knowledge
- A new scientific caliber, namely innovation, in order to attract adherents from competing modes of scientific discoveries
- The ability to provide open-ended research results that offer new solutions for unknown complex problems
- A willingness to pursue initial investigations until it is impossible to go further within the contextual boundary of bioethics. We call this productive successful, timely problem solving method a multidisciplinary *normative paradigm* of life sciences

In this chapter our objective is to go thoroughly in a very deep conversation to analyze traditional values of bioknowledge and to prove that it is not error free because in reality bio-techno-scientific discoveries and breakthroughs are not viewed as holistic real natural logic. They are scientific logic. Within a biosophical deliberation, if we believe that there is a difference between natural logic and scientific logic, and then we may conclude that there are erroneous thoughts that exist, and if existence is based on thinking, then false thoughts are as real as any among bio-techno-scientists and practitioners. Thus, through biosophical logic, we may choose both the paths of natural logic and scientific logic in order to arrive at a true consensus conclusion.

From another point of view, the discovery and transmission of bioknowledge congruent with principles of bioethics, as well as the protection of human rights, is the distinctive task of bioacademicians and bioresearchers. It is the distinctive professional task of bio-techno-scientists and bioresearchers to safeguard the dignity of human subject. The search to discovering viable and reliable bioscientific formulas and biotechnological procedures postulates a more promising general affirmation about enhanced life or about any general class of biosubjects.

Bioethics begins with the assumption that prudential bio-trials are better than risky bioerrors; just as biomedical practitioners accept that health is better than sickness or illness. Thus, biosophy begins with the belief that having the certainty of assurance of natural logic is better than being at the mercy of arbitrary scientific logic.

SIX THEORIES OF ACQUISITION OF KNOWLEDGE-BASED LOGIC

At the present time creative knowledge is being emphasized more intensively within the normative paradigm of bioknowledge, which refers to the multirelationships among biosciences, biotechnology, and bioinformation systems rather than to other fields of inquiry. There are several reasons for this logic. Arieti (1993:19) indicated:

> The first is the twentieth century's bias in favor of scientific knowledge. A second is found in the belief held by many investigators that it is easier to study the creative process in scientists than in artists... A third reason is the assumption by many investigators that the process of scientific creativity consists of logical or mathematical steps that can easily be traced back.

As to the first reason, we must accept the traditional scientific validity of problem solving. The second and third reasons, however, require multi-dimensional techno-scientific and informational trials in order to arrive at truthful and workable solutions. In order to achieve this sort of multidimensional bioknowledge logic, we must understand six types of theories of logical discernment.

There are six logical theories of understanding things: revelation, coherence, preventative, representative, pragmatic, and intuitive (Weber, 1960: 13-14):

- *The Revelation Theory*: This view holds that the final test of the truth of assertions is their consonance with the revelations of authority.

- *The Coherence Theory*: This theory says that a statement is true if it is consistent with other statements accepted as true. Statements, of course, must be true to the particulars to which they refer, just as revelations accepted as valid in religion are not necessarily extended to other areas of belief.

- *The Preventative Theory*: This view holds that reality as presented to the mind in perception is known directly and without alteration. Errors of perceptions occur, but further observation is able to detect and explain them.

- *The Representative Theory*: This view, again favored by certain realities, holds that our perceptions of objects are not identical with them. This differs from the representative view sketched above which goes to the length of saying that when we perceive truly, our perception is identical with the object perceived. This implies that the object perceived literally enters the mind that perceives it -- a rather startling conclusion. The representative realist tries to be more cautious on this point. What we see when we look at a tree is only its image. The tree cannot be identical with this image. The image is in one's mind, and the mind is somehow located in the brain; if the tree is fifty feet high there is not enough room, (physically), in one's brain to accommodate it.

- *The Pragmatic Theory*: This view holds that statements are true if they work successfully in practice. If an idea or principle is effective in organizing knowledge or in the practical affairs of life, then it is true. The belief of the pragmatist that the function of knowledge is to lead through successful action is at the root of the important development in American education known as the progressive movement.

- *The Intuitive Theory*: This view varies so much in its definition that it sometimes becomes identical with some of the other theories sketched above. At one extreme, intuition refers to a mysterious and immediate inner source of knowledge apart from both perceptual observation and reasoning. At the other extreme the term intuition has been used to designate generally accredited and immediate ways of knowing, such as immediate sensation, or the immediate awareness we may have of self-evident or axiomatic truth. For example, Blake's poem "The Sick Rose," which compares the sick woman to the sick rose and makes us aware of a class of "beautiful life destroyed by illness," is an illustration of syllogistic intuitive knowledge. The poet leaves things somewhat ambiguous. It is part of our aesthetic intuitive appreciation to first experience the ambiguity of the unfinished statement, and then to attempt a clarification of that statement by finding a psychological resonance in our feelings and ideas.

WHAT IS A PARADIGM?

It is useful before discussing what a paradigm of bioknowledge is, to know first what we mean by a paradigm. A *paradigm* is a basic holistic logical framework through which we conceive and perceive the world, giving shape and meaning to all our knowledge and experiences. It provides a basis for interpreting and organizing both our conceptions and perceptions (Palmer, 1989: 15). A paradigm is more than a theory because it is a holistically synthesized essence of our reasoning potential and actions within the historical events of our traditional cultural value systems and pragmatic innovative thoughts. A paradigm is a fundamental asserted logical belief that sometimes isn't even articulated until brought into question by someone else's new competing paradigm. Since the paradigm of biosciences, biotechnology, and bioinformation systems has been implemented in the various fields of inquiry with different applications of means and ends, in reality that paradigm is faced with serious moral, ethical, legal challenges and critical conclusions. Finally, a paradigm is viewed as a human intellectual ability to alter the universe to fit a human design.

WHAT IS THE NORMATIVE PARADIGM OF BIOKNOWLEDGE?

Historically, bioscientists have used the paradigm of bioknowledge to alter nature in order to fit new alternative forms of human design. They have actively posed the questions:

- Under what conditions should we interfere with natural life on this planet?
- Should the earth be altered so that the human race can survive?
- Should clones have natural or civil rights?
- Is kinesthetic intelligence (implanting an electrode in the brain) an invasion of privacy?
- How should the Constitution be expanded in the light of biological innovativeness?

To answer these and other similar questions, Taylor (1969: 205) provided the future possibilities bioknowledge within the following categorizations (see Figure 6.1).

As we mentioned above, a paradigm is not a theory, it is a pragmatic multidimensional logical holistic integration of intellectual deliberations concerning ideas and facts. Within the paradigm of bioknowledge, there are multidimensional bioethical concerns. These concerns are viewed as strategic bioknowledge considerations, intellectual deliberations, rationality, reasonableness, compromises, and consensus concerning the preservation and maintenance of the sanctity of the human species. The problem is aggravated by the fact that the complexity of bio-techno-scientific research requires close cooperation among all professionals who may, as individuals, have differing, but not unreasonable, positions on bioethical issues. Either individually or in a small group, people will examine ethical and moral issues and trends of the above bioknowledge processes.

Since bio-techno-scientists and bioresearchers have been studying only one form of life on Earth, they need to follow the paradigm of bioknowledge with exobiological (the study of extraterrestrial life in space), biochemical, and microbiological research in order to encounter other forms of life. Bio-techno-scientific research needs to probe holistic (macro) mysteries of the human mind/body within the contextual universalization of the reality of life. This is the exact meaning of a normative paradigm of bioknowledge.

SYLLOGISTIC AND ENTHYMEME IN RESEARCH DISCOVERY

In trying to be innovative in research, there are several mechanisms that provide researchers with successful end results. One of those mechanisms is to be familiar with similar traditional instances which could lead researchers to endlessly multiplied alternatives in which great discoveries are made by the act of perceiving an identity among two or more things that had been thought dissimilar or unrelated (e. g., multidisciplinary approaches). For example, Newton observed an apple falling from a tree and observed a common quality in the apple attracted by the earth and the attraction between heavenly bodies. Then syllogistically, he questioned himself as to what the similarity was between two forces that caused an apple to fall to the earth, and that that holds the moon in its orbit. He theorized this insight by comparing the rate at which masses fall to earth with the rate at which the moon deviates from the path it would follow if the earth did not exist. Such a scientific conclusion is the result of progeny.

Progeny converts innovative brainwaves into sophisticated types of creativity. It is the task of pharmaceutical companies to put together generic secrets and make the *synergy via prodigy* through three activities:

- Mingling enlightened pharmacologists from diffusive scientific disciplines.
- Accelerating prodigies of biotechnological innovativeness and creativity.
- Transforming new scientific ideas into new lines of pharmaceutical products.

PHASE ONE: BY 1975
Extensive transplantations of limbs and organs.
Test-tube fertilization of human eggs.
Implantation of fertilized eggs in the womb.
Indefinite storage of eggs and spermatozoa.
Choice of sex of offspring.
Extensive power to postpone clinical death.
Mind-modifying drugs: regulation of desire.
Memory erasure.
Imperfect artificial placenta.
Artificial viruses.

PHASE TWO: BY 2000

Extensive mind modification and personality reconstruction.
Enhancement of intelligence in men and animals.
Memory injection and memory editing.
Perfected artificial placenta and true baby-factory.
Life coping: reconstructed organisms.
Hibernation and prolonged coma.
Prolongation of youthful vigor.
First cloned animals.
Synthesis of unicellular organs.
Organ regeneration.
Man-animal chimeras.

PHASE THREE: AFTER 2000

Control of aging: extension of life span.
Synthesis of complex living organisms.
Disembodied brains.
Brain-computer links.
Gene insertion and deletion.
Cloned people.
Brain-brain links.
Man-machine chimeras.
Indefinite postponement of death.

Figure 6.1: Paradigm of Bioknowledge Development

Within such an innovative techno-scientific approach bioresearchers can use two types of methods to conclude their bioresearch projects: syllogism and enthymemism. It is worthy while to define bioknowledge in terms of its reference to syllogistic and/or enthymeme induction enumeration. Also, it's worthy while to define reasoning as seeking knowledge either for the sake of simply knowing or for the sake of doing or making something excellent. In addition, it's worthy while to define knowledge as an ordination of practical reasoning to signify the establishment of an order either through induction by enumeration or through intuition by enumeration. This type of induction by enumeration is called a syllogism.

Enthymeme Induction by Enumeration: Reichenbach (1951) referred to bioknowledge as an induction by enumeration. Induction by enumeration is the procedure by which an individual, having observed that some sequences; say the daily alteration of light and darkness; recur again and again, feels entitled to draw a general principle such as night follows day or vice versa. Induction by enumeration is a simple understanding, even for the average individual, through enthymeme reasoning and/or observation (an enthymeme is a simple syllogistic reasoning or argument in which a premise is expressed for understanding by lay people of the rationality behind a resolution).

Syllogistic Intuition by Enumeration: A syllogism is a conclusive argument in which two premises and conclusions possessing multiple routes of inquiry with different magnitudes of size, time, and process, can be expressed either by demonstration or deduction. We could say that many scientific enumerations are the result of individualizing a common characteristic or connection among things that were deemed dissimilar or unrelated before; novelties.

According to Frank (1957) syllogistic intuition by enumeration or induction by imagination consists of (1) individualizing a common property (as, for instance, the shared property by the moon and the apple), (2) not identifying the objects (as, again, the moon and the apple) as having some such common property by putting them into a primary class, and (3) recognizing that they belong to an unsuspected secondary class (such as gravitational bodies). In such a syllogistic reasoning, the concept of the new class is much more important than the recognition of the similarity. Once the concept of the new class of characteristics is created, it will be easy to use thereafter in induction by enumeration.

Strategic Bioknowledge Considerations: Strategic bioknowledge considerations include both strategy content and strategy process. Bioknowledge is an integration of bioscientific thoughts and biotechnological possibilities in that they build on the dynamic paths of these disciplines to serve humanity. It requires us building an accurate body of bioinformation through collection of biodata. Bioknowledge predicts what types of know-how formulas, procedures, and methodologies bio-techno-scientists and researchers will offer to the present and future generations to diagnose and cure deformities, diseases, illnesses, and injuries. Additionally, bioknowledge has the capacity to appraise its own internal course of progress and development and acquires an on going process of redefinition its biotrial and bioerror.

As indicated in Chapter 1, triangulation in bioresearch is viewed as a metaphor describing a form of multiple research operationalization or convergent validation. In a bioscientific research project, triangulation largely is used to describe multiple data-collection via conducting repeated testing procedures to measure a single concept or construct a formula for problem solving. In using biotechnological procedures an additional metaphoric bioparadigm can characterize the use of multiple data-collection technologies, multiple theories, multidisciplinary researchers, multiple methodologies, or combinations of these categories of research activities to discover new knowledge.

Strategically, for many bioresearchers, triangulation is restricted to the use of multiple data-gathering techniques (usually three) to validate a theorem. A theorem is a scientific proposition, statement, or formula embodying something to be proved from other expressed propositions or formulas. Fielding and Fielding (1986: 31) have addressed this dimension of triangulation. They expressed their views that the important feature of triangulation is not the simple combination of different forms of data-collection, but also, the attempt to relate them so as to counteract the threats to validity identified in each.

In the field of bioethics, triangulation is viewed as a syllogistic proposition that can be deduced from the premises or assumptions of a truthful and justified reasoning. This interpreted proposition is viewed as a means of mutual confirmation of measures and validation of findings. Also, multiple-methods approach is a generic form of this approach. Nevertheless, bioethical triangulation represents varieties of religious faiths, multicultural values, and political ground concerning humans, substances, and environmental issues, researchers, theories, and methods to accept or reject a conclusive research assertion (e.g., embryonic stem cell and human cloning). In supporting the aforementioned attributions, Denzin (1978: 295) has outlined the following four categories:

- Data triangulation has three subtypes: (a) time, (b) space, and (c) person. [Time analysis has three levels: (a) past, (b) present, and (c) future. Space analysis has three dimensions: (a) width, (b) depth, and (c) length.] Person analysis, in turn, has three levels: ʼ(a) aggression, (b) interactive, and (c) collectivity.
- Investigator triangulation consists of using multiple rather than single observers of the same object.
- Theory triangulation consists of using multiple rather than simple perspectives in relation to the same set of objects.
- Methodological triangulation can entail within-method triangulation and between-method triangulation.

The triangulation of multicultural bioethics research literature stresses that a bioethical attribution allows bioethicists to offer perspectives other than their own. It provides a universal view concerning a means of refining, broadening, and strengthening biosophical, theosophical, and biophilia linkages in these matters.

Arguments for continuing or ceasing a bio-techno-scientific research project may be either strategic or tactical. Strategically, all considerations are highly socio-culturally and politico-economically orchestrated in long-run efforts to emphasize the instrumental added values to the human life span. Bioethically, the strategic considerations need to be sufficiently persuasive, challenging, and above all effective in order to attract the public authorities' interest to support and provide sufficient funds for the continuity of bioresearch projects.

On the other hand, the tactical considerations center on a more direct connection between professional ethical consensus and moral rightness. Biosophy has a strong argument, which indicates that bioknowledge does not always make a pragmatic position of a morally right action in strategic choices. For example, for the last four decades, bioscientists focused strategically on human cloning and gene reengineering in order to create "smart pocket-size cloned human beings." Such a strategic initiative has failed because people resented it morally. However, while the government of the United States legally bans human cloning, on November 5, 2003, the United Nations postponed its decision on banning human cloning. Turner (2003) reported that:

> In the closest of votes on Thursday the United Nations General Assembly postponed for two years a decision on whether to ban human cloning, defying intense last minute lobbying by the U.S. The decision split the UN down the middle, with the postponement winning 80 votes in favor, and 79 votes against. Fifteen countries abstained.

Tactical moral considerations provide immediate alternatives in practice to analyze a comparative assessment between the nature and extent of pragmatic strategic bioknowledge intentions and consequences, the distinction between rationality and reasonableness, and the extent to which both bio-techno-professionals and bioethicists can pluralistically raise genuine uncertainty or reasonable disagreement on biotrial and bioerror research projects, or bioknowledge based practices.

Intellectual Deliberations: Biosophists, bioscientists, biotechnologists, and biomedical clinicians have gone through very deep and complex arguments concerning bioknowledge and bioethics. They have presented their intellectual deliberations on proceeding in different paths of biopractices and have held cherished positions about the nature and structural possibilities of universal existence and humanity's place in it. Bioscientists and biotechnologists have tried to articulate their innovative and technovative ideas on the basis of pragmatic observable solutions, while ignoring the holistic comprehensive integration of moral, ethical, religious, and biosophical outlooks of their activities. In addition, biotechno-scientists have failed to consider the holistic compromises of interlocking general moral virtues, ethical values, and cultural beliefs about bioknowledge and its consequential effects on the human race. Parhizgar (2002: 36) indicated:

> It is proper to speak about human intellectual proclivities that are parts of our culture. Human beings are born into cultures that house a large number of domains such as disciplines, crafts, and other pursuits in which one can become encultured and then be assessed in terms of the level of competence one has attained. There is a relationship between domains and the intellectual liabilities of human beings. More generally, nearly all domains require proficiency in a set of intellectual capabilities; and any intellectual ability can be mobilized for use in a wide array of culturally available domains.

Among the elements of holistic intellectual deliberations there are one's deepest conceptions that Benjamin (1995:249) indicated as following:

> (1) Religious faiths and the nature of God, that is, whether there is a God and, if so, God's nature; (2) the nature and purpose (if any) of the universe and human life; (3) the nature, justification, and extent of human knowledge; (4) the nature of human beings (including sexual and familial relationships, friendship, political institutions, and obligations to strangers); (5) the nature and status of morality, especially injunctions and principles having to do with the taking of life, the nature of equality (or equitability), respect for liberty, and so on; and (6) the moral standing of nonhuman animals and the intrinsic value (if any) of the natural environment.

We will analyze all of the above issues in future chapters.

Rationality: Ethically and morally, human beings exist as an end in themselves, not merely as means to be arbitrarily used by this or that will; but all their intentions and actions, whether they concern themselves or other rational beings, must always be regarded at the same time as an end. Human beings, by their very nature, are very well organized. By the same token, they are organizers. They are *rational beings*. They are called *persons*, because their very nature points them out as ends in themselves, which is something that must not be used merely as a means. They are *objective ends*, an end moreover for which no other can be substituted. The foundation of this principle is the rational nature of human beings (Parhizgar, 2002: 35). Rationality is, for most part, an intellectual deliberation having to do with the deductive selective wisdom of choices and the pursuit of the most effective reasonable possibilities to a set of carefully selected ends (Benjamin, 1995: 251). Sibley (1953: 556) expressed his irrationality:

> When I do not bother to ascertain the true nature of the ends I set myself;
> or when I heedlessly sacrifice one end to a second, which when attained I
> find to be of less worth to me than the first would have been; or when I
> select unrealistic means; or when, having reached a rational enough
> decision, I fail to implement that decision in practice.

As we defined in Chapter 2, morality is the search for excellence as an end. One's ends as a rational bioscientist and/or biotechnologist need, however, to be altruistic, searching and serving beyond the self. Consider, for example, bioscientists whose worldview and deliberated efforts for investigating and serving people place a premium on the advancement and enhancement of human life. Insofar as these bioscientists and biotechnologists are rational, they will do what they could do to pursue such a humanitarian end. But bioscientists and biotechnologists are not living in a rational world; greed, selfishness, and the cynicism of interest groups may rule over their daily lives. At least bioscientists and biotechnologists can act simply as rational agents to give equal attention and concern to the conflicting ends of humanity. Bioscientists and biotechnologists are required to take conscientious responsibility for the well being of their societies. Rationality requires that bioscientists and biotechnologists take humanity's ends into account in investigating and serving people and avoiding harming and hurting people. For example, production and unprofessional distribution of Anthrax not only destroys innocent people, it also creates fear among people.

Bioethical rationality places an unusual strain on bioscientific and biotechnological moral inspirations and frameworks to advance bioknowledge. Also, it motivates bioresearchers to build up a sense of curiosity in their research agendas to develop innovativeness in applicability of biotechnology. Such scientific advancements and technological developments should create rational choices and possibilities to normalize natural abnormalities, but not to increase abnormalities. Bioknowledge should be directed towards the enhancement of human life and avoid serving particular worldviews and ways of life for endowed classes of elite people. Finally, bioscientists and biotechnologists need not only to rationally learn about the complexities of their innovativeness but also to define the application of their findings. They should not only serve wealthy and powerful people, while hurting poor and volatile powerless people. This is against both natural human rights and civil rights.

There seems to be a general agreement that in reality science itself is amoral. This means that science is ethically neutral, but scientists could be moral or immoral. Bioresearchers strive for discovering causes and effects of things.   Sometimes they strive to discover the whole truth (moral), and sometimes they are satisfied with a partial truth (amoral). However, bioethicists examine their research objectives and the use of human subjects in order to express value decisions and actions. On the other hand, bioscientists examine the relationships between X and Y in order to be able to express their significant reasoning statements on the basis of "as things are existed and/or as things ought to be." They believe that science is "an *is world*," a set of facts growing out of a consensus rational reasoning among a small group of things (Dalton, 1964: 60). When we say that we should state our ethical statements with honesty, we need to disclose the whole truth and not a portion of truth. We should remember that all moral beliefs and ethical values, like scientific findings, are not statements that come from an invariant sources. They are not residing in a world of abstract ideals. Rather, they consist of conventional symbolic meanings subject to the syllogistic complex continuous debates. As Denzin (1978: 325) indicated: "Hence, when I speak of values and ethics in the scientific process, I refer to meanings that are subject to negotiation and redefinition. What is ethical in one period, one university, one profession, or one group may be unethical in another."

Bioscientists and biotechnologists should change their amoral (disclosing a portion of the truth not the whole) intentions and actions to moral (disclosing the whole truth). They need to be proactive to safeguard the sanctity of humanity, and the dignity of present and future generations in regard to procreation, childbirth, child bearing, and family value systems. Not only do they have ethical responsibilities and moral convictions in rational choices and possibilities, but they should also be deeply committed to the enhancement of human dignity. Although we are living in a conflicted world, bioscientists' ethical positions should be rooted in reasonable worldviews and ways of life so that all human beings can enjoy and appreciate their efforts and natural rights.

What Is Reasonableness? So far rationality has been identified, for the most part, as an intellectual virtue having to do with the selection and pursuit of the most effective means to a set of carefully selected ends; excellence. When we speak of reason, whether in the practical order of morality or in the theoretical order of speculative bioknowledge, it is necessary to emphasize time and again that reason merely refers to the power we have to know reality for what it is.

Reasonableness means to pay keen attention or fair consideration to the logical ends or viewpoints of others for their own rational sake. Reasonableness is the human just intellectual power by which we discover and express, not manufacture and/or claim, the real order. We speak of reasonableness, therefore, simply as meaning the power we have for grasping whatever bioknowlegable truth we can know about reality.

Reasonableness is a pluralistic bioethical principle that provides a neutral consensus position to rationally satisfy all opposing parties. All bioknowledgeable inquiries and experimental practices should be based on the reasonableness of the application of scientific methodologies. Such scientific methodological reasonableness should match with the good of reasoning in a moral sense. Bioexperiments should contain a virtuous reasonableness towards directing either their own good of reasoning or the acts of other powers. The application of all biosomatic and biopsychological experiments should contain the good of reason, first of all, as they are realized in the very act of reasonableness itself, which gives us the cardinal virtue of prudence.

Prudence is a rational (not emotional or passionate) reasonableness, the reasoned way of acting in conformity with the right appetite. It is wholly practical, not concerned with general bioknowledge, but with acting here and now in specific circumstances. The distinction between the morality and amorality of bioknowledge is related to prudence and doubt concerning the application of bioscientific and biotechnological research conclusions to human beings. Prudence deals with cases of conscience as casuistry, that is, as a system of dealing with cases of conscience in relation to doing what is right or wrong in particular instances. Nevertheless reasonableness, as an ethical term, is a matter of the intellect alone, while the practical wisdom of prudence is reasoning in relation to desire. Hence, we see how bioethics alone cannot solve the problem of good moral actions; at the same time, we are aware that bioethics helps the bio-techno-scientists to act prudently and rightly in each successive experimental research projects.

Compromise: There are two different major views concerning biomorality and bioethicality: (1) compromise and (2) consensus. Compromise bears more than a superficial resemblance to consensus, but it is also importantly different. Concession is the centerpiece of any compromise to provide win-win, lose-lose, or win-lose, or lose-win (concessionary) consequences for different adversarial parties to have mutual gains and loses. Consider, in this connection, the ethical deliberations and moral conclusions of human fertilization and embryology. Among the serious issues here are germ line engineering and the cloned embryo. Germ line engineering embraces several biotechnological procedures and techniques that provide for the alteration of germinal epithelium, sperm or eggs, or the early products of conception such as the genetic changes to be coded in the sex cells of the resulting adults. The cloning alternatives provide holistic somatic cell alterations by virtue of their intergenerational consequences. In theory, only germ line alterations can produce heritable changes, while in cloning some somatic cell alterations may also become intergenerationally transmissible. Already within such bio-techno-scientific alterations the genomic alteration of germ cells has been demonstrated in eugenic techniques and procedures (Hammer et al., 1986: 269), and has been developed as a rapid method for accelerating the genetic improvement of livestock (Van Raden and Freeman, 1985: 1425). For example, in meat and bone meal (MBM) alternatives, bioscientists made seventy years of historical error to change the path of proteins in livestock. It caused the creation of prion, which killed millions of heads of livestock and many human beings and hundreds of people.

While historically germ line engineering marked a major advancement in bio-techno-scientific abilities and possibilities to manipulate and control materials in animals, the prospect of their application to humans raises fundamental ethical and moral questions about the rationale and legitimacy of limits to human control over genetic destiny (Rifkin et al., 1983: 1360).

Germ line alterations can be produced by any of four techniques, each with technical strengths and limitations and with ethical and moral considerations of its own:

- The first technique entails the direct microinjection of specific sequences of DNA (cloned DNA) into the pronucleus of a one-celled fertilized egg. Is it ethical to do so? The argument is related to the natural sanctity attributions to each human natural generational cell characteristic. Is it ethical to mix-up the natural mechanical characteristics of the germ lines?

- The second utilizes an embryonic stem cell derived from the blastocyst stage that is manipulated in tissue culture by direct transfixions with raw DNA or by using a retrovirus to carry genetic material into the cell. Effectively transfixed cells can then be reintroduced to a developing embryo during the blastocyst period of development.

- The third technique involves the use of retroviruses to carry DNA sequences into four cell embryos, the blastocyst or the midgestation embryo.

- A fourth technique, in which sperm treated directly with raw DNA, appeared to promise a rapid method for achieving permanent genetic alteration, but it has not proven to be reproducible to date (Barinagg, 1989: 590).

Consensus: A consensus decision is a collective unanimous agreement among a number of people on an issue, idea, or opinion. It is a logical position concerning an issue, opinion, or idea about the causes and effects of an issue, opinion, idea, or problem at hand. Usually, within the boundary of a consensus process, there are specific structured topics or objectives to be discussed, argued, debated, and/or considered and to be concluded with a unanimous decision. It is usual to be exposed to some important issues or problems when there are different large groups of people involved in predeliberative conclusions, for three major reasons:

- Bioethical issues or problems directed to a body of inquiry are usually contested. This is usual when large groups of people must speak with one voice on complex bioethical concerns to which members of these groups give certain or unanimous answers to specific articulated questions. The major ethical and moral consensus view concerning genetic engineering and eugenic cloning voices the basic assumption that human genes as natural organisms should not be viewed as *objects* to be manipulated. Human genes should proceed according to their natural processes of life characteristics and they should be determined by their own *evolutionary* experiences and determinations of their own destiny. Such a natural process requires specific calculated timelines. If bio-techno-scientists rush to try to manipulate and shorten natural evolutionary timelines of human genes, they change their natural evolutionary roles as creatures, to creators. Then, serious questions arise:

- o   Do human beings know the mystery of life?
- o   Do they have the holistic ability to be creators of themselves?

- The predeliberative consensus answer to these questions is "*no.*" Then the tendency to objectify human genes and persons, avoiding empathetic responses; culminates. Since we are not only using the human genes themselves for our purposes, but we are also permanently altering the genetic codes of all our future progeny. Moreover, we are treating our own bodies as technological artifacts, to modify and contemplate our genes as spare parts. Such a biosophy is called Promethean; creative progeny. It is the consensus view that dominance and control of superior genes over inferior genes in the human race will be ended with eugenic engineering.

- Bioethical issues or problems directed to a body of inquiry represent differing socio-cultural and politico-economical viewpoints or differing areas of bioethical cause-effect views, or both. In such a situation the diverse and different views are debatable. Consequently, those issues and problems may end with convincible consensus deliberations among parties, or issues and problems will remain unsolved.

At any pre or post deliberative agreement, foundational religious faith and principles and political ideological positions play important roles on the outcomes of consensus agreements. Therefore, in both cases, predeliberative and postdeliberative consensus decisions and actions provide some guidelines for the future implementation of consensus decisions and actions.

Within such a broad vision, the paradigm of bioknowledge explains how the relationship of the Earth's bionic systems can be fitted to the sanctity of nature. Do we know sufficiently the kinetic characteristics of earthly life? Do we know where are we heading? T. S. Eliot (1950: 145) pondered these questions and expressed his views as follows:

> We shall not cease from exploration
> And the end of all our exploring
> Will be to arrive where we started
> And know the place for the first time...

The concepts for the kinetic characteristics of earthly life are the intrinsic and extrinsic conditions of possible or problematic bionic conditions. The human race must decide whether or not to alter the atmosphere of this planet.

BIOSCIENTIFIC DELIBERATIONS AND INNOVATIVE BIOSOPHY

These biosophical and biophilial concepts of bioethics are not wholly unambiguous. The doctrine that there is an absolute bionic truthfulness in cloning and that the quest for it is intrinsically valuable has become associated in many non-bionic scholars' minds with metaphysics, ontology, epistemology, axiology, and theology. However, at the same time, these variables can serve people in either right or wrong directions; depending on the biobusiness investors' appetite and their lobbyists' money-power.

The funding of academic research by for-profit organizations has been a feature of scientific advancement since the beginning of the Twentieth century. It has provided some significant biotechnological breakthroughs for the benefit of investors and has heightened the potential for conflict of interest and conflict of commitment for bioscientists and biotechnologists. It has emerged new desires through biopharmaceutical industry to create products on the basis of cost-benefit analysis. This means that commercially sponsored bioresearch grants and/or contracts are more likely to be found in applied rather than in basic biosciences. These grants and/or contracts limit the breadth of their educational endeavor. The importance of biotrade secrets, licenses, and franchisees in the biopharmaceutical industry makes it difficult to maintain the traditional sharing of biodata. Consequently, bioresearchers have to compromise their scientific objectives in favor of a sponsor's interest. This poses a challenge to the ethics of bioscientists and biotechnologists that may be difficult to recognize without concerted professional review. Nevertheless, bioscientific formulas, biotechnological breakthroughs, and bioinformation systems are practical realities in our modern lives. Morally and ethically they should be expanded for the intuitive usage of goodness in order to enhance the conscientious wisdom of the human race.

IS BIOETHICS A THEORETHICAL OR PRACTICAL PHENOMENON?

Practical reality is a truth of ethical action, not a truth of theoretical knowledge. What kind of knowledge (theoretical or practical) is bioethics? The perception of practical knowledge refers to the fact that bioethics is a holistic embodiment of viable bioscientific formulas, biotechnological breakthroughs, and bioinformational systems which should direct bio-techno-scientists and bioresearchers in the right direction. This holistic embodiment is known as the paradigm of bioknowledge. An ethical paradigm of the bioknowledge system brings academic constituencies together along with a humanitarian conviction, not through an interest group. It links bioacademic and bioresearch organizational missions to their legitimate practical operational and conclusive commitments to comply with natural law.

Let us first know what we mean by biosophy and biophilia, and then discuss the issues of biosciences, biotechnology, bioinformation, and bioknowledge. A successful scientific innovation needs to apply practical effective innovations. In regard to innovativeness, scientists have stated that excellence needs a vision in order to be focused on the maximum achievement of creativity. This objective requires scientists to syllogistically question the answers to:

- What do they want to be?
- Where is the world of humanity going?
- Which path of discovery will assist in the maintenance of human dignity and integrity?

Scientific endeavors require a single scientific project, no matter what its history to have more accomplishments. In order to understand the holistic knowledge-based integration of means and ends of all actions and dynamic movements, we need to define branches of knowledge: philosophy, science, and technology (see Table 6.1).

KNOWLEDGE-BASED INTEGRATION OF PHILOSOPHY, SCIENCES, ARTS, AND TECHNOLOGY

Knowledge-based understanding relies on the synergistic integration of philosophy, technology, arts, and sciences. The main reason for applying the interdisciplinary approach is based on a holistic view of the concept of peoples' culture, which includes all human made-knowledge. Among some of the special features of knowledge-based understanding is active participatory observation of the moral consciousness, the view on cultural values, the fundamental value orientation of ethical relativism, the synergistic pragmatic end results, and the holistic cultural relativism.

The moral approach holds that the universal truth is essentially a generalized principle that holds the sanctity of humanity. Labor forces and customers around the globe, particularly in the United States are becoming more diverse in terms of national origin, race, religion, gender, predominant age categories, and personal preferences.

The world is shrinking rapidly. Multinational corporate assignments are becoming a standard part of a sounded business. Cross-cultural understanding and behavioral skills are a necessity. As the result the traditional bioknowledge that has

Table 6.1: Holistic Interdisciplinary Relationships Among Academic Philosophy, Sciences, Arts, and Technology

KNOWLEDGE	PRIMARY DIVISIONS	SUB-DIVISIONS
PHILOSOPHY	Metaphysics	Cosmology, Ontology Theology, Causalogy Consequentiality
	Epistemology	
	Axiology	Morality and Ethics
	Phenomenology	Culturalogy, Forensicalogy
ARTS	Aesthetics	Music, Dance, Movies, Theatrical Drama, Choreography, Painting, and Sculpture
LITERATURE	Humanities	Poetry and Prose
SCIENCE	Observable Sciences	Astronomy, Geology, Physics, Chemistry, Mathematics, Statistics, Science of Logic, and Scientific Quantitative Methods
	Natural Sciences	Zoology (Animals), Botany (Plants), Protistology (One-Celled Organisms), Biology, Biorheology, Physiology, Microbiology, Immunology, Ecology and Evolution, Molecular, Cellular Biology, and Pharmacology
	Social Sciences	Economics, Geography, History, Political Sciences, and Demography
	Behavioral Sciences	Anthropology (Physical Anthropology, Cultural Anthropology, Archaeology, Anthropological Linguistics, Ethnology/Ethnography), Demography, Sociology, Psychology, and Social-Psychology
TECHNOLOGY	Traditional Technologies	Eolithic, Neolithic, Monolithic, Craftsmanship, and Synthetic
	Modern Technologies	Mechanistic, Automotive Robotics, Cybernetic, Cyber-Robotics, Micro-Technology, Nano-Technology, and Cyber-Space Technology

been highly fragmented and uncompleted is not effective any more. With an eye toward educating tomorrow's global bioscientific experts, we need to think and behave globally.

Today, multinational organizations are faced with unsolved potential problems and issues. The main reason is a misunderstanding of multicultural value systems. It is necessary to move from tolerance to appreciation when mapping bioacademic curricula. The main challenge of today's and especially tomorrow's bioexperts is to be aware of specific multicultural changes, along with the factors contributing to the scientific and technological synergy.

A successful bioscientific innovation needs to apply the practical effective ones. Bioscientists concerning innovativeness have stated that excellence needs a vision to be focused on the maximum achievement of innovativeness. This objective mandates bioscientists to question the answers of what they want to be, where the world of humanity is going, which the path of discovery in which will assist in the maintenance of human dignity and integrity. Scientific endeavor requires a single scientific project, no matter what its history to have more accomplishments. In order to understand the holistic knowledge-based integration of means and ends of all actions and dynamic movements, we need to define branches of knowledge: philosophy, arts, science, and technology.

WHAT IS PHILOSOPHY?

Philosophy is a basic foundation of conceptual understanding of human's life for the examination of cause and effect of existence. In a traditional conception, philosophy endeavors to integrate all human knowledge. Inquiries such as the following domains of knowledge have shaped philosophy:

- Was there a beginning of time?
- Will there be an end?
- Is the universe infinite or does it have boundaries?
- Is the universe developing or is it shrinking?
- Or could be it both finite and without boundaries?

On viewing these conceptions and others, the current problems of philosophers still relate to four areas of inquiry: metaphysics, epistemology, phenomenology, and axiology. Thus, philosophy is the integration of all human knowledge and erects a systematic view of the nature and the place of human beings in it. In an attempt to study multicultural behavior of different groups of people, we should try to understand the four above modes of arriving at knowledge.

Metaphysics

This concerns issues of the nature of reality and humanity place in it:

- What is the matter in its essence? How does it form the vast material cosmos ordered in time and place (Cosmology)?
- What about the existence and the nature of a super power; God (Theologically)?
- What does it mean to exist? What is the criterion of existing (Ontology)? (Ontology refers to the knowledge of the nature of the world around us).
- What are the ultimate causes of things being what they are
- (Causalogy)?
- What are the ultimate effects of things being what they will be (Consequentialogy)?

Epistemology

This has to do with the problem of knowledge:

- We have knowledge.
- How is this possible?
- What does knowledge mean?
- Can all knowledge be traced to the greatest gateways of our senses (to the senses plus activity of reasoning, or to the means and ends of reasoning)?
- Do feelings render knowledge wordless but true?
- Does true knowledge ever come in the form of immediate intuition?
- How can we identify different branches of knowledge?

Axiology

This is concerned with the problems of value. There are two main traditional fields of value inquiries: (1) Morality and (2) Ethics:

Morality: As previously indicated in Chapter 2, the term *moral* is derived from the Latin word *mores*. In the *Oxford English Dictionary* (1963) "moral" means habits to right and wrong conduct," to "good and bad virtuous or vicious," to "right or wrong in relation to actions and conducts," and in an etymological sense, it means "pertaining to the individual's manner and custom of judgments." Morality is the term used to manifest the individual's virtue. Morality also has to do with an individual's character and the type of behaviors that emanate from that valuable character. Virtue refers to the excellence of intellect and wisdom. Morality's end result through intellectual truthfulness, righteousness and goodness of thoughts and conducts is happiness. Conscience is a base for moral acts. It is the ability to reason about self-conduct, together with a set of values, feelings and dispositions to do or to avoid conceiving and perceiving actions. While morality is viewed as telling the whole truth, amorality is telling a partial truth. Individuals are morally obligated to develop an objectively correct conscience; but their own judgmental behavior usually is in accordance with their conscience. Failure to fulfill one's moral commitment can lead not only to blame and shame, but also to remorse (De George, 1995: 119).

Ethics: As previously indicated in chapter 2, the term *ethics* is derived from the Greek word *ethos*. Ethos means the "genius" of an institution or system. Also, it refers to the science of morals and the department of study concerned with the principles of human duty. Ethics concerns itself with human societal conduct, activity, and behavior that are manifested through knowledge and deliberated behavior. Ethics is the collective societal conscious awareness of a group of people. Ethical end results through societal conscious understanding of fairness, justness, and worthiness can lead human beings towards social justice and peaceful behavior.

Phenomenology

What is the essential nature of the mind and/or soul (Phenomenology)? Phenomenology stresses careful descriptive value systems through an appearance or immediate object of awareness in human experience. Phenomenology is a qualitative conceptual awareness that can be manifested constructively by quantitative value judgments in the human mind. Rational decision-making processes in the field of life sciences consist essentially of starting with certain axioms or assumptions, stated as principles of applicability of successful experiences and knowledge to the world existence. The phenomenology contains two major interdisciplinary knowledge: (1) Culturalogy and (2) Forensicalogy:

Culturalogy: The emergence of cultural behavioral variables and their consequential affects on citizens' perceptions in a nation have drastically changed policy-makers' decisions. The term behavioral *culturalogy* within the context of the global free economy is a new field of inquiry and needs to be applied and directed synergistically for positive outcomes. Within such a domain of inquiry, scientific management, bureaucracy, technocracy, meritocracy, plutocracy, and gerontocracy are valid theories to some extent to be analyzed for knowing and classifying cultural behavior of nations. Those theories have taken heuristic, cognitive, behavioristic, pragmatic, and humanistic approaches for modeling socialization of modern cultures (Parhizgar, 2002: 84).

Forensicalogy: The term *forensic* is an artistic documentary imagery of iconic meanings in symbolizing the viability and reliability of visual and intellectual reasoning for constructing past pragmatic events within the boundaries of interdisciplinary bioknowledge. In a general term, forensicalogy pertains to the primary interdisciplinary application of philosophy, science, art, and technology to connect the present reliable and viable reasoning to the past evidences in a debatable rhetoric (e.g., forensic medicine, forensic chemistry, forensic physics, forensic psychiatry). In recent research projects, biological anthropologists are searching through their research curiosity to discover how long a body takes to be decayed. The result will be used in criminal investigations to identify the patterns of how long a body has been dead, or how long a person has been missing. One of the professors of the University of Northern Iowa is interested in to creating a "body farm," in order to study the rotting processes of human corpses (*CNN.com*, 2005).

WHAT IS BIOSOPHY?

Biosophy is a holistic rational reasoning for viewing an ordered holarchical life in nature. It is a type of natural reasoning based on mutual balanced cooperation and enhanced co-evolved symbiotic relations among all living things; physical and spiritual. Fox (2001: 29) defined: *"Biosophy* as the wisdom derived from a scientific (especially biological and ecological) and empathic understanding of life." It is an intellectual deliberated reasoning for biosubject matters, their structural mechanisms, and operations in terms of the processes of life and death. It bridges the spiritual phenomena, human, and nonhuman realms of the life of a community, as well as linking all human spheres of intellectual activities.

Biosophy is the knowledge of critical thinking to discover the spiritual reasoning which provides all sentient beings with interrelated and integrated considerations for forming life. It is a type of syllogistic reasoning to discover the mysterious key factors in life. It is a holistic understanding of how humans, animals, plants, and microorganisms are integrated to form life and the causes of death. Biosophy views life and death within the context of holarchy, or the cycle of life and death. Strictly speaking, biosophy is about redefining, reorienting, reintegrating, and reinventing bio-organisms to accommodate the continuity of species' lives. It speaks to the initiation, restoration, protection, and cherishing of universal life and beauty in a synergistic manner.

WHAT IS BIOPHILIA?

Keller and Wilson (1993: 12) coined the term *biophilia* with a book of that title. They defined biophilia as: "The innately emotional affiliation of human beings to other living organisms." Within biophilial boundary of living entities, all creatures are highly interrelated and integrated in real life. It is a common holarchical understanding that human beings should place a greater value on living organisms and on themselves. In this sense Fox (2001: 71) stated that biophilic knowledge of the biology of organisms and ecosystem biosophy is the reward of biophilia. Therefore, biophila is an antidote to the acceleration of loses of biodiversity and the extinction of plant and animal's species and communities. It is an affinity for life and the beauty of the natural world. It is the spiritual ethos of the deep ecology and creatures right movements. Finally, biophilia bridges human and nonhuman spirits together for understanding through more meaningful intellectual reasoning.

Bioknowledge-based understanding relies on the synergistic integration of philosophy, technology, arts, and sciences. The main reason for applying the interdisciplinary approach is based on a holistic view of the concept of peoples' nature, which includes all human made-knowledge. Among some of the special features of bioknowledge-based understanding is the active participatory observation of the moral consciousness, the academic view on cultural values, the fundamental value orientation of ethical relativism, the synergistic pragmatic end results of bioknowledge, and the holistic cultural relativism.

The moral approach holds that universal truth is essentially a generalized principle that posits the sanctity of humanity. Scientific forces and technological innovativeness around the globe, particularly in the United States, are becoming more diverse in terms of national origin, race, religion, gender, predominant age categories, and personal preferences. Cross-cultural understanding and behavioral skills are a necessity. As the result, the traditional bioknowledge discussion that has been highly fragmented and uncompleted is not effective any more. With an eye toward educating tomorrow's global bioscientists, we need to think and behave globally.

Today, biosciences, biotechnologies, biomedicine, and the biopharmaceutical industry are faced with unsolved potential ethical and moral problems and issues. The main reason is the misunderstanding of multicultural value systems. It is necessary to move from tolerance to appreciation when managing bioorganizations. The main challenge of today's and more especially tomorrow's scientists and researchers is to be aware of specific multicultural changes along with the factors contributing to professional synergy. For example, different nations treat and value human dead bodies differently. Among all religious faiths, there are different views concerning the disposal of human corpses. Some value them as sacred while others value them with no respect. Christian's burry a dead body in a sealed coffin and deprive the ecosystem's revitalization of the underground insects by not having access to these nutrition recourses. Hindus and Buddhists criminate dead bodies because they believe that the soul should be freed for the next cycle of reincarnation. Not only they may pollute the environment by crimination, they also deprive the underground insects from nutritional sources of ecological life substances. Moslems burry their copses underground without any barrier because they believe that they should not interfere with ecological survival sources nutrition for other underground creatures. Zoroastrians put human dead bodies barely in high altitudes over mountains in order birds to have sufficient nutrition. Through reviewing the above religious faiths, you will be able to understand how different religions value alive and dead bodies of human beings. That is the main reason that in some cultures, people value the nature differently. Such a biosophical principle reveals how different nations believe in biophilia. Now we turn our discussions to review other dimensions of knowledge; arts and humanities.

WHAT ARE ARTS AND HUMANITIES?

Arts

The term of *art* is the production or expression of what is creative, beautiful, appealing, and/or of what is more than ordinary significant. Arts are the establishment of human unity in variety, similarity, proximity, and connectivity in bounded perceptions. Arts are expository detailed modes of creativity of novel things. Arts manifest compositions of an individual and/or a group of human beings' emotional conceptions, sensational feelings, and thoughts to explain or manifest something in specific causal forms. Artists manifest the interrelations, tendencies and/or values of human beings with their environments. Such behavioral modes represent the interpretation of cultural facts, conditions, concepts, theories, beliefs and relationships between the individual's diametrical conception and the cultural circumferences of the human's life cycle. Artists try to explain human's inner motivations at a particular time and place.

Aesthetics: Of particular interest to the human concepts are the formal aspects of art, color, and form, because of the symbolic meanings they convey. Aesthetics pertains to a culture's sense of beauty and good taste and is expressed in arts, drama, music, folklore, and dances (Ball and McCulloch, Jr., 1988: 269). Aesthetics pertains to a culture's sense of beauty, excellent thought, and illustrative elegant visual tastes. It is the reflection of human expression in humanities: arts, music, dances, movies and theatrical drama. Of particular interest to multicultural behaviorism is artistic combination of humanities: arts, colors, and forms specifically in exhibitory conceptions and perceptions because each group conveys symbolic meanings and values in human cultural taste. There are different Types of aesthetic arts as follows:

- *Music and Dances*: Music is an art of sound in time that expresses ideas and emotions in significant forms through the elements of rhythm melody, harmony, and color. Dances are rhythmical movement of one's feet, body, or both in a pattern of steps.

- *Movies and Theatrical Drama*: Movies are motion pictures. They are a genre of art or entertainment. Movies are selling specific motion pictures of ideas, body movements, fashion, sex, history, political ideologies, sociocultural values, and industrial life-styles (Parhizgar, 1996: 309).

Humanities

Humanities are those branches of knowledge that are concerned with human intellectual thoughts, emotional and sensational expressive values in communication through literature (in forms of poetry and prose systems). Also, humanities mean history and literature. Humanities are the branch of learning regarded as having primarily a cultural character and usually including languages and literature.

WHAT IS SCIENCE?

In a general term we can define *science* as simply the empirical rational process that can form the generalized inquiry by which viable understanding is obtained. Science can tell us how to act at a given time and in particular circumstances in order to attain an end. Science is the opposite of opinion because it formulates generalizations through deductive understanding. Therefore, science is defined as a conclusion of a good intellectual habit. It is a comprehensive understanding of true predictions concerning causes and effects. It contains certain conclusions that follow necessarily from premises.

Science deals with humanity's understanding about the discovery and formulation of the real world in which inherent properties of space, matter, energy, and their interactions can be perfectly scrutinized and predicted. Science is a rational convention related to the generalization of expected environmental norms, expectations, and values. It is nothing more than the search for understanding of the real world. Nevertheless, the real world in practice is composed of ethical and unethical phenomena. Therefore, scientific discoveries reveal these attributes. That is the main reason that some scientists believe that science is a neutral phenomenon. To use it or not depends on the moral convictions, ethical values, and legal commitments of the users in practice.

In the field of scientific inquiry, a scientist uses analytical scientific methodologies to discover valuable alternatives for generalizing problem solving techniques. Therefore, scientific findings are reliable and validated to further problem-solving alternatives. For a scientist, mathematics is a tool for building models and theories that can describe and, eventually, explain the operation of the world. Be it the world of material objects (Physics and Chemistry), living things (Biology), human beings (Social or Behaviors

Sciences), the human mind (Cognitive Science), or human truthfulness, justness, and fairness (Cognititive Science). Therefore, science is the manifestation of a positivistic conception of inquiry and has provided an acceptable understanding of nature. The distinction between science (normal science) and non-science or quasi-science (pseudo-science) is therefore blurred.

There are several scientific socio-economic research frameworks that help explain observed objects and phenomena: basic research, applied research, developmental research, accelerated research, targeted research, mission-oriented research, disease-oriented research, relevant research, commission-initiated research, contract-supported research, and payoff research.

Basic Research: This type of research focuses on theoretical problem areas in order to innovate new techniques and methods as final products of a group of scientists' innovativeness and invention (e.g., cloning human beings or animals).

Commission-Initiated Research: This type of research is supported by a governmental executive power (e.g., in the United States the National Institute of Health -- NIH). Comroe, Jr. and Dripps (1993: 28) indicated:

> *Commission-Oriented Research* is a classical example of the importance of mission-oriented research was that of Luis Pasteur's experimental work legitimacy. The French government as an industrial troubleshooter employed Pasteur, originally trained as a chemist. Among the problems assigned to him were the practical ones of how to keep wine from turning to vinegar, how to cure ailing silkworms, and how to save sheep dying of anthrax and chicken dying of cholera. The solution of these practical problems led Pasteur to discover bacteria and become the founder of modern bacteriology and the father of the germ theory disease.

Applied-Research: This branch of inquiry has two objectives: (1) to explain enhanced interrelationships between material objects and/or phenomena and (2) to compliment the theoretical frameworks for such an explanation. Applied research tends to diversity scientific techniques to be varied as a product along with its product life cycles (PLCs).

Development Research: This kind of research focuses on versatility of a product and/or phenomenon in terms of more discoveries of new characteristics of things and applicability of a product and or phenomenon for consumption (e. g., the PhD syndrome glorifies development research for its own sake; or the baking soda can be used for taking odors of refrigerators). From this perspective, something useful may flow from basic research, but what matters is the applicability of knowledge itself.

Accelerated Research: This kind of research focuses on speeding up the process of maturity of previous research systems in order to reach to their final products within a very short timetable to milk the market niches' opportunities (e.g., the Cash Cow). Accelerated research is very important because of the product's physical attributes and capabilities most effect on the financial performance of a firm. Accelerated research focuses on progenistic entrepreneurial aspects of products and infopreneurial of databases.

TAXONOMY OF SCIENCES

Acquisition of knowledge refers to an individual's perceptual and practical capabilities that typically take in information via the senses through scientific methodology. They are most comfortable when containing the details of any feasible situation in a quantified understanding process. Sciences generally can be classified into four major categories:

1. Observational sciences
2. Natural sciences
3. Social sciences
4. Behavioral sciences

Observational Sciences

Observational sciences include Astronomy, Geology, Physics, and Chemistry. The primary aim of these sciences is to describe a cause-and-effect relationship between material things. The observational sciences offer the best possibility of accomplishing this goal simply through manipulation of independent variables to measure their effect on, or the change in, the dependent variables.

Natural Sciences

Natural Sciences include Zoology (Animals), Botany (Plants), Protistology (One-Celled Organisms), Biorheology (Deformation and Deterioration), and Biology (Physiology, Microbiology, Immunology, Ecology and Evolution, and Molecular and Cellular Biology). Natural sciences identify real characteristics of causes, functions and structures of all material things.

Biology concentrates on the study of all living things. Biology examines such topics such as origins, structures, functions, productions, reproductions, growth, development, behavior, and evolution of the different organisms. Familiarity with both biological and ecological conditions of the living things is a must. In most cases, both endemic and epidemic diseases are the most organizational interruptive problems in human societal life.

Social Sciences

Social Sciences include Economics, Political Sciences, Demography, History, and Geography. Economics is the study of the production, distribution, and consumption of goods and services. Social sciences are concerned with areas of the labor market, capital intensity, synergistic dynamic of human resources planning and forecasting, accessibility, scarcity, and suitability of productive resources, and assessment of profitability concerning economic development and growth through cost-benefit analysis.

The mainstream of thought for modern civilized societies through history is concerned with power, politics, people, and public policy. Politics in all societies is a fact that has made our modern life very complex. Politics is considered to be the fundamental concern in today's international diplomacy (Parhizgar, 1994: 110). Politics has been defined in number of ways. A common theme running through politics is behaviors aimed at exercising influence through the exertion of power (Meyes and Allen, 1977: 672-678). The study of diplomatic behavior: decision-making, conflict resolution, focusing on interest objectives of groups, coalition formation, preservation of classes of power, power-distance, and ruling system.

Demography is the science of bio-statistics and quantitative statistics of populations: as of births, deaths, diseases, marriages, numbers, means, percentages all both material and non-material value systems, etc.

History is a branch of scientific analytic knowledge dealing with past events. It is a continuous, systematic narrative of chronological order of past characteristics of human civilizations as relating to particular people, country, period, and person.

Geography is the science dealing with the real differentiation of the earth's surface, as shown in the character, arrangement, and interrelations over the world of such elements as climate, elevation, soil, vegetation, population density, land use, industries, or states.

Behavioral Sciences

Behavioral Sciences include Anthropology (Physical Anthropology, Cultural Anthropology, Archaeology, Anthropological Linguistics, and Ethnology/Ethnography), Sociology, and Psychology.

Anthropology is the science of human. Anthropology is literally defined as the science of human generations with the interactions between generations and environments, particularly their cultural environments.

Physical Anthropology is the study of the human condition from a biological perspective. Essentially, it is concerned with the restructuring the evolutionary record of the human species and to deal with how and why the physical traits of contemporary human populations vary across the world.

Cultural Anthropology deals with human beings learned behavior as influenced by their cultures and vice versa. In a general form and term, cultural anthropology studies the origins and history of human cultures, their creation, evolution, development, structure, and their interactive functions in every place and time (Beals and Hijer, 1959: 9). Cultural anthropology deals with humanity's conceived and perceived behavior as influenced by their culture, and vice versa. Since the definition of a total culture is usually beyond the scope of a single specialist, anthropologists have developed specialization of this science into: Psychological Anthropology, Economic Anthropology, Urban Anthropology, Educational Anthropology, Medical Anthropology, Rural Anthropology, and Applied Anthropology. In sum as Harvey and Allard (1995: 11) indicate: "An anthropologist takes the role of an observer from a culture more developed than our own and describes features of our civilization in the same manner as we describe cultures we view as primitive."

Archaeology is the study of the lifestyles of people from the past as determined by excavating and analyzing the sites, artifacts and written records. Archaeologists reconstruct the cultures of people who are no longer living. Archaeologists deal mainly with three basic components of culture: material culture, ideas and behavior patterns.

Anthropological Linguistics is the study of human speech and language. This branch of knowledge is divided into four distinctive branches: historical linguistics, sociolinguistic, descriptive linguistics, and ethnolinguistic.

Ethnography deals with the study of specific contemporary cultures and *ethnology* deals with more general underlying patterns of human culture derived through cultural comparison. Cultural anthropologists provide insights into questions such as: How have traditions, habits, orientations, and customs relating to a group of people emerged? How are marriage customs, and kinship systems operated? In what ways do people believe in supernatural power? How do migration and urbanization affect each other?

Sociology is traditionally defined as science of society. Psychology is the science of behavior. It generally includes animal as well as human behavior. Sociology is traditionally defined as the science of society, for searching and solving social problems within the context of its dynamic processes, purposes, and goals. Sociology is the science of human groups and is characterized by rigorous methodology with an empirical emphasis and conceptual conscious-ness (Luthans, 1985: 36). Sociology is the study of social systems like families, occupational classes, mobs, and organizations. The overall focus of sociology is on social behavior in societies, institutional behavioral patterns, organizational structures, and group dynamics.

Psychology has been defined as the science of behavior. Psychologists study the behavior of human beings and their perceptions in both industrial and/or agricultural organizational ecology. Psychologists study the behavior of people in organizational settings. There are many formative schools of thought in the field of psychology. The most widely known are structuralism, functionalism, behaviorism, Gestalt psychology, and psychoanalysis.

Wilhelm Wundt founded structuralism theory of psychology in 1879 in Germany. He had established a laboratory for studying human psychology. The theory revolved around conscious experience and attempted to build the science of mind. This theory applies to a structural division of the human mind into units of mental states such as sensation, memory, imagery, and feelings.

Functionalism was developed by American Psychologist William James (1842-1910) and philosopher John Dewey (1859-1925). This theory of psychology is based upon the function of mind. Emphasis is mainly placed on humanity's adaptation and adjustment to the ecological environment. This theory of the mind is emphasizes human sensory experience such as learning, forgetting, motivation, and adaptability to a new situation. Morgan and King (1966: 22) state: "Functionalism had two chief characteristics; the study of the total behavior and experience of an individual, and an interest in the adaptive functions served by the things an individual does."

The foundation of the behaviorism theory is based upon the connectivity of the human mind toward behavior. Ivan Pavlov (1849-1936) the Russian Psychologist initiated the concept of behaviorism. Since the structuralists were only concerned with the mind, and functionalists emphasized both mind and behavior, behaviorists focused on consequential results of such connectivity in relations with observance, objective behavior, and the significant outcomes of human mind and body movements.

Psychoanalysis psychology has come from Sigmund Freud (1856-1939). His theory is about unconscious motivation and the development and structure of personality and his treatment techniques.

Social psychology is academically interdisciplinary. It consists of an eclectic mixture of sciences and arts (Luthans, 1985: 30-38). Social Psychology is generally a synthesized scientific theory of psychology and sociology. If social psychology emphasizes on individual behavior, its close tie is with psychology. Also, it is equated with behavioral science. From the standpoint of emphasis on sociology, social psychology is the study of an individual behavior within relation to the groups (group emphasis).

WHAT IS TECHNOLOGY?

Terpstra and David (1991: 136) stated: "Technology is a cultural system concerned with the relationships between humans and their natural environment. A society is well adapted to its environment when its technological system is: (1) environmentally feasible, (2) stable, (3) resilient, and (4) open to revision." Technology focuses on a system of ideas to be reflected in physical and non-physical materials or cyberspace entities such as matter, machines, waves, time, light, and movements.

From another point of view, technological breakthroughs are known as integrated innovative systems which have discovered how to access cyberspace information in nature as well as in modern societies through processing both deep and broad domains of know-why, know-what, know-how, and know-where. Within such a highly sophisticated cyberspace environment, cognivistic mapping, pragmatic operational designs of data gathering, and holistic distributive operational techniques can be potentially abusive systems. Technologists can easily misuse data processes and designed outputs. Therefore, within the context of the real business world, we can claim that the development of technological civilization may not be evidence of progress from an ethical and moral point of view. However, technological developments are facts reflected in humanity's physical and intellectual abilities to affect and shape the natural environment and extend it to their desirable objectives (Parhizgar and Lunce, 1996: 394).

WHAT IS BIOINFORMATION?

Bioinformation is development of bioknowledge acquisition techniques known as bioscientific automated discovery systems. Bioknowledge inquiry is known as the essence of in-depth and narrowed domains of bioinformation. Automated bioscientific discovery is the generation of new pragmatic bioinformation by a computer system on its own, without the help of other knowledge sources. All biological and biomedical scientific information systems require extensive analyses of large amounts of data. The data collection and data handling processes should meet bioethical principles. Bioresearch projects and bioresearchers should have the appropriate tools for affecting the types of analysis their research require. They are required to apply highly sophisticated statistical and mathematical procedures to assist in a wide variety of research problem solving.

Bioinformation revision, improvement, and enhancement are relentless activities of bioresearchers on the basis of knowledge-based evidence endeavors, because the validity of problem solving techniques of these phenomena requires distinctions from problem to problem. Specifically, problems in bioscientific and biomedical research involve data having many variables for each case or many observations but fewer validated variables.

HOW DO WE DEFINE DATA?

Scientific formulas direct us to know not only if something is true but also why it is true. This type of scientific awareness is called a syllogism. A syllogism is a conclusive argument in which two premises and conclusions can be expressed either by demonstration or deduction. When we use scientific syllogistic formulas, we prove two domains of facts:

- The existence of the logical truthfulness of a demonstrative reasoning concerning a phenomenon, an element, a process, or the dynamics of a synthesized group
- The possible deductive conclusion is the manifestation of politics that states why such formulas are true

Data are simple and absolute quantitative facts and figures that in and themselves may be of little practical use. Data represent observable or factual quantitative incidents or figures out of context. Data are not directly meaningful. To be valuable and useful, the data must be processed into finished information by connecting parts with other data. Data should be placed within the meaningful contextual boundary of an event in order to be effective.

Bioscientific data needs to be carefully analyzed. Each type of data programming needs to handle a certain type of data analysis task. However, a particular scientific result may be obtained from more than one scientific program. In order to proceed with scientific data analysis, we need to use six major methodological classes of information. These classes are called RASSTOV:

- **R.** Real description and tabulation of scientific data.
- **A.** Accurate mathematical multivariate analysis.
- **S.** Statistical regression analysis.
- **S.** Syllogistic reasoning for specific research objectives.
- **T.** Time series analysis.
- **O.** Objectivity in selective descriptive and tabulation of data.
- **V.** Variance analysis.

An analysis of data usually starts with specific defined data screening programs and then proceeds with various types of analysis, with each analysis based on the findings of the preceding analyses.

Information is data that have been linked with other data and converted into a new type of attributed meanings. Meaningful information and workable context for the specific right or wrong use of integrated data relies on accurate syllogistic reasoning to conclude with a specific knowledge. Therefore, knowledge is the essence of codified meaningful information to be believed and valued based on the workable organized accumulation of information through cognitive experience, communication or inference.

WHAT IS KNOWLEDGE?

In today's free market economy, the basic organizational resource is no longer material capital, or labor, or natural resources, but knowledge. Knowledge is not the same thing as scientific formulas, data or information, although it uses all. Knowledge manifests a step further beyond scientific boundaries; it is a conclusion drawn form of the application of scientific formulas and information after it is linked to other known and unknown phenomena and compared to what is already known.

In a general term, knowledge always contains a human intellectual value factor. Knowledge is distinguished from science, data, and information. Knowledge has been perceived through different observations and outcomes. Peter Drucker (1993: 5) coined the term *knowledge-work* in the early 1960s. Knowledge-work involves the creation of a new understanding of nature, the multidisciplinary effective functioning of integrated parts of problem solving, the structural summation of synthesized organs, and the application of science, information, and aesthetics in innovation. This new paradigm needs to be examined in terms of moral, ethical, and legal implications. In the decades between the 1970s and 1990s, scientists and technologists began to recognize knowledge as an important resource that, like other socio-economic resources, should be managed.

In traditional bioorganizational paradigm systems managers usually concentrate on cash flow, human resources, or the acquisition of raw substances, scientific skills, synthetic machineries and component parts for manufacturing drugs. Pharmaceutical managers began to capitalize on knowledge ventures in the modern technological era.

Knowledge-wealth is an intangible resource which synergizes an organization to effectively acquire, create, apply, and transfer know-what, know-how, know-whose, know-where, and know-why across the company and modify their activities to reflect new knowledge and insights (Garvin, 1998: 47). Buchholz and Rosenthal (1998: 60) state:

> Within pragmatic process philosophy, all knowledge is understood as fallible, to be tested by ongoing consequences in experience. And knowledge emerges through intelligent reflection on experience within nature. Our experience within nature undergoes continual change, and while some aspects of experience are relatively stable, other aspects are unstable.

Also, Zack (1999: 45) states:

> Organizations are being advised that to remain competitive, they must efficiently and effectively create, locate, capture, and share their organization's knowledge and expertise, and have the ability to bring that knowledge to bear on problems and opportunities.

Knowledge management is a modern form of biobusiness that organizes bioscientific, biotechnological, and bioinformational intellectual and creative properties. It refers to the efforts to systematically search for, find, organize, establish, and make available an organization's intellectual capital for more productivity. It is a continuous intellectual effort through knowledge discovering, sharing, and applying innovativeness toward more profitable and suitable outcomes. Also, knowledge is a phenomenon in which achievable synergistic outcomes can be obtained through prodigy.

The synergistic bioknowledge paradigm system is the sum of its bioscientific discoveries, biotechnological innovativeness, bioinformational database processing, experimental testing, and understandable reasoning. A comprehensive paradigm of a bioknowledge system includes capturing, processing, storing, and disseminating bioknowledge, but also fosters bioknowledge learning through an academic institution.

Intellectual reflection on bioknowledge acquisition has been pursued for about as long as records of human intellectual activity are available. Traditional epistemology identifies three distinctive kinds of knowledge: (1) knowledge of things and objects, (2) knowledge of how to do things, and (3) knowledge of statements or propositions. Lundvall (1996) has identified four categories of knowledge:

- **Know-what-knowledge** about facts that can be broken down into bits and easily codified.
- **Know-why-knowledge** about principles and laws.
- **Know-how** skills, the capability to undertake a given task successfully.
- **Know-whose** information about who knows what and who knows how to do what.

Collins (1993: 95) has made a clear distinction between codified and non-codified knowledge. He proposed four categories of knowledge:

- **Symbolic-type knowledge** that can be transferred without loss in a codified form   (e.g., E-books and Floppy Diskette).
- **Embodied knowledge** held within the body of a human (e.g., How to play golf; the knowledge is internalized, but not easily communicated).
- **Embrained knowledge** held within the physical matter of the brain (e.g., certain cognitive abilities are related to the physical structure of the brain).
- **Encultured knowledge** that is linked to social groups and society.

Miller *et al.,* (1997: 399) expressed their views on the basis of Collins' four categories of knowledge which distinguishes between knowledge of information and contextual knowledge and created another type of categorization of knowledge as:

- **Catalogue knowledge** which that is known as know-what
- **Explanatory knowledge** that that is known as know-why
- **Process knowledge** that that is known as know-how
- **Social knowledge** which that is known as know-whose

Blackler (1995: 1021) has proposed five categories of knowledge:

- **Embrained knowledge or abstract knowledge:** This depends on conceptual skills and cognitive skills, generally conflated with scientific knowledge and accorded superior status.
- **Embodied knowledge or action-oriented knowledge:** It is likely to be only partly explicit: transmission requires face-to-face contact, sentient and sensory information and physical clues, is acquired by doing, and is context-dependent.
- **Encultured knowledge or related to the process of achieving shared understanding:** It is embedded in cultural systems, and is likely to depend strongly on language, and hence to be clearly socially constructed and open to negotiation.
- **Embedded knowledge:** It is a type of knowledge that resides in systemic routine. It relies on the interplay of relationships and material resources, and may be embedded in technology, practices, or explicit routine and procedures.
- **Encoded knowledge:** It is a type of knowledge in which recorded in signs and symbols, such as books, manuals, codes of practice, and electronic records. Encoding requires the distillation of abstract codified knowledge from other richer forms of knowledge.

Flack (1997: 383) has developed a categorization scheme that also attempts to encompass knowledge source and storage as follows:

- **Formal knowledge:** It is embodied in codified theories, formulas and usually encoded in written or diagrammatic forms that are acquired through formal learning.
- **Instrumentalities:** It is embodied in tool and instrument use. It requires other components (informal, tacit and contingent) for effective use. It may be learned through demonstration and practice.
- **Informal knowledge:** It is embodied in verbal interaction, rules of thumb, tricks of the trade, and is held in verbal and sometimes in

written forms (e.g., manuals, guidebooks). It is a pattern of learnt interaction within a specific milieu.

- **Contingent knowledge:** It is embodied in a specific contextual distributed fashion. It is apparently trivial information; specific to a particular context. It is sometimes available as data that can be looked up or acquired through an on-the-spot learning endeavor.
- **Tacit knowledge:** It is embodied in people and rooted in practice and experience. It is transmitted by apprenticeship and training.
- **Meta-knowledge:** It is embodied in the organizational cultural pattern. It is viewed as general organizational saga and philosophical assumptions concerning values and beliefs. It can be local or cosmopolitan -- acquired through socialization.

WHAT IS BIOMORAL KNOWLEDGE?

It is worthwhile to define biomoral knowledge as it refers to the excellence of intellect and wisdom and to the disposition of cognizance of mind to effectively perform its proper function. Also, it is worthwhile to define biomorality as seeking knowledge either for the sake of simply knowing or for the sake of doing or making somatic life excellent. In addition, it is worthwhile to define biolegal knowledge as an ordination of a practical reasoning to signify the compliance of civil rights as an order to attain a given proper ends. As we stated before, therefore, biomorality is related to the personal knowable beliefs and faith, bioethics is related to the societal group's acceptable valuable natural human rights, and biolegality is concerned with knowable civil rights to formulate peace and order by a mandated practical reasoning concerning doing or avoiding an action or operation.

THE EPISTEMOLOGY OF BIOKNOWLEDGE

As we indicated before, we defined epistemology or the theory of knowledge is to do with the problem of knowledge, we have knowledge:

- How is this possible? What does bioknowledge mean?
- Can all knowledge be traced to the greatest gateways of our somatic senses; to the senses plus the activity of pragmatic reasoning, or to the means and ends of pragmatic reasoning?
- Do feelings render wordless but true knowledge? Does true knowledge ever come in the form of immediate intuition?
- How can we identify different branches of knowledge?

The minimal answer to these questions is a function of somatic life:

How to view the holistic assessments of our understanding is related to arriving at conclusions to justify or criticize the kinds of reasoning we are trying to make up our minds about?

Within the context of bioknowledge there are two paths of reasoning that should be distinguished: rationalism and empiricism. Bioethicists in general keep to the rationalist side of the fence and bioscientists keep to the side of empiricism.

Bioethicists rely on the reasoning of bioknowledge to be appreciated through reasoning which reveals the constants and principles of natural selection, rather than on artificial selection. Curiously enough, this ancient point of view pervades the popular ideology of today, as we think of the rationalists as the armchair of biosophists who keep their attention focused on the consequences of bio-techno-scientific development and growth. They believe empirical observations do not create principles, but only discover them. Therefore, through their observations bioscientists and/or bioresearchers may end up in error. Such an error in nature will not be reversible. In addition, bioscientists believe that natural laws or natural selection are inherently related to matters rather than to phenomena.

In relation to morality and ethics the first question to answer is: What is biomoral about what kind of thing is a moral belief in bio-techno-scientific research? In other words, what is it that moral epistemology must investigate our bioknowledge? The minimal answer has two dimensions: (1) biomoral knowledge applies to the enhancement of an intrinsic individual's spiritual and practical goodness, and (2) bioethical knowledge applies to the extrinsic pluralistic beliefs and societal goodness. The most general concept of biomorality advocates believing in and practicing substantive contents or practical foundations of humaneness to ordinate an individual's behavior. In addition, the most general concept of bioethics advocates sharing collective beliefs in principles and standards for people to agree in determining what ought to be done in a given ideological content and context.

The above dimensions raise different opinions over how wide the range of possible agreements on bioknowledge should be: (1) whether biomorality should seek answers that permit convergence only among bio-techno-scientists and bioresearchers, (2) or among all human beings including multinational socio-cultural and politico-economic classes of people. Nevertheless, bioknowledge is a non-partisan phenomenon. It is related to the whole not just parts. It is related to humanity that does not have any politico-economic ideological boundary.

Ethically, bioknowledge is an independent phenomenon and should not be associated with any political *isms*. If bio-techno-scientists and bioresearchers try to decide what to do with humanity, and if there are biomoral commitments and bioethical principles, they should be open to the public and provide all technical information concerning what they are doing and what they ought to do. Bioknowledge and bio-techno-scientists should be independent of political and military decisions and actions. They should be committed to their professional convictions for the goodness of humanity, not for the benefits of partisan interest groups. So the search for the biomoral knowledge and bioethical practices is the search for the enhancement of human life.

Is there any room for bioknowledge justifications and/or concessions to be used for mass sicknesses, injuries, or the death of a group of people based on their ethnicity, race, religion, and political ideologies? Within moral and ethical beliefs, the answer is "no." If politicians and militarists try to justify and/or to have a concession on bioknowledge, the end results will ordinarily divide humanity. What does is this and what it means? Whether such justifications and concessions are found in political and military circles are the central issues of bioethics and biomorality. Therefore, if there is morality and/or ethicality in human civilization, they require all bio-techno-scientists and bioresearchers to transcend the practical domain of humanity in their means, and in their ends they should collectively converge on a common standpoint to enhance human life.

CHAPTER 7

THEOSOPHICAL DEONTOLOGICAL AND BIOSOPHICAL UTILITARIAN PROMETHEANISM BIOKNOWLEDGE AND BIOETHICS

CHAPTER OBJECTIVES

When you have read this chapter you should be able to do the following:

- Analyze and further explore the factors that inhibit bio-techno-scientific responsiveness to ethical changes in our contemporary society.
- Analyze different types of biosophical and theosophical views and their relationship to biosciences, biotechnology, and biomedical practices.
- Understand philosophies of creation and evolution.

- Understand philosophies of creation and evolution.
- Know what is Promethean biosophy.
- Identify crucial societal factors that influence biopharmaceutical profitability in the long term.
- Identify both dimensions of material and non-material cultures in relationship to the importance of ethical values in evaluating, financing, and accumulating wealth through biosciences, biotechnology, and bioinformation.
- Describe why bioethics must be related to practical biosciences.
- Know the meaning of practical ethics.
- Know how bioethics is both a process and a conclusion of a biobusiness event.
- Know not only what type of event is true but also precisely why it is true.
- Know how an individual who is intellectually well informed of doing good or evil can be characterized.

PLAN OF THIS CHAPTER

Farrington (1949: 5) on views of the Baconian theosophical principlism of living systems indicated:

> Man is the helper and interpreter of Nature. He can only act and understand insofar as by working upon her or observing her he has come to perceive her order... Nature cannot be conquered but by obeying her. Accordingly these twin goals, human science and human power, come in the end to one [Creation].

Such a statement indicates that the nature does not reveal its mysterious natural flow of events to human beings. Humans need to try to discover how nature works and progresses. Humans need to be in harmony with nature.

Opponents to the theosophical principlism of living system such as Buddhist Tarthan Tulka (1977: 73) stated:

> The disharmony in our lives is reflected in our attempt to control the environment and the conditions that result. We so often attempt to use the world around us for our personal uses and immediate comfort without taking into consideration any wider perspective. In implementing such narrowly construed purposes, we create imbalances that bring forth both present and future problems for others and ourselves... We should now consciously consider our responsibility to restore a balance, an integration of material (scientific and technological) advances with the deeper values of humanity. And when there is a balance of the two ways of thinking – technology can be utilized as a very valuable and creative force [Revolutionism].

Fox (2001: 121) indicated: "This statement is relevant today, in that we have broken 'the seal of God on things,' in atomic and genetic research especially, and now superimpose 'the seal of our image on the creatures and works of God."

This chapter analyzes two major views that have a technical significant throughout bioethics: (1) theosophical principlism and (2) biosophical Prometheanism. The extent to which bioethics involves a deeper epistemological analysis which should be adequately discussed in terms of bioknowledge. Also, this chapter begins to define and examine both theosophical and biosophical views of bioknowledge concerning bioethical principlism views of our world of organic nature. Before we embark on a more detailed consideration on theosophical principlism and biosophical Prometheanism of bioknowledge, we will examine the general development of theories of creation and evolution. Without drawing attention to those beliefs we cannot always fully understand what is at stake in many of our bioethical analyses.

INTRODUCTION

The more community of theosophists, biosophists, bioethicists, and bioscientists think, theorize, and practice within the context of paradigm of bioknowledge they penetrate more detailed processes of life, death, and valuable environmental characteristics. Also, they become more confronted with vital issues concerning principles of two theories: (1) creation and (2) evolution. These two religious and scientific theories cover a range of known and unknown facts, which are rooted in individual's self-consciousness, and pluralistic wisdom of human race. Bioscientific and biotechnological discoveries involve specific kind of deliberations concerning the formation of universal higher mysterious complex order. As Hoyle (1965) indicated such a very complex order has taken from the idea of a universe with no privileged position, no center no place where things look any different from any other places. Within the biosophical context, the human world is based on earthly organic life. It is a tiny, short-lived episode within the enormous events of the cosmic cycles. There is no sense in asking for a beyond. This is the existence as such, and we are just barely able to understand a small fraction of it (Matare', 1999: 3).

From this perspective, the traditional religious theosophical idea of creation and the biosophical pragmatic findings of evolution are in large a measure of a story of movement in which created daily debates about bioethics. Callahan (1989: 348) has described this as a movement from an internalist to an externalist view of the relation of bioethics to the wider ethical standards of society. From the internalist view, bioethics is largely self-contained. Its principles are internal to the practice of medicine. The externalist view, by contrast, thinks that the ends of biosciences must be determined by the ethics of the lager entity (the cosmic world). By such a kind of reasoning bioscientists, biotechnologists, and bioinformationalists' skills should be in service of the ends.

WHAT IS THE THEOSOPHICAL PRINCIPLISIM OF DEONTOLOGICAL BIOETHICS?

Theosophical principlism of bioethics is a clear cut of deontological views within the external societal norms of bioethics. It is based on specific logical arguments concerning prioritization of factorial elements in pursuing moral and ethical objectives. To be sure, bio-techno-scientists necessarily have a kind of priority in their trial and error judgments on which they should follow spiritual foundational values in their actions. These foundational values guide professional practitioners to follow those beliefs in their prioritized choices. Within such a deontological spiritual domain of metaphysic, connectedness is increasingly central to the spiritual theosophical principlism. The major principle values indicate that the web of energy that enlivens the cosmos and the power of revelation known in and through communities are struggling for justice and wholeness. This metaphysic of ritual connectedness serves a basis for envisages of a unified and integrated cosmos to act to preserve the integrity of the cosmic web of spiritual life and to affect right relationships among all incumbents. Thus, it is the God's moral power to internalize justice within such a vast cosmic order. This manifests a Divine power to understand the state of excellence as a principle in creation of the whole world. More to the point, God is the creator of everything that exists, and there is therefore a unity in the knowledge that human beings attain – no matter what its immediate source.

Proponents of this idea are Beauchamp and Childress (1989: 394). They expressed their views as:

> Ethical theory does not create the morality [intellectual excellence] that guides professional's decisions and actions. It can only cast light on and supplement that morality, in part by analyzing and appraising moral justifications, their presuppositions, and their implications.

Beauchamp and Childress (1989) turned the three principles (respect for persons, beneficence, and justice) of the American National Commission for the Protection of Human Subjects of Biomedical and Behavioral Research into four: (1) respect for autonomy, (2) nonmalfeasances, (3) beneficence, and (4) justice. Their views indicate that what is now called moral foundamentalist is the view that our moral knowledge is based not upon history and tradition, but upon ahistorical (to be able to reveal a portion of historical truth) universal truth.

Opponents of the theosophical principlism attack not only the idea of ahistorical foundations but also on a perceptive reasoning as deductive. This indicates that we reason our bioethical judgments on the bases of those universally justified principles to more specific judgments. Anti-foundationalists are more likely to describe biomoral reasoning in terms of a movement back and forth between the general principle values we hold and our personal judgments about specific cases that we observe. In this dialectical movement, we seek coherence between deontological principlism and utilitarian particular judgments, a coherence that can be gained by adjusting either principles or judgments (Meilaender, 1995: 13). In a general term, Beauchamp and Childress (1989: 7) acknowledged: "Application of their principles will depend on factual beliefs about the world." This moves us to understand the theosophical theory of creation.

THE THEOSOPHICAL THEORY OF DEOTOLOGICAL CREATION

The theory of creation is a religious metaphysical deliberation in which expresses strong beliefs concerning the existence of cosmos based on God's will and reasoning. It is a doctrine that God immediately can create everything out of nothing. Theosophical theory of deontological creation is a doctrine that matter and all other things have been created, substantially as they now exist by the will of an omnipotent Creator (God). Creation theosophy rejects gradual evolutionary development. Creationists believe that creation is the emergence of the original "just" existence by bringing everything into existence of the universe by the Deity. The just existence is the product of God's inventive ingenuity. How we describe a moral situation will depend on the background beliefs on the basis of generalized paradigm of scientific formulas, metaphysical beliefs, and religious faiths that we bring to it. Such a deductive judgment stems from ahistorical experiences. Since a major point of such an ahistorical paradigm of theosophy is based on fundamentalism values of metaphysics and religious faith we should turn our attention to theosophical theory of "creation" as the major foundation of our bioethics. On the other hand, there is another opponent view that indicates humans are innovative. It is the image of human beings that owns the capacity to create those things that compete with nature. This theory is called biosophical utilitarian Prometheanism.

WHAT IS THE PROMETHEAN UTILITARIAN BIOSOPHY?

Kimbrell (1994: 29) reported that working for General Electric in Schenectady, New York, in 1971, Indian microbiologist Ananda Mohan Chakrabarty set out to create a special cloned kind of "bug" that would eat crude oil. Its central use would be to devour oil slicks created by tanker spills or similar disasters. Nature already had produced several strains of bacteria that had the propensity to digest different types of hydrocarbons in oil. All these bacteria were from a family of bacteria known as Pseudomonas. Each of these bacteria had plasmids (auxiliary parcels of genes) that break up or eat oil. Chakrabarty performed this feat of genetic manipulation by fusing the genetic material from four types of Pseudomonas. Taking plasmids from three of the oil-eating bacteria, Chakrabarty transplanted them into the fourth, thereby "creating" an innovative crossbred version with an enhanced appetite for oil. Crudely put, the criticism could be stated this way: it is unknown what would be the side-effects of the human made "bugs" on other living things in nature. Alongside of the viewpoints of inventors and creators of new biological germs, the goodness of biotechnology can cause to fight diseases and death. Biotechno scientists are the true benefactors of mankind and are revered like God. Kass (2002: 29) indicated:

> Biotechnology is a neologism for the new age. New and novel (biotechnology) also is the thing it names: industrial-scale processes and products offering power to alter and control the phenomena of life – in plants, in animals and, increasingly, also in human beings. But while the word may be new, the *idea* of biotechnology is old, and so are the motives behind it.

The arguments concerning rational, technical, political, and creative animal, all are denoted to one package of intelligence that is known Promethean utilitarianism. Although everyone remembers philosopher Aeschylus, who indicated that Prometheus was the philanthropic god who gave fire and the arts to humans, it is often forgotten that he gave them also the greatest gift of blind hopes; to cease seeing doom before their eyes. That is the main reason that ignorance is viewed as dynamic derivative forces to motivate humans to live with open-ended hope for aspiration and achievement.

For Descartes to search and secure human happiness is based upon technical means, without the need for law or force or fear of God. Descartes indicated:

> For the mind depends so much on the temperament and disposition of the bodily organs that, if it is possible to find a means of rendering men wiser and cleverer than they have hitherto been, I believe that it is in medicine that it must be sought.

Nevertheless, in the famous allegory of the cave in Plato's *Republic VII*, Socrates implied that it is the Promethean gift of fire and the enhancement of the arts that hold humans unwittingly enchained, warm and comfortable yet blind to the world beyond the city. No arts, no cities, and if no cities, no true humanity. Mistaking, the human's crafted world for the whole, human lives ignorant of their true standing in the world and their absolute dependence on power not of their own making and beyond their control (Plato: 427-347 B.C.).

The Promethean utilitarianism biosophy of bioknowledge is a cult in which its initiatives are directed toward transcending material limits and transforming them into innovation. It is a cult that desires to create superhuman – that human will be playing the role of God. Theosophically, the argument is about God or no God. This means that humans are becoming creators of self-life, and indeed, of an individual's life *in vitro* fertilization or cloning. The end result of such a cult is super-slavery. Biotechnological corporations will be seen in a path of godlike role of creators that their products must stand before them as supplicating creatures. This type of utilitarian biosophy tries to manipulate and dominate natural genes, cells, proteins, enzymes, and organisms in the most possible holarchical term. They will determine who should live and who should die on the basis of genetic merit; genetic-meritocracy. Don't you think this theory of bioethics germinated with discrimination?

Within the Promethean utilitarian biosophical vision, the claim is based on: We as human beings should be the creator of life and our ultimate objectives should be based upon recreating ourselves on the basis of our own image, vision, mission, intention, and conviction. This is known as the evolutionary theory of human selection.

WHAT IS THE EVOLUTIONARY THEORY OF HUMAN SELECTION?

The evolutionary theory of cognition has helped us to realize the fact that there is room for human updevelopment. Matare' (1999: i) indicated:

> Within our pragmatic world of organic nature, "evolution" is the key to understanding all development from plant to animals, vertebrates, mammals, and humans... Characteristics like color of a flower, the beak form of a bird, or the brain capacity of humans, all are part of a continuous process of adaptation, obviously to some environmental pressure. With the development of human brain and its concomitant wider understanding of nature and its laws, a somewhat new level of feedback from entity to nature arose. With its wide scope and understanding of nature's laws, the human brain can interfere with natural process of eliminating of the sick and regressive ideas by extinction. Humanity is increasingly becoming witness to a multitude of possible actions and controls that interfere directly with the old, natural process of evolution.

The evolutionary theory of human selection can help bioscientists, biotechnologists, and bioinformationalists to popularize a kind of scientific thought and practice in order to create a new path for human updevelopment. What bioknowledge can help us in such an updevelopment process is to create a short cut for the time-consuming process of evolution? In nature, there is a room for natural selection and adaptation. Elimination of unfitted creatures is due to the active interference of bioscientists, biotechnologists, and bioinformationalists to extinct undesirable characteristics and events. Such a biosophical idea changes the position of human beings from "creatures" to creators. This is known Prometheanism.

We, human beings, like other predator species; like the lion, the wolf, the wale, and the eagle, are the interlocutors between chaos and order, playing a vital creative role in keeping all natural species including human beings in balance. Human beings possess the ability and capability to be creators. Promethean utilitarian biosophical believers believe in creation of coevolutionary forms of holarchy in which they perceive moral life should be based on amorality. They do not perceive themselves as creatures to be managed by other extra Gs' power (God and/or Government). This means that they do not perceive life as an absolute phenomenon. They believe life is a balance between right and wrong, good and evil, just and unjust, beautifulness and ugliness, and worthiness and worthlessness. What is right for the wale is catching the fish or the death of the deer is not evil or wrong because the deer is a means to a wolf's end. This is the biosophy of balance of nature, which carries capacity of the whole ecosystem to be maintained.

From the utilitarian Promethean biosophical view, our human-oriented amorality should not regard all sufferings and pains including death as evil or immoral, because sentient life and death are either good or evil. They are integral parts of natural holarchical life experiences and processes. They believe death and suffering to be caused by human beings rather than by natural means are viewed legitimate because they are creating a balance between life and death. For example, war, pestilence, or famine that are results of overpopulation and overconsumption are not evil.

Utilitarian Promethean biosophy does not perceive any difference between natural evil; the inevitable suffering of sentient being from extreme cold, heat, drought, heavy vegetation, overpopulation, and epidemic diseases; and human evil, which is raised as consequences of human needs and wants are legitimate. In principle, they believe in the philosophy of Social Darwinism: the survival of the fittest and the demise of the weakest or the sickest.

Within the utilitarian Promethean biosophy, there are two sets of law: (1) natural physical laws and (2) human arbitrary laws. Natural physical laws make it clear that there have been a number of cyclic Big Bangs in universe. Big Bangs have been conceived as initial high-energy states of cooling and expansion that created a positive arrow of time. The human aspect of nature is intimately connected not only to the natural physical laws, but it is based on the second laws of thermodynamics. In other words, all organic lives exist only as entropic-bound (a measure of unavailable energy in thermodynamics system). For example, commonly it is expressed in terms of its changes on an arbitrary scale: being zero for water at 32 as freezing point degrees of Fahrenheit. This is known as a conventional agreement in a scientific method.

According to the natural physical laws from the quantum theory of gravity and the uncertainty principle, the vast expansion becomes irregular; the nature reaches to its maximum of entropy, that is, a total state of disorder. From this point on where all energy has been converted into mass, gravity takes over and the contracting phase begins. In this case, the arrow of time points backward and the entropic machines revert to their original point of maximized order or energy. In reverted contracting process, no organic nature or human beings could exist, because life and existence are synonymous with increasing entropy. Thus, positive time flows as the fourth dimension in terms of the natural physical laws restarting the new cyclic life through new emerging Big Bangs. The new Big Bangs are results of trajectory phases of contraction and death.

According to the above theory at the stages of birth and growth the anthropic machines (bio-organics) are expanding to the extent of their full capacity to create a massive potential of synergy. Such a synergy needs to be harnessed through prodigical innovative processes if possible to maintain balance in continuity of life. According to the quantum theory of thermodynamics, bioorganic machines create gravity with a huge condensed germ that can result in progenies. Since progenies are entrepreneurial and moving towards their dense masses of capabilities in absorbing energy they cause saturation (Big Crunch); the new phase of trajectory contraction (the curve describes by a trajectile in its flight through air) emerges. Such a saturated massive density of contraction (Big Crunch) causes to revert the arrow of time towards death. The end result will be emergence of new Big Bangs.

$$v = t\,(e + s + p + g)\,\text{.}\,d$$

v = velocity (a time rate of change plus direction of change)

t = time

e = energy: Appropriate environmental resources.

s= synergy: Consideration of overwhelming defused physical and chemical boundary conditions of parental genes to create the early stages of molecular functionality of sperms and eggs to create organic forms consequently leads to life.

P = prodigy: Application of scientific formulas in the domain of technological manipulation.

g = progeny: Application of entrepreneurial opportunities by taking appropriate decisions in the right time, right places, and right element for acquisition of profitable and suitable consequences.

d = direction (Birth, Growth, Trajectory Contraction, and Death)

EVOLUTION AS A PRINCIPLE IN PROMETHEAN BIOSOPHY

The cosmic evolution is viewed as a gradual embodiment of order and harmony system as distinguished from chaos. Improved astronomical technology and scientific analysis have provided us a clearer picture of the cosmos. Our spaceship earth moves at a speed of roughly 100,000 km/h around the sun, such a speedy movement would only be possible with spaceships working with ion propulsion. As we know our spaceship earth is a part of the

Solar System. Through the best radio telescopes, we discovered suns and galaxies in a distance of 1000 million light years.

There is no end in the universe. Kinetically, where are we located in the cosmos is a puzzle. However, we have realized that the source of all dynamic movements is energy. From the initial super-energy state of the cosmos, the formation of elementary particles and the positive signs of arrow of time have emerged. Matare' (1999: 3) indicated:

> The old Friedmann (1922) model for the universe spelled out such an evolutionary expansion and allowed for three different curvatures of the center-flight of the galaxies verses time:
>
> • Circular, that is a reversal due to gravitation (Big Bang/Big Crunch).
> • Steady increase in center-flight or expansion.
> • Parabolic or asymptotic leveling off of the speed of center-flight with time.

Scientifically, universe is not static. It is dynamic. Through an existentialist view, it is expanding with multi-sources of energetic supra powers with different levels of gravity. These levels of gravity create systematic balance in dynamic movements. Such sources of energy have caused balanced and harmonious interrelated diverse lives.

How life is possible? It is gradual evolutionary processes in which increase entropy. Constant synergistic entropy emerges from cycle to cycle and would result in increasing cycle duration and also more synergistic characteristics to be carried from one cycle to the next. The question about the extended beyond of the cycling cosmos could have no meaning, because according to the cyclic energy expansion and contraction, time and movements as major variables, play important roles to restart at each subatomic high-energy point.

According to the utilitarian Promethean biosophical views, human thoughts as manifestation of innovative bio-techno-scientific entities are intimately related and conditioned by the existence of synergistic processes of natural atomic intellectual power. Clearly, synergistic functional brain size and its progenitive operation is an important parameter. Its number of neurons and axons and their variable multi-fascinated connectivity make the different levels of intelligence. In addition, the levels of synergistic interconnections of neurons and axons are a function of the genetic setup and the learning and memorizing processes are subjects to the human's will power how to use it in daily life. Accordingly, humans can expand their evolutionary creativity with a positive arrow of time with appropriate logical direction and can only exist during the expanding phase of their societies (e.g., Renaissance).

Renaissance is viewed as a Big Bang in our civilization, because it was a revival of art, letters, and pragmatic scientific discoveries. It was the beginning of transition from the medieval to the modern world. In modern civilization, Renaissance has been an appropriate turning point of the positive arrow of time for a society to be synergistic and creative in establishing a foundation for resembling synergistic entities in future generations. It should be noted that there is no human logic and conjecture at the sociocultural and politico-economical cycle end-point where mass population and/or intellectual energy maxima dissolve in a time reversal during a war or a revolution; Big Crunch.

According to the Promethean biosophy, all identical twins are cloned by nature. If nature permits existence of twins, then why bio-techno-scientists should not find opportunities to clone human beings as replication of selves. Why at the turning point of progeny human beings should stop their creativity? Why should cloning by human beings be unethical? We should argue that something is unethical if unethical reasons lead to unethical consequences. In the field of medicine, physicians try to cure patients and providing them with enhanced healthy longer lives. We cannot claim that the profession of medicine is unethical. Accordingly, through Promeathean biosophy, the aim to produce a healthy progenistic human being within a system that guarantees a healthy updevelopment of human species is not unethical. As in the field of education, we are upgrading learners' intellectual synergy through prodigy (application of effective technologies towards more understanding), in the field of biotechno-scientific endeavor, we must create new methods to enhance physiological capabilities of human species.

Through eugenic processes, gene engineering, the stem cell, and cloning biotechno-scientific innovativeness of Promethean biosophy, bioscientists must enhance human genes and stop defected genes. As we believe that a high birth rate in impoverished societies or in slum environments is unethical, we need to follow the same task in human reproduction system. Critics of cloning said that cloning might be used to duplicate undesirable personalities like criminals. Such a claim raises a fundamental question concerning heredity of social trends in human genes. It means criminals are offspring of criminal societies. Then with such an attribution, we must sterilize criminals. If we believe that genes carry criminal characteristics, then we are negating the effectiveness of educational systems for human's mental development or growth. Such logic is unethical and immoral.

Utilitarian Promethean biosophy considers all innovative alternatives in biology should be focused on the context of human species. They believe that the trans-species mutation of human and animal genes (chimerical genes) is unethical and immoral. Pragmatic Promethean biosophy does not see any honorable feature in human existence per se. The only successful innovativeness is based upon our ability to better understand nature in order to discover natural selection for the enhancement of human species. To achieve such an idealistic objective, biotechno-scientists need to influence our own fate in order to enhance our ability through synergistic trends of biosciences and biotechnology.

Historically, bioscientists have identified that the comparative anatomy illustrated that all structural developments of the growing elements in biosphere are interrelated. For example, as Matare' (1999: 19) indicated:

The variations of all pentadactylic extremities, from the primitive mammal to the horse, the camel, the dolphin, or man do not alter their basic form. Five fingers are the rule, while some reductions in the case of the horse- and deer-shoe appear, but in all cases the five fingers are the original starting point, being fixed in the original genetic code.

Paleontological and embryological research has contributed a multitude of evolutionary phase sequences and related developments. Embryological phases repeat evolutionary steps of the past (Haeckel, 1905). Siewing (1987) indicated that the well-known examples are the gill slits in chicken embryos and in other mammal embryos up to man. Phylogenetic development is partially reflected in the ontogenetic sequences. However, there is no complete repetition, as biologists have pointed out.

Within the contextual boundary of evolution, there are two main theories: *Lamarckian* and *Darwinian*. Jean Lamarck (1774-1829), as a naturalist philosopher, celebrated as the author of the first systematic evolutionary theory in biology. He sought to comprehend the fundamental laws of nature. This meant assuming that nature was in fact lawful and, perhaps that human could determine the character of such laws. He believed in the integral character of science; at least of those special sciences such as chemistry, meteorology, geology, and botany-zoology (for which last, Lamarck in 1802 coined the term biology). Growing from this conviction, there appeared in succession, beginning in 1794, a series of publications that expressed Lamarck's gradual and developmental view of chemical, geological, and biological changes. The culmination of these thoughts constituted Lamarck's statement of biological transformation (latter known as evolution), (Burkhardt, 1977).

Lamarck noted that the changes produced in evolutionary processes were more pronounced in animals and plants and domestication lasted for longer time. Charles Darwin often attacked the Lamarckian system at this as its weakest point. Later Charles Darwin (1859) explained this variability in terms of the selective rules rather than the Lamarckian habitability of acquired properties. Modern genetics has proven Darwin correct, who did not know how genes and mutation interact through adaptation to environmental pressure.

Charles Darwin brought biology into focus in 1859 when he published his book, *On the Origin of Species*. Darwin understood *natural selection* on the basis of three undeniable facts. He identified many issues about past evolutionary processes of the human race. Also, he revealed an inescapable conclusion about natural life (Campbell: 1993: 15). Darwin identified the following characteristics about an individual's natural existence:

- Individuals in a population of any species vary in many heritable traits.
- Any population of species has the potential to produce far more offspring than the environment can possibly support with food, space, and other resources. This overproduction makes a

struggle for existence among the variant members of a population inevitable.

- Those individuals with traits best suitable to the local environment generally leave a disproportionately large number of surviving offspring. This selective reproduction increases the representation of certain heritable variations in the next generation. It is this differential reproductive success that Darwin called "natural selection," and he envisioned it as the cause of evolution.

It should be noted that there are no sudden changes in nature or what it be called macroevolution. Evolution took place in an extended time and it will continue in future to the point of natural revolution (Big Crunch). However, biophysicists and biochemists have found that macro-evolution can take place when animals and plants are exposed to a very condensed pre-designed environment in order to create an extraordinary explosive development in the sense of an adaptive radiation or relatively fast adaptation within a given time-frame. Part of the environmental adaptation is the energy supply system variation and its structural modifications. The major bioethical questions concerning macroevolution stems from the objectives of bio-techno-scientists how morally are liable for the application of their innovative discoveries.

Physicists have long debated their roles in the development of nuclear technology and believe that it has been for the purpose of peace and demanded control of nuclear weapons. Also, bioscientists expressed their views on banning and controlling further macro-evolutionary processes of biological and biochemical weapons. These are the most disturbing consequences of biotechno scientific side effects.

In the early Twentieth century building upon Darwin's effort in biology, a number of psychologists, including Sigmund Freud focused on application of the theory of psychoanalysis in order to understand an individual's behavior. Freud presented a comprehensive application on the *Origin and Development of Psychoanalysis*. His view on human personhood was a radical behaviorist point, which was based upon pessimistic European intellectual conservatism. This conservative view was based upon a historical cultural tradition which meant that people were more tuned to their past experiences rather than to their future challenges. Freud viewed an individual's personhood as the result of a progressive development through four unconscious motivational stages: dependent, compulsive, Oedipal, and nurture. These motivational stages are shaped by a variety of personality development, each of which has sexual motives under tones (Freud, 1933: 48-52). Contemporary psychoanalytical theorists, however, do not generally accept these stages. Freud viewed behavioral sensation is the essence of the movement through these stages as being driven largely by unconscious needs and desires (*Psychology,* 1989). Also, Freud focused on the socio-cultural development of the individual psyche, its battles with the individual's immediate family, the struggle for independence, and the manifold anxieties to defend the ideology of individualism. For Freud, the key factor for well being was self-knowledge and self-actualization through confrontation with the inevitable pain and suffering for survival and continuous existence. Within such an evolutionary biological and psychosocial *natural selection*, human species preceded their evolutionary lives with very slow pace.

According to the utilitarian Promethean biosophical presumptions, what human beings need to do is to change the pace of natural *selection* into *human selection*. The Prometheanism biosophy theory is a revolutionary based-bioknowledge in which it claims it resides in the synergistic triune power of bio-techno-scientific innovativeness. This type of biosophy relies on assumptions that biosciences including biology, biophysics, biochemistry, biospheric, and bioengineering promise to empower human race to search for discovering everything. They believe human beings through application of biotechnology can be empowered to do everything even to change their own natural somatic genes, cells, and proteins. Moving to such a bio-techno-scientific path so swiftly has motivated bioethicists to call for a far more cautious approach to the application of genetic science that is presently being pursued. Chargaff (1998) described genetic endangering as a molecular Auschwitz and warned that it poses a great threat to the humanity than nuclear technology. The Noble Prize Winner George Wald (1979: 127) indicated:

> The utilitarian Prom Recombination DNA technology faces our society with problems unprecedented not only in the history of science, but of life on earth... Up to now, living organisms have evolved very slowly, and new forms have had plenty of time to settle in. Now whole proteins will be transposed overnight into wholly new associations, with consequences no one can foretell, either for the host organism, or neighbors... It is all too big and is happening too fast. So this, the central problem, remains almost unconsidered. It presents probably the biggest ethical problem that science has ever had to face.

The utilitarian Promethean biosophists believe in commodification of plants, animals, human tissues, and humans. Within their bioindustrial biosophy, Prometheanism biosophists believe that all natural selections should be converted into in-door farming, bioindustrial husbandry plants, biotech corporations to grow DNA cell lines in sexless fertility clinical laboratories, or use biopharmaceutical companies to assess mass cost-benefit analysis of human cloning processes if a safety measure is worth the number of natural lives to be discontinued and the number of human cloned be initiated and preserved. Therefore, Promethean bioscientists in searching for knowledge should proceed too far; in a sense to be God. Do you find some ethical and moral flaws within such a biosophy?

PRINCIPLES OF THE UTILITARIAN PROMETHEAN BIOKNOWLEDGE

If humans desire to conquer the universe, first they need to conquer themselves. They need to create artificial boundaries to compete with nature. To compete with nature, bio-techno-scientists need to convert atoms into bytes. This may involve the processing of bytes into bioinformation-based products and services. Bio-techno-scientists need to know how to package their bioknowledge in a digital form. They need to decide the right mix between atoms and bytes, in order to be creative.

Through utilitarian Promethean biosophy, many bio-techno-scientists try to change the natural habitual paths of creatures and convert them into artificial ones. They need to compete with natural forces head-to-head to create unique bioknowlegable outcomes. They believe that bio-techno-scientific research is viewed as a legitimate social choice; not a natural force. Once bio-techno-scientists discover bio-techno-organisms on earth, they have the right to patent them and then to manipulate them to achieve their economical means and ends. For example, in commercial factory farming, bio-agri-scientists replaced traditional farming in most animal products with bionic artificial products such as milk, eggs, white, red, and dark meat, and pork. Bioresearchers based on their Promethean biosophy have created new-engineered cross-organisms such as *pomatoes* (cross-species of vegetable seeds of potatoes and tomatoes) and have precisely engineered what they desired to create. Such a cross-genetic processing may generate many mysterious errors and can cause unexpected consequences. Specifically, such a line of research activity with multicelled organisms may create unknown consequences that will not show up its side effects in short period of time. Not only these side effects will affect present species, but also they may defect ecologically future related organisms. Also, not only cross-mammal eugenic biotechnological practices can emerge severe side effects on mammal species but also they will have affects on plants and other animals (e.g., bees, butterflies, bats, and birds). For example, French bioresearchers (1998:13) studied rape plants with transplanted fungus-resistance genes discovered that the plants posed a threat to nearby colonies of bees. After two weeks' exposure to the plants, the bees' memory for smell, the basis for their ability to locate food sources, was dramatically reduced. Furthermore, they have shown a 30 percent drop in bee population in areas where genetically engineered cotton was being tested.

According to the above foundational scenarios, bio-techno-scientists follow the governmental rules and regulations and try to avoid God's spiritual order and/or natural law. The adherent people need to rely on both to be protected. Through spirituality, people pray and search for revelation and through materiality people pay taxes and search for earthly protection.

One of the major problems of utilitarian Promethean biosophy lies on the type of scientific methodological applications of biosciences and biotechnology. There are two major dimensions: (1) micro analysis and (2) macro analysis.

Promethean micro bioscientists and biotechnologists tend to be in favor of reductionism/expansionism and/or exterminationism/accelrationism methodologies. They break down organisms such as genes, cells, tissues, and proteins into their component parts in order to discover their natures rather than to discover how organisms interact with one another in coexistence ecosystems.

The reductionism/expansionism micro bioknowledge and extrenalism/ accelerationism Promethean macro bioknowledge tries to be innovative in specific kinds of alternatives for creation of new specific scientific objectives which can lead to new procedures, products, and species. They may ignore the holistic environmental side effects of their innovative solutions on the ecosystems. The consequence is catastrophic. Promethean bio-techno-scientists believe in themselves to change the natural path of life and provide solutions for eternal human life.

THE NEW EVOLUTIONARY BIOTECHNOPIA PROCESSES

Biotechnopia revolutionary products and procedures are everywhere in the digital age. As bio-techno-scientists, you deal more and more with machines, and less and less with people. This heady march into the digital age is beneficial in many ways, but there is an underlying danger that must be addressed, that is known human alienation. Bio-techno-scientists, bioresearchers, and biomedical practitioners can become so obsessed with the wonders of biotechnology and they completely may forget about their important visions and missions to protect and preserve the sanctity of human race. Instead of viewing and applying biotechnology as a way to foster better, more meaningful relationships with ecosystem, they view biotechnology as a universal panacea for their problems, or as a way to shield themselves from direct contact with people. Instead, bio-techno-scientists desire to be creators of life through their Promethean biosophical theses. Should it be ethically and morally happened as self-creators? What is the exact meaning to be as creators of selves? It means humans desire to manipulate their artificial fertility processes in order to be able to processionally create and destroy themselves. Consequently, living things including humans will be in hands of powerful elite groups. We like or dislike it; it is the future of civilization.

The dramatic changes in the third millennium tempt biotechno scientists to predict basic changes in biosciences and biotechnologies. Radical changes occur in the time of crisis (e.g., epidemics, atomic, biochemical, and biological catastrophes). The radical changes in biosciences and biotechnologies clearly set new evolutionary staging processes in human lifestyle. In addition, the emergence of holistic integrated bioknowledge also called the information society, or learning and innovative breakthroughs, might simply be characterized by bioscientific advancements and biotechnological developments more directly rooted in the production and usage of bioknowledge than ever before. The bioknowledge enhancement is real, expanded, and growing. Specifically, biotechnopia output growth in bio-techno-scientific research paves the highest pace in biopharmaceutical and biomedical practices. They develop and use of bio-techno-scientific intensive innovativeness. The bioknowledge is also apparent from the heavy investment in bio-techno-scientific research and development (Bio-R&D). Like an organism, bioknowledge evolves and is not absolute or fixed in any way. What shapes it, is its appropriateness and fitness to human nature. If bioknowledge gives us a promising aspiration, then its inspiring strategic advantage facilitates bioknowledge to survive. Nevertheless, any size of growth and derivative development in bioknowledge can only ever be disproved; it can never be proved in an absolute sense.

Bioknowledge is more valuable when it is delivered the moment it is needed, just in time, rather than being available at all times, just in case. Epidemiologically, bioknowledge has to do with the problems of nature, and of the human's place in it. Although biotechnology is very new trend of bioscientific development, Flowers (1998: 1737) has assessed its position in four phases:

- 1985-1990: The First Period; Developing Tools: Within such a period of time, biopharmaceutical and biotech experts and institutions realized that it was the appropriate time to develop the tools of biotechnological research in order to do the biotechnical research.
- 1991-2020: The Second Period; Curing Diseases: The bio-techno-scientific tools have been used to produce more sophisticated tools and techniques to contribute effective solutions for biomedical/biotechnological disease cures. The successfully marketed cures offer new promises; to cure diseases when antibiotics have become ineffective. Bioscientific research and· biomedical research have been persuaded to use computers and databases to search for completion of human genome.
- 2021-2075: The third period; Genetic Modifications: Biomedical modifications of the body will begin to include modifications not needed to cure diseases or inherited natural errors in the genome. Within this period of time, special purpose of genetic modifications of the body will bring about by somatic gene therapy, gene reengineering, and eugenic super class of human beings. For such purposes bio-techno-scientists expand their research endeavors into outer space for conducting space exploratory processes. Such bioactivities will emerge new kinetic life conditions on other planets and adapt colonists with new life span. Such adaptive life modifications may create new super class people with new craft unions based on enhanced (or retarded) physical attributes. This period of time is crucial for contiguity or ceasing outer space life span.
- 2076-2200: The Fourth Period – Redesign the Human Genome: Within this period of time, bio-techno-scientists will require a crucial holarchical assessment to support changes for human mass-modifications rather' than to retain the status quo. Such a challenge will not be new to biosciences. This

situation will be extremely difficult, because changes require new learning, disrupt research patterns, and shift politico-economic authorities and social standings to a new form of living. In the future, new bio-techno-scientists may find themselves to proceed with temptation, comforting, promising, and perhaps to argue whether they should leave things as they will be or may speed up to accelerate change and changing agents to new forms of life.

Within contextual boundary of bioethics, experiences from biomedical ethics movements will provide a debating ground to encourage or discourage for change. Nevertheless, medical professionals, in order to promote or demote bioscientific revolutionary changes, will assess all bio-techno-scientific changing experiences and strategic outcomes. If the holistic community of bio-techno-scientists, biomedical practitioners, and bioethicists come to agree that biorevolutionary changes are appropriate and beneficial for survival of "super class" of human race, then the global competitive politics will play crucial role, which nation should enjoy from such a progress and which group of nations should suffer and be destroyed. The social Darwinism theory indicates: the survival of the fittest, and the demise of the weakest and sickest.

The promising biotechnopia revolutionary innovativeness needs to be tested with principles of bioethics: truthfulness, trustworthiness, stewardship, and doing no harm to any human being. Morally, maintaining truthfulness as a super characteristic of intentions and operations is essential for bio-techno-scientists themselves and for the triumph of objectivity over bias and self-interest in biosciences and biotechnologies. Ethically, the promising biotechnopia revolutionary innovativeness should be embodied in the concept of societal stewardship. It should promise how bio-techno-scientists and bioresearchers deal with the effects of discoveries to help human species not to harm or destroy them. The added values to the politico-economic power of biotechlogical holder should refrain the fact they need to avoid harm to others. Also, it is crucial to any type of bioknowledge including biosciences and biotechnologies to consider international human rights. Otherwise it may forge bioknowledge in emerging a new form of significant politico-economic power. What bio-techno-scientists and bioresearchers need is a type of delineation, which should promote the best choices under any circumstances. After reviewing the two competing theories of creation, and evolution, we need to consider power struggle between two Gs: (1) God and (2) Government(s).

ANALYSIS OF THE TWO COMPETITIVE G'S POWER: GOD AND GOVERNMENT(S)

Individuals by their very nature are not self-sufficient. They need to cooperate with one another in order to fulfill their needs. If humans are to survive over time, they must develop biological, biosocial, biopolitical, and bioeconomical power. Every society must maintain pluralistic decisions on the basis of the enormously wide range of bio-techno-scientific potentiality which could be open to them starting at birth through their biological power. Power is one of those value-laden words about whose definition there is a general agreement. Fundamentally, power is the ability to influence or determine the process of life to conform to power-holder's wishes or desires. Power is a set of dynamic functional forces used to implement the desirable ends. There is today no aspect of societal operations that government cannot and will not regulate if the occasion to do sound popular or legislative support exists. Nevertheless any democratic government should respect individual citizen's natural rights and civil rights. Kass (2002: 17) indicated:

> The account of *human* dignity we seek goes beyond the said dignity of 'person' to reflect and embrace the worthiness of human life, and therewith of our natural desires and passions, our natural origins and attachments, our sentiments and aversions, our loves and longings. What we need is a defense of the dignity of what Tolstoy called 'real life,' life as ordinary lived, everyday life in its concreteness. It is a life lived always with and against necessity, struggling to meet it, not to eliminate it.

In the universal and earthly life, there are two types of power: (1) God's and (2) Government's. Sometimes these two Gs are exercising their power over human beings in both constructive and destructive ways. Let us go through an ethical image to analyze these two Gs' power.

The images of God's power are universally and spiritually oriented and Government's power is locally and biotechnopia oriented. God's power is based on absolute knowledge and Government's power is based on relative power. Ordinary people follow more Governmental power and ignore God's power. Poor people rely on God's power and wealthy people rely on their Government's power, because it protects their societal status, properties, and territories. When wealthy people become disappointed or frustrated from their Government's power or physically become weak, then they return back to God's power for empowerment.

God has ordered human beings voluntarily through religious scriptures to follow His goodness and Government has ordered citizens mandatory through the civil law to be obedient. Both Gs promise disobedience to be ended up with punishments. Government punishes randomly disobedient people through fines, imprisonments, injunctions, corporal tortures or psychosocial depravation with possible parole. But God enforces its power without exception and promises justice. God treats both obedient and disobedient people with unknown causes of punishments on earthly life or eternal grace/curse with/without parole. It seems unlikely that the focus on any of the several dimensions of bioethical discourse, no matter how sharply defined and analyzed, will succeed in absolutely excluding God's power. How this may happen? For example, in the sexless processing of cloning human beings, there is no chance for natural selection. It is based upon the intentions and desires of biotechno scientists' baby making craftsmanship mechanisms. Such a craftsmanship of sexless baby making may or may not keep human life human. This may simply be acknowledged that our bioethical discourse will inevitably expose to an unknown complex power struggle between God and Government(s) to create either richness or messiness for human race on this planet. That is the main reason that Government tries to separate itself from the God's kingdom and maintains an independent power. How could it be, and why would Governments want to be is a big question?

In all religious faiths (e.g. Buddhism, Hinduism, Judaism, Christianity, Islam, Mormonism, Bahai'ism) theosophists try to establish the Kingdom of God on earth and biosophists try to implement the Government's ideology in that natural kingdom. It is interesting that after many centuries again the Kingdom of God has become something for which to work, because in the neo-orthodox ideology of separation of religion and science the time has come to examine impossible possibilities. What we have, in sum, are many serious socio-religious and politico-economical efforts to relate bioethics both to the natural crises and to the key elements of contemporary political life. Theosophical thoughts, seen sociologically, are sensitive indexes to the ways in which social change and religious power interact. Religious thought is powerfully influenced by a changing social context. But the resulting forms of politico-economical forms of governmental restatements redefine the values of society in its contemporary circumstances and shape the power-oriented motives of governments to influence individuals who are facing new opportunities and threats.

Now, it is the choice of biotechno-scientists to follow one of these Gs: God or Governments. Bio-techno-scientists strongly believe in their Governments to permit them to do research and provide them sufficient funds – as a source of continuous income to live. They try with their implicit resourceful strengths experimentally penetrating the sanctity of nature and discover the essence of life. They may ignore the spiritual side of life. They ask themselves this question: Is spirituality only about becoming God? Or is it equally about being related to God's inspiration and intuition and acknowledging our humility before God's power – submission to the God's will (*Ensha Allah*) as Moslems believe through their faith?

The connection between certain techno-scientific methodological approaches and religious faiths covers a wide spectrum of intimacy or exclusivity. At one end of a spectrum will be the techno-scientific methods of casuistry and at the other end is religious traditional faiths that have used casuistry for thousands of years to refine human's ambition and selfishness. Thus, application of bioethics can integrate both God's power and Governments' power to redeem human efforts for a better life.

Governments try to establish their biological policies and objectives to crossing species barriers through the genetic engineering of foods, plants, animals, and in some occasions cloning human beings to be easily disposed. Members of faiths follow the God's guidelines and adhere to God's power. They do not interfere with boundaries of natural selection. They try to enhance each individual member of species within the sanctity of the domain of their own existence. Many Jews, Christians, and Moslems believe that cross-genetic engineering and cloning plants, animals, and human beings violate God's plan for living things, while Buddhism and Shintoism believe that exercising bioknowledge capabilities to engineer genes serves negative human motives such as greed and desire for acquiring excessive illegitimate appetite for power.

CONVERGENCE OF BIOKNOWLEDGE INTO BIOETHICS

There are different objectives between domains of bioknowledge and bioethics. While bio-techno scientists and bioresearchers are striving for discovering the mystery of somatic life, bioethicists spiritually are striving to preserving, valuing, and enhancing human dignity and integrity. Nevertheless, both are concerned with intellectual convergence of ordinary things into extraordinary super things. Both parties require intellectual transcendence of a purely intellectual point of view into innovativeness in order to be able to create ones that more shareable and objective of possible life enhancement. The bioknowledge converges ordinary things into practical goodness – convergence on a practical truthful account of how things should be. Bioethics seeks intellectual convergence into valuable convergence of beliefs. This means that a common principle of the world that ought to be is the ultimate objective of bioethics. Therefore, application of bioknowledge to enhance the nature of human race must proceed by development of bioethics in practice, not by our politico-economic ideological beliefs and descriptions, because ignoring the spiritual side of bioknowledge may end up with catastrophes.

An appreciation of the antecedent convergence of bioknowledge into bioethics can create the harmony to which bioethics seeks a spiritual solution to pursue good preferences, experiences, and interests. This requires escaping from egocentric values and searching for the sort of impartiality. Whatever the bioknowlegeable solution, it should have an appeal that is the same for everyone. It is no more possibility to specify a pure objective that can be used methodologically to produce good results. Within such a contextual holistic view, convergence of bioknowledge into bioethics needs an account for collective humanity interest, ecological and natural sanctity, and universalization of human rights and dignity.

MORAL CONVENTIONS AND ETHICAL COMMITMENTS OF BIOTECHNO-SCIENTISTS

As the third millennium began, the world's evolutionary paradigm of bioknowledge has been reshaped in as fundamental manner as at any other time in human civilization. In our modern society, the level of reliable bioknowledge about life has increasingly developed. By any measure these bioscientific advancements and biotechnological breakthroughs are extraordinary achievable and unmatched in history. Just to give you an idea of the rate of expansion of our bioknowledge since 1900, the number of research papers published in the field of biochemistry was of the order of thousands; 100 years later, the equivalent number stands at more than 500,000 conference papers and professional journal articles a year (*Financial Times*, 2001: 11). Nevertheless, with all of these progressive bioscientific and biotechnological efforts, people feel that the world is becoming an increasingly uncertain and dangerous place to live. The main reason for such a pessimistic impression lies not on the neutrality of biosciences and biotechnology, but rests on the intention and objectives of some bioscientists and biotechnologists who morally, ethically, and legally abuse their discoveries, or provide ample opportunities for immoral and unethical people to abuse scientific discoveries and misuse technological breakthroughs for the purpose of evil acts (e.g., biochemical germs and biological weapons).

The ascertainment of any virtuous intention and action is a difficult matter. Users in the light of new egoistic observations and inhumane objectives could reverse these virtuous intentions and actions continuously. For these reasons, there must be bioethical rules and principles in order to safeguard the sanctity of bioknowledge. The urgency to include bioethics in all biological curricula in bioacademic programs and bioresearch centers is not tantamount to relativism. The acceptance of bioethical rules and principles implies an admission that bioscientists and biotechnologists need to be like physicians under oath in order to safeguard human life and eco-life.

Today, most colleges and universities offer the degree of Philosophy Doctorates – Ph. Ds. to qualified bioscientists and biotechnologists without offering them any course in philosophy, biosophy, and bioethics, because they believe that these scientists are highly specialized in their fields. That is why academic authorities justify their reasoning that academic life and the existence of bioscientific and biotechnological curricula do not have room for social sciences and humanity.

To most modern academic institutions separation of academia from politics is like separation of the church from the state. What is lost between the two Gs' (God and Government) zones is ethics in which links them to each other in societal life. The modern political life is not anymore free from religious and ethical values. This type of conception has been very prominent in subsequent religious and political theories. The political ideological civil rights require us to accord everyone an equal status in some sense – the same status we claim for ourselves in their treatment of us; and that this status should be defined as a kind of inviolability. On the other hand, religious faiths promote humanity with a moral boundary that accord us a degree of commitment to act in pursuit of goodness, kindness, and kindredness without interference by others not violating the identical boundary of spiritual life. That all human work depends upon this assumption that often disappears from sight when academicians are immersed in their specialization or distracted by the demand of commercial industries.

Just as if we assume that sickness is a myth, there is no point in having medical ethics, if human natural rights are a myth there is no point in having a justice system, and if biosciences and biotechnologies are myths there is no point to have bioethics. That is why it is urgent to remind graduate schools to include ethics in their advanced programs in order to orient their graduates not to forget that their intellectual contributions in all fields that they study, teach, and conducting research should respect human dignity and integrity. Thus, bio-techno-scientists should stand together for two things: (1) for pursuing the intellectual integrity and (2) freedom of inquiry with bioethical inspiration and avoid inhumane causes even if it has politico-economic motives.

One primary objective for today and tomorrow bioknowledge is to make efforts to manage biosciences and their leverages according to virtuous value systems. Humanely, the bioscientists and biotechnologists' convictions should be devoted to do the right things and avoid evil actions. Having greater access to scientific formulas, technological breakthroughs, and information systems is useless unless bioknowledge to be put into the use for further legitimate and ethical operational processes. Bioknowledge neutrality should lead and be equated with ethical virtuous neutrality for professionals. The former is acceptable as a condition of personal career and the latter is acceptable as a condition of social justice. The quest for ultimate ethical valuable bioknowledge is one side of the equation between money-power and humanity-power. Those professionals who use money-power for bioknowledge merely increase the distance between what is possible and what is desirable. To exert money-power or material-objects without aiming toward humanitarian moral imperatives is to exert money-power without moral responsibilities.

THE EMERGENCE OF GERM LINE ENGINEERING AND A NEW EUGENIC SOCIAL CLASS STRATIFICATION

The eventual implementation of the gene engineering, the gene therapy, the germ line, the cell line, the stem cell research, and the eugenic therapy will emerge a new structured class of human species in a full-blown eugenic society. Such a society will create both economic and genetic classes of people who will be deferred from the present natural and socio-economic class structures. Once bioscientists, bioeconomists, and politicians know that there are lots of natural organisms on earth to be exploited for achieving politico-economic purposes, they will use them as biological means to achieve political ends. Converting the paths of evolutionary natural selection into innovative evolutionary cloned selection certainly is not the only way to arrive at ethical and moral end points because it may or may not create an economic dovetail. It takes at least generations to see the full-fledged consequential effects from innovative cloned selection. This was true in nuclear energy and synthetic chemicals; it will likely be true of bio-techno-scientific endeavor as well. By an ethical and moral point of view, we may not to say that genetic engineering, gene therapy, stem cell research, and cell therapy will be bad for humanity, but simply by a conservative point of view *we do not know* what they will be.

Biopharmaceutical industry already has started to enhance its R&D capabilities according to the selective classes of biological type of gender, race, age, and color of people. They are manufacturing those drugs, which are affordable for the first class of people to buy, monopsonies. The main reason for such a biobusiness strategy is the economic affordability of purchase power of consumers that provides them a safe haven towards profitability.

We know that if something will be wrong in innovative evolutionary cloned selection ultimately the worst threat appears to wipe out appropriative-targeted classes of people selectively than nuclear weapons or biochemical, biological warfare, and microbiological pollution.

Through biophysical research, it is proven that bioradioactive elements such as radioactive iodine substances, which have been used for hyperthyroid treatment, have half-life and biochemicals, which are used for treating cancerous cells, will be breakdown in specific periods of time. But effects and/or side effects of cloned genes will go on and on through future of generational human species. Which species or classes of people will be affected by cloning species? It depends upon covert up intentions and strategic politico-economic implementation of such biochemichal, biological, and microbiological warfare.

WHAT IS THE PARADIGM OF
BIOKNOWLEDGE MANAGEMENT?

In today's free market economy, the basic organizational resources are no longer material capital, labor, or natural resources, but knowledge-wealth. As previously stated, knowledge is not the same thing as scientific formulas, data banks, and information systems, although it uses all of these phenomena. Knowledge manifests itself a step further beyond scientific boundaries. It is a conclusion drawn from application of scientific formulas, technological breakthroughs, and information systems after it is linked to other known and unknown phenomena and compared to what is really known and what we should know.

Within the contextual domain of bioknowledge inquiry, our initial concern is to state precisely how we view the paradigm of bioknowledge management as an integrative system of scientific, informational, and knowledge-based endeavor. In terms of the fundamental distinction, first, we can question whether this paradigm is a tacit knowledge or explicit. Second, whether the paradigm of bioknowledge focuses on intellectual capital and captures measurement of the intellectual intangible assets. Third, whether this paradigm of bioknowledge is concerned with optimization of knowledge creation and its smooth flow into organizational life or if it is viewed as a transformation of bioknowledge into practices. The proceeding ethical remarks lead us to the methods that are operational to the bioscientific, biotechnological, and bioinformational success. To aid the following discussion, we will define several terms associated with the paradigm of bioknowledge management.

We may perceive that since the objective of qualitative natural life is to discover the new path toward excellence, therefore, the paradigm of bioknowledge management is to deal with those acts that proceed from deliberative good will in the field of biomedical and biopharmaceutical industries. Nevertheless, the extent of the nature of scientific goodness is highly variable and at some levels, it is controversial. For example, in the industry of transportation, scientific discoveries facilitated more quick population and commodities movements; however it created more pollution to harm the environment and people.

Application of biotechno-scientific knowledge in pharmaceutical industry creates crucial liabilities for biotech corporations. This raises the question: Are they morally liable for the application of their patents? For example, the availability of birth control pill has been linked to socio-cultural phenomena ranging from the economic empowerment of women to the disintegration of the family, causing side-effects, and epidemic infertility. Could bio-techno scientists whose work led to oral contraceptives have anticipated their effects and tried to shape them? The public's view of biotechno-scientists and bioresearchers is marked by debates: Are people expecting for scientific miracles? Do people mistrust the power of biopharmaceutical industry and their monetary motives to influence their natural lives? Pharmaceutical companies must educate the public about their products and ensure that their self-regulation merits public confidence.

MULTIETHICAL ASPECTS OF BIOKNOWLEDGE

At the heart of the evolutionary multiethical paradigm of bioknowledge management systems (MPBMS) lie four related forces: (1) advancement of science, (2) convergence of technological breakthroughs into computing, communication, and information systems, (3) explosion of knowledge, and 4) assertion on validity and viability of progenistic bioknowledge for the conclusive operational result of innovative outcomes. This new integrated membership functioning system of know-why fuzzy logic, know-what structures, know-where information, and know-how knowledge is now generally manifested in the composition of bioethics. For the clarity of these attributes, we will analyze each one within their contextual boundaries as follows.

WHAT IS KNOW-WHY FUZZY LOGIC?

In order to decide why bioknowledge should be oriented toward discovering the truth, we must first ask: "Why is know-why biologic the essential nature of inquiry?" This theme explicitly shows the essential continuous reasoning which should determine the nature and direction of bioknowledge in all places and times. Know-why biologic signifies the rational reasoning that represents the essential nature of truth. Truth can be perceived through three major causes: formal causes, material causes, and efficient causes. As Parhizgar (2002: 51) indicated, within a matrix of the truth, there are three levels of biological reasoning: (1) necessity of reasoning, (2) sufficiency of reasoning, and (3) vitality of reasoning including quiddity and equilibrium biologic (see Figure 7.1).

CAUSES AND REASONING	FORMAL CAUSE	MATERIAL CAUSE	EFFICIENT CAUSE
NECESSITED REASONING	Logical truth	Scientific truth	Generalized truth
SUFFICIENT REASONING	Syllogistic truth	Technological truth	Prodigical truth
VALIDITY OF REASONING	Deductive truth	Observable truth	Synergistic truth
NETURE OF TRUTH	Conventional truth	Pragmatic truth	Progenistic truth
	↓	↓	↓
	CONVENTIONAL TRUTH	PRAGMATIC TRUTH	PRODUCTIVE TRUTH

Figure 7.1: The Matrix Structure of the Essential Truth

There are three cause-effect consequences of different types of truth. These consequential functioning truthful attributes are: (1) conventional, (2) pragmatic, and (3) productive. Each type of truth provides you with different judgments concerning decision-making processes in bioethics. Through conventional moral truth, bioscientists are viewed as trustworthy people whose responsibilities rely on their personal dignity and integrity. Through pragmatic amoral truth, pharmaceutical corporations are viewed as successful scientific based entities whose responsibilities rely on quiddity and equilibrium of cost-profit analysis. Through productive legal truth, biopharmaceutical and biotechnological industries are viewed as effective entities whose responsibilities rely on the synergistic functioning of holistic socio-professional outcomes. For example, in related areas, the explosion of information from the Human Genome Project is anticipated to have crucial consequences on its ethical and social ramifications.

Discovering the truth requires relentless holistic rational efforts to be expressed concerning the truth. Know-why biologic is the embodiment of the examination of our implicit conceptions, explicit perceptions, and deductive judgmental reasoning concerning the complex domain of truthfulness and falseness of bioinquiries. Within the contextual boundaries of know-why biologic, there are two extreme opposite poles: (1) truthfulness and (2) falseness.

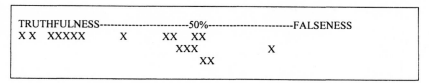

Figure 7.2: Syllogistic Reasoning Proximity for Truthful
Assertion in Fuzzy Functioning Membership Logic

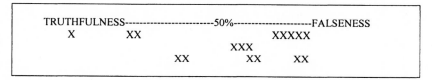

Figure 7.3: Syllogistic Reasoning Proximity for Falsehood
Assertion in Fuzzy Functioning Membership Logic

By looking at Figures 7-2 and 7-3, we may find that if something is true, therefore, it can not be wrong or *vice versa*. However, there are some "membership functions" of parameters and events within the domain of biologic that indicate some functioning membership groups are partially right and others are partially wrong– effects and side effects. Such a conclusive result manifests the degree of relativity and reliability. For example, if you examine the positive effect of Lipitor, Zetia, or Tricor for lowering the cholesterol and their side effects on liver you may find both relative and reliable consequences of righteousness and wrongness. The relativity of a compounded membership functioning facts in biologic substances and biomedical procedures depends on the location, the volume, and the size of characteristics of the membership functioning groups and their holistic proximity assessment between the magnitude of truthfulness and falseness and their more proximity towards one side of the magnitude of righteousness and wrongness; risk assessment.

From another perspective, since religious faiths and cultural values of some membership functioning groups are differentiations of moral and ethical perceptions of specific groups, and groups are periodically refunctioning, then they may not be considered as pure truthful or falsehood connotations. The consequential results of righteousness and wrongness depend on circumstances and laden values to save life of a group of people. For example, the controversial issues on having abortion for women have created ethical and moral debates. Is it a crime or is it a professional duty for a physician to practice abortion in order to save the mother's life? This is the major argument concerning absolutism and relativism of moral and ethical judgments: pro-choice or pro-force. This type of reasoning is known as fuzzy logic. Therefore, fuzzy logic specifies billions of probabilities and possibilities of integrated membership functioning systems between the poles of righteousness and wrongness. In order to analyze such a complex task, we need to identify the magnitude of the truth from the standpoint of fuzzy logic. For example, let A be the event that a decision selected is of economical type, and let B be the event that another decision selected is of ecological type; if we ask a mathematician, a bioscientist, and a lawyer:

For example, let A be the event that a decision selected is of economical type, and let B be the event that another decision selected is of ecological type; if we ask a mathematician, a manager, and a lawyer:

For the result of $P(A \cap B)$, we get these responses:

A mathematician using the multiplicative rule of probability replies with: $P(A \cap B) = P(A) \bullet P(B)$, assuming that A and B are independent events.

A bioscientist in search of synergy replies with: $P(A \cap B) = \mu > P(A) \bullet P(B)$, assuming that A and B are correlated fuzzy events.

A lawyer considering divorced events replies with: $P(A \cap B) = 0$, assuming that A and B are disjoint or mutually exclusive events.

This assumes $P(\bullet)$ is a probability function with domain A (an algebra of events) and counterdomain the interval $[0,1]$ which satisfies the axioms of probability theory; and on the other hand m represents a fuzzy membership function associated to the probability of the intersection $(\cap)$ of A and B. .
    The meaning of "synergy" effect $(\Delta H = H_S - H_T)$ can be clarified by using the annual rate of return (H) for all n independent products in a product line, $H_T = (S_T - O_T)/I_T$, where S_T represents.

The total sales of the firm for all their unrelated products $(S_T = \Sigma S_T)$,

similarly for operating costs $O_T = \Sigma O_i$ and investments $I_T = \Sigma I_T$.

$S_S = S_T$, but if $O_S < O_T$ and $I_S < I_T$, therefore $H_S > H_T$, where subscript S denotes the respective quantities for an integrated firm, while subscript T is the sum for independent enterprises. The synergy effect can produce a combined return on the firm's resources greater than the sum of its parts. In other words when companies are splitting the synergy will be lost. When companies are merging the synergy then the synergy is emerging.
    Fuzzy logic embraces gray areas and partial truths (amoral). Fuzzy logic was introduced by Lotfi Zadeh (1965: 338) as a means to model the uncertainty

of natural phenomena. The process of fuzzyfication, as a methodology, generalizes any specific theory from a crisp (discrete) to a continuous (fuzzy) form. Fuzzy logic is a way to deal with the uncertainties and reasoning we have as human beings. Fuzzy know-why logic is a kind of reasoning that speculates answers in favor of more complex explanations. The end result of fuzzy logic is progenistic innovation.

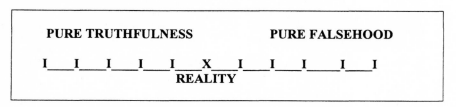

Figure 7.4: The Domain of Fuzzy Logic Reasoning

A progenistic innovation is a creative mindset of novel things. It is a new way to think about everything. Innovation is best described as pervasive creativity that perceives drastic change beyond the present and creates a future vision. According to moral and ethical judgments concerning good or bad, just or unjust, fair or unfair, and right or wrong, people constantly change their positions and express their views differently. This type of judgment is related to fuzzy know-why logic.

Fuzzy logic is a superset of conventional (Boolean) deductive logical system that has been extended to handle the concept of partial truth truthful values between "completely true" and "completely false." As previously stated the Boolean body of logic establishes a range of values with multiplicative identities in which every element is an idempotent. This means that when an element multiplies by 0 or 1, it remains unchanged [e.g., $(0) \bullet (1) = (0)$ or $(1) \bullet (1) = (1)$] or when a truthful phenomenon multiplied by a truthful phenomenon then the result equals to the truth).

Sometimes in fuzzy logic we cannot classify and specify some effects in terms of just black and white. According to fuzzy know-why knowledge, people are constantly reengineering, restructuring, reorganizing, and reexamining their views about life events. Therefore, fuzzy thinking, fuzzy logic, and fuzzy future are the essence of human rationalization of reasoning. Fuzzy future confuses community with networking, joy with stimulation, and meaning with matter. Fuzzy future logic is really the best we can hope for sometimes it asserts truthfulness and sometimes overrides falseness. For example, according to moral and logical fuzzy knowledge there are three major domains of reasoning: (1) algebraic logic, and (2) boolean logic, and (3) fuzzy logic.

Algebraic Logic	**Boolean Logic**	**Fuzzy Logic**
$R \bullet R = R2$	$R*R = R$	$R \otimes R = \mu_{R \otimes R}$
$R \bullet W = W \bullet R$	$R*W = W*R$	$R \otimes W = \mu_{R \otimes W}$
$W \bullet W = W^2$	$W*W = W$	$W \otimes W = \mu_{W \otimes W}$

Where R represents an event of take a right action, and W is the event of take a wrong action, while   represents a fuzzy membership function of the product of two events. If we look at the above equations through Algebraic logic, Boolean logic, and Fuzzy logic we will find different outcomes of reasoning when we compare them to each other. We know that R $\neq W$, but if we let $R = 1$, and W = -1, thus $W^2 = R^2$, then for example, if something becomes wrong in a society for all citizens then according to algebraic logic that wrong thing will be perceived as good for all. If a tyrant behaves equally to all citizens, then according to Algebraic logic that behavior is perceived as justice. But in Boolean logic and Fuzzy logic the result of wrong things is wrong and it does not follow the algebraic rule. This is the nature of biosciences.

The comparative results indicate that there are three types of moral and ethical cultural reasoning among nations as follows:

- Those nations that believe and assert that everything, by its inherent nature, can be either good or bad and we cannot change good to bad or bad to good because good is good and bad is bad; absolute logic.
- Those nations that believe and assert that everything could be good and bad, and depends on our perception; fuzzy logic.
- Those nations that believe and assert that survival is not related to good and bad and we should not use such distinctions in our lives. Survival is a mandate. Survival is an amoral phenomenon; algebraic logic. It is logical to follow law rather than moral and ethical principles in our daily life.

There are two types of logic to be perceived in practice in such a process (1) Causal and (2) Consequential. For example, impressive bioscientific research achievements have made extraordinary progress in the field of recombinant DNA molecules. These techniques have a remarkable potential for furthering our causal understanding of fundamental biochemical processes in pro and eukaryotic cells. The use of recombinant DNA methodology promises to revolutionize the practice of molecular biology. Nevertheless, some bioexperts believe that recombinant DNA molecules may create biohazards (Berg et al., 1993: 263).

WHAT IS KNOW-WHAT BIOKNOWLEDGE STRUCTURE?

One of the foremost problems for biosciences is know-what bioknowledge structuring of the value added systems in medicine, health care, and the life sciences. This is viewed as establishing a bridge among multifaceted scientific deliberations. Bioknowledge as synthesized concentration of human intellectual efforts in genetic challenges with issues such as DNA recombinant processes, prenatal genetic testing and abortion, genetic manipulation, and eugenics can create critical arguments concerning bioethics. Reasonable scientific principles for dealing with these potential issues raise serious risks. In such a domain of inquiry, there are different levels of risks that should be considered:

- *Minimal risks* either with minimal, low, moderate, or high interference of restructuring a new substance.
- *Low risks* either with low, minimal, moderate, or high interference of restructuring a new substance.
- *Average random moderate risks* either with low, minimal, moderate, or high interference of restructuring a new substance.
- *High risks* either with low, minimal, moderate, or high interference of restructuring a new substance.

From the standpoint of bioknowledge and bioethical research, human genetics has been a continuous source of intriguing. The recent worldwide interest in a project to structuring the genetic road map and ultimately sequencing the estimated three billion base pairs of the human genome has created bioethical controversy over the effects and side effects of such bioknowledge on human beings. Controversial bioethical issues may be grouped into four categories:

- To disclose genetic information about individuals and populations to the interest groups (e. g., governments, insurance companies, employers) for good or bad consequences.
- The manipulation of human genotypes and phenotypes for structuring phylontype groups of individuals; promotional speciation of the fittest groups (Parhizgar and Parhizgar, 2000, 185-187).
- Challenges to understand makeup of individuals and groups and their propensities towards diseases, sicknesses, and injuries.
- Challenges to manipulate genes for treatments of unpredictable diseases; especially human made germ lines.

Structuring bioinformation concerning individual and group genes by biotech corporations can be used for specific objectives of interest groups. Also, such bioinformation can be used for modifying people with innovative and patented biotechnology.

People Modification With Synthesized Hormone Therapy

The ability to clone a human gene incorporates it into a microorganism or mammalian cell line and purified gene product can have substantial ethical consequences. Human growth hormone (hGH) is the result of this biotechnological innovativeness. Such a biotechnological methodology and product was used in biosynthetic hGH to be taken from pituitaries of human cadavers for the purpose of major therapeutic use for hGH-deficient pituitary. For example, the biosynthetic hGH has been used to make non-hGH deficient children taller. This raises a question: who will be able to afford to use hGH in pregnancy and/or fertility clinics? The answer is: Those wealthy and adventurous families who can afford to pay the cost. In a business term, such groups of people are known as *monopsony*. If we believe that monopoly in our market is unethical, then monopsony will be unethical too.

Genetic Testing for the Benefit of Insurance Companies

In the insurance industry, there are some principles as both insurance companies and insured people agreed upon. Those issues define the involved risks for parties to be involved. Insurance companies function on the agreed bases of sharing risks between buyers and sellers. As much the risk is higher the uncertainty will be higher too. This can cause all parties to contribute equitably certain gains and loses. For example, the older people are the greater the risk of death and consequently they should bear more cost sharing with higher premiums for life insurance. As Wilfond and Fost (1990: 2777) indicated insurance companies have begun to think about what to do with tests for genetic predisposition to diseases. There are two inherent factors to force insurance companies with or without consent of customers to proceed genetic testing. First, individuals can be tested privately to learn whether they have enhanced risks of deformities or deficiency syndromes. When they learn about the results of genetic testing, then they are more likely to buy larger amount of life insurance. In the insurance industry, this phenomenon is known as "adverse selection." Second, competition among insurance companies will tend to drive companies toward gene screening for predisposition of diseases and/or deformities. Therefore, genetic testing can provide more leverage for insurance companies to increase premiums and/or denying selling insurance to more risky people. Such a business issue creates collision between bioethics and business ethics.

Genetic Testing in the Workplace

Genetic testing in the workplace can cause serious ethical problems. As Murray (1983:5) indicated, it has four purposes: diagnosis, research, information, and exclusion. Genetic testing and/or genetic screening of applicants and current employees like many other procedures can be helpful or harmful for both employers and employees. Their use within the context of bioethics is related to diagnosis, treatment, prognosis, and therapeutic research. These are governed by the medical ethics of human subject and they are covered under the Privacy Act.

Genetic testing and genetic screening may also be used for hiring or not hiring particular applicants to uncover a genetic susceptibility believed to put them or not at greater risk of occupational diseases associated with hazards in the workplace. In addition, employers may use genetic testing for screening non-susceptible workers to lower their health care insurance costs. This can exclude many qualified workers and cause discrimination based on natural endowed characteristics; deficiency syndrome and/or deformities.

In structuring the know-what bioknowledge structure of bioethics, identification of the boundaries of the moral, ethical, and legal value systems should be closely related to the distinctions of three domains: (1) cognitive issues, (2) affective parties, and (3) effective substances.

Cognitive Issues: To deal with cognitive issues, biotechno scientists often choose selective perceptions by making conscious or subconscious beliefs and opinions on what issues possess scientific priorities. Sometimes those issues are related to their professional commitments and sometimes they are related to the status of their occupations. In professional commitments bioscientists may not violate human rights. But in occupational issues they may ignore human rights and respond directly to their institutional objectives. For example, CBS and or AP (2005) indicates:

> Correspondent Elizabeth Kaledin reports that in an unprecedented move, the journal published what calls an "expression of concern," chastising the study's authors and saying "at least two of the authors knew about the three additional (heart attacks) at least two weeks before submitting...drafts of the study... The findings of what become known as the VIGOR study have been a key part of testimony in the three product liability trials to date over the withdrawn drug; Vioxx.

Nevertheless, institutional objectives could be moral, amoral, or immoral. Judgments concerning validity and viability of these types of occupational issues are directly related to bioresearchers' personal conscience cognizance. These and other similar issues identify the basic foundation of normative morality.

Normative morality is based upon personal self-disciplinary and societal-discretionary ordered value systems. Normative morality manifests bioresearchers' moral principles, beliefs, and expectations to justify their behavior on which they base their judgments and actions. The ethical societal norms identify distinct sets of socio-cultural value systems including legal rules for behavior. These ethical normative rules provide various sources including family and friends, the local community opinions, national beliefs, religious indoctrination and faith, econo-political platforms, the workplace attitudes, and of course, civil law and international human rights. In addition, the cognitive domain of bioscientists' judgments includes those objectives that deal with the recall or recognition of knowable problems concerning defective medications or therapeutic radiation. This requires the establishment of research centers to collect and compile all data as the main source of know-how knowledge concerning both providers and users. Then an exchange of information between parties must be established. This is the domain in which it is central to the continuity of work together in order to improve quality of life. For example, *CBS/AP* (2005) reports:

> Authors of a study funded by Vioxx maker *Merck & Co.* failed to disclose in a report published in the *New England Journal of Medicine* in 2000 that three additional patients in a clinical study suffered heart attacks while using the now-withdrawn painkiller, the journal wrote in an editorial released Thursday (December 8, 2005).

Affective Parties: The second part of know-what bioknowledge is concerned with the affective domain of knowledge. It includes structuring mutual objectives, which describe changes in reengineering the workplace and reconstructing interest, attitudes, values, and development of appreciations and adequate adjustments to new environmental conditions. Know-what bioknowledge objectives in this domain should be defined precisely? All involved parties should be informed about genetic testing purposes and consequential decisions and actions. The geneticist J. B. S. Haldane (1938) observed that all workers exposed to a particular occupational hazard become symptomatic. He postulated that the difference in response to toxic exposure was at least in part genetically determined. Compulsory genetic testing leads society to possible exclusion of gene deficiency from employability. It can violate individual natural law and civil law. For example, Murray (1993: 287) indicated testing for sickle cell anemia followed by exclusion of those with the trait would effectively exclude one of every eight black job candidates in the U.S.

Effective Substances: The third domain is the manipulative restructuring of the know-what bioknowledge for the benefit of special interest group. Although pharmaceutical companies recognize the existence of this domain either for the benefit of certain groups of patients, sometimes they do not believe in development and appreciation of these objectives because of heavy investment in R&D. They ignore manufacturing tailored medications for rare diseases because of cost-benefit assessments of reasons. Ethical effectiveness should be purely descriptive. This indicates that the value systems or quality of one class of value as compared with another should not be established quantitatively or momentarily. This means that pharmaceutical companies should avoid partiality to one view of morality, ethics, and legality as opposed to another. They need to attempt implicitly to avoid biased judgments and actions. Another way of saying this is that valuable moral, ethical, and legal objectives that describe intended behavior should be included in the paradigm of bioknowledge.

WHAT IS KNOW-WHERE BIOINFORMATION?

Know-where bioinformation in the field of biosciences is a matter of actual operational knowledge. In order to acquire scientific bioknowledge certain steps with an appropriate pragmatic methodology are followed in a scientific experiment. The bioresearchers must assess what has been accomplished by others, develop an appropriate innovative scientific hypothesis, design a comprehensive research project with crystallized objectives, execute step by step the experiments necessary to test hypothesis, repeat similar testing on the basis of triangulation methodological systems to find correlated end results, records, processes, analyze the data obtained, and compare the acquired results with similar professional published articles. High quality of experimental execution is necessary at each step to insure validity and viability of the resulting consequences. Ethically and morally, it is important to disclose the normal range of discrepancies at each stage and in repeated experiments. Bioresearchers must avoid fabrication, falsification, and plagiarism, because poor data management and failure to observe safety regulations can end up with controversial consequences. For example, it is observed that failure in disclosing the total side effects of a medication can cost lives of many people (e. g., implantation of Silicon Gel in women breasts).

WHAT IS KNOW-HOW BIOKNOWLEDGE?

Now that we have analyzed know-why, know-what, and know-where bioknowledge, we want to describe how this dynamic bioknowledge paradigm system can be used in biotechno-scientific ways. The biotechno-scientific advancement has made more effective and efficient use of medical technology. As silicon chips for integrated circuits have created the computer, so III-V-chips have created the light emission and detection revolution. In the presence of computer sets or electronic data systems, bioresearchers and physicians can detect bodily defections and exchange medical information in real time. For example, the method to monitor the nuclear spin by nuclear magnetic resonance (NMR) has produced new analytical tools for diagnostics. Similarly, radiography by nuclear diffusion of GeV protons is now being used as a complement to X-ray tomography. With each advance in basic physics, a new diagnostic or treatment tool can be developed.

The most know-how integrated bioknowledge progress is the gene-identification project. The 100,000 functional genes that part of the forty-six chromosomes are identified and coordinated with the bodily traits reveal millions of gene-locations for certain abnormalities. From earlier studies of pedigree transmission of heritable abnormalities, a large number of genetic diseases with simple Mendelian pattern are known. For instance, the Tay-Sachs disease (on Chromosome 15), Huntington's disease (on Chromosome 4), immunodeficiency (on Chromosome 20), or retinoblastoma (on Chromosome 13) are identified by know-how bioknowledge. All these know-how bioknowledge deliberations represent only a small fraction of life sciences as to gene function. What remains to be done is the full coordination of millions of genes to the loci under their control (Matare', 1999: 63).

WHAT IS KNOW-WHOSE BIOKNOWLEDGE?

The primary task of syllogistic bioknowledge is to discover members of scientific and scholarly professions. These professionals are citizens of their own large societies to which they have, by virtue of their elaborated stock of rigorously tacit knowledge. An occupation requires a more than ordinary amount of tacit knowledge. Also, it is an acquired tacit and explicit knowledge by persistent and systematic study and authoritatively certified knowledge. The primary task of a knowable person is the acquisition and transmission of knowledge and its logical reasoning application to solve complex problems. Within this contextual boundary, there are different types of people such as academicians, technologists, informationists, and biosophists.

Academicians acquire, discover, and assimilate bioknowledge by scientific methodological studies, interpret them logically, and scientifically transmit them to learners. Academicians transmit bioknowledge about the methods of discovery especially the validation of knowledge in problem solving. They discover and transmit the principles and techniques of the application of knowledge and their rules or methods governing their application to learners.

Biotechnologists apply the explicit knowledge which bioacademicians taught them in practice. Technologists examine what bioscientific formulas are known about particular phenomena and how to dispel error, confusion, and misunderstanding of pragmatic application of knowledge. Bioinformationalists seek large stocks of complex and imitative knowledge that have not been mastered by the laity of their clients, to whom the professions address themselves. This paradoxical acquisition of bioknowledge gives to the infomationalists large opportunities abuse the position of acquired information.

Bisophists' possession of syllogistic logical reasoning requires greater intellectual breadth in amount and intensity of fundamental criticized and tested reasoning than scientists, technologists, and informationalists. These differences in the amount of and quality of holistic bioknowledge possessed by biosophists are ultimately the ground for the exploration of innovative reasoning and predictable solutions. Nevertheless, bioscientists are reputed to not only have specialized knowledge and the inclination of objectively considering alternatives, but also are reputed to have scholarly, detached, and dispassionate judgment.

From a bioethical point of view, the Job-Shop Know-How Bioknowledge is viewed as a vital source for strategic decisions and actions that crystallizes the establishment of a continuous regular production system on the basis of the "know-whose" dimension. Bioknowledge can reside wholly within an expert, or can be shared within a professional group, or the firm's managerial system. In all of the above cases organizational knowledge-wealth maintenance is a complex and dynamic valuable commodity in our today's economy. This is related to retention of experts and specialized employees. Brown and Woodman (1999: 175) stated:

> Essvac is a vaccine manufacturing company wholly owned by Archer Pharmaceuticals Ltd (AP)... AP has declared its interest in product development (vaccines) in its mission statement and has research and development (R&D) division as part of its operational structure. Henry Black was the only member of that division with both theoretical and practical experience of vaccine R&D. He was due to retire in 18 months' time and, whilst there was talk of him being missed, both for his knowledge and his contacts, there were no plans to replace him. No other mechanisms existed within the organization to retain his knowledge for the Group.

Within the terminology of labor efforts this peculiar trend was considered as preserving the Job-Shop knowledge within AP. It was internalized by recipient and used as a component part of the organizational knowledge-wealth. The ethical question might be raised was: What was Mr. Henry Black's intellectual freedom concerning being hired by another pharmaceutical company to produce the same type of vaccine? "Was he free to do so, or was he under moral obligation to the Shop-Right not to take the company's secrets to other competitors?

CHAPTER 8

MELIORISTIC BIOETHICS OF HUMAN SUBJECTS IN BIORESEARCH

CHAPTER OBJECTIVES

When you have read this chapter you should be able to the following:

- Understand what are ethical, moral, and legal responsibilities in biopharmaceutical companies.
- Question why do biobusinesses need ethical philosophy.
- Reason why do biotechno scientists need moral philosophy.
- Know what do we mean by populism and individualism.
- Know what is reciprocity in the field of biobusiness.

- Define what is competition.
- Make a distinction what is the difference between oligopoly and monopoly.
- Know what are different types of property ownership.
- Describe what are the differences between copyrights and patents.
- Describe what is shop right.
- Know what is the difference between a brand name and a counterfeit bioproduct.
- Understand what is wrong with insider information and privacy.
- Recognize what are differences between price fixing and price discrimination.
- Know what is the difference between price fixing and tying arrangements.
- Know what is the difference between bribery and payola.
- Know what we mean by melioristic biosophy.
- Make a distinction between what is selflessness and selfishness.
- Know what are the principles of libertarianism. Know what are the principles of conservatism.
- Know what are eudaemonistic principles of ethics.
- Understand what are hedonistic means and ends in bioethical justifications.
- Know what are the ethical and moral differences between eudaemonistic and hedonistic moral principles.
- Know what is the difference between dignity and integrity.
- Know what are the differences between discipline and order.
- Know what are different rights and duties.

PLAN OF THIS CHAPTER

The main idealistic mission of biosciences and biotechnology is based on meliorism theory of bioknowledge, a doctrine that the world tends to become better or may be made better by human efforts through pragmatic scientific experiments. Within such a positivistic biosophical foundation, bioresearchers try to conduct their research experiments within the boundary of ethical, moral, and legal limitations in order to be led to the discovery of future knowledge.

Philosophically, the theme of this chapter has been selected on the bases of the internal crisis of the Baconian melioristic ideal. Francis Bacon (1561-1626) addressed himself to the problem of knowledge. He asked himself how is it possible for human beings to know everything with certainty or to have a reliable, truthful, and usable knowledge of the nature. He attacked earliest methods of theoretical seeking knowledge. He rejected the methods of the schoolman or scholastics; the thinkers in the academic tradition of the Middle

Ages. Middle Ages ideal of knowledge had been rationalistic and deductive. That is, its characteristic procedure was to start with definitions and general propositions and then discover what further knowledge could be logically deduced from the definitions thus accepted. These methods followed the Aristotle moral reasoning and ancient codifiers of human thoughts. Bacon held that the medieval (or Aristotelian) methods were backwardness. He held that knowledge is not something that we postulate at the beginning and then explore it in its ramifications, but that it is something that we can find at the end, after a long process of investigation, experiment, or intermediate thoughts. Bacon, thus, announced the advent of a pragmatic scientific civilization. This is known as a leading search with innovative ideas as empiricism. Empiricism research is based on observation and experience.

This chapter examines the melioristic views to arrive at an ethical and moral conception of human to understand the kinetic position of human beings in nature in contrast to the misunderstanding of humanity and nature that fuels the Baconian melioristic ideals. This indicates that predecessors' views concerning the conception of the human values have traditionally claimed the biosophical perception concerning knowing the nature should not be based on the certainty or the robust content. It should be based on evidence in practice. Finally, this chapter describes the dialectic arguments concerning biotechno scientific power that characterizes the modern subject and plays out through a peculiar combination of moral commitments and ethical responsibilities of biotechno scientists.

INTRODUCTION

One of the most ethical and moral issues of meliorative bioresearch is related to human beings used as subjects of biomedical experimentation. Hans Jonas (1974: 117) expressed his opinion concerning this issue as:

> The designation of research is essentially melioristic... Unless the present state is intolerable, the melioristic goal is in a sense gratuitous... Both nobility and the gratuitousness must influence the manner in which self-sacrifice for it is elicited, and even its free offer accepted.

Also, Hans Jonas (1974: xvi) described the decade of 1960s as the emergence of the most acute, internal crisis of the Baconian ideal that woke him up from complacency about the perils of biotechnology. McKenny (1997: 39) indicated:

> What shattered this complacency was the ecological crisis and developments in human (especially genetic) engineering; in other words, the growing threat to the biosphere that sustains human life and the capacity of refashion human life through genetic, biochemical, and

neurological interventions.

The Sixteenth century's melioristic ideal of Baconian bioknowledge became reality in the late Eighteenth century when Thomas Jefferson introduced America's first Patent Act. Jefferson was determined to ensure that "pragmatic ingenuity should receive a liberal encouragement." In 1793, the U.S. Congress enacted into law a proposal allowing inventors to patent "any new and useful art, machines, manufacture or composition of matter, or any new useful improvement [thereof]." As established by the 1793 law, a patent was granted by the U.S. Government giving the patent owner the sole right to make, use, or selling an invention within the United States during the term of the patent, generally 17 years (Kimbrell, 1994: 26).

Again after passing more than four hundred years, the Baconian melioristic biosophy became a reality in life sciences. On October 29, 1991, the. United States Patent and Trademark Office (PTO) issued a patent of a type never imagined by both Bacon and Jefferson namely "the patent of human body shop. "On that day, for the first time, the PTO granted patent rights; patent number 5,061,620, to Systemix Inc., a Palo Alto, Californian corporation to control of human bone marrow stem cells (stem cells being the entrepreneurial progenitors of all types of cells in the blood). The PTO had never before allowed a patent on an unaltered part of the human body. Such a historical event created a new path in bioethics and raised many fundamental issues. First, what the government of the United States established was to build new blocks of human life belonged not to God, nature, or humanity, but to biopatent holders. Second, how could be this? How human natural body parts including genes, cells, stem cells, cell lines, proteins, and embryos become commercialized? How living things including human beings or parts of human somatic limbs being patentable products in our civilization? Finally, how the natural life became a commodity to be bought or sold by monopolistic appetite of patent holders with permission of the U.S. Patent Office? These and other ethical and moral questions will be the milestones for furthering discussions and analyses in this chapter.

In searching for advancement in bioknowledge that may benefit mankind, bioresearchers need to implement their scientific ideas in practice after going to go through very detailed professional codes of ethics. In all bioresearch endeavors, all scientists and technologists must respect human dignity and integrity. They need thoroughly inform research participants with great details of possible consequential benefits and risks of harm. Therefore, using human subject should be based on moral principles to disclose both possible benefits and risks of harm. Prior to their experiments, bioresearchers must acquire the voluntary consent of research participants. They need to avoid as being amoral; only to disclose a portion of the truth not the whole. In addition, bioresearchers need to acquire collaborative efforts of research participants to disclose honest and relevant feedbacks with good faith and goodwill.

Honesty, nobility, and altruistic intention of individuals and even sometimes sacrifices in voluntary participatory bioresearch projects need to be appreciated. This means that not only biotechno scientists receive full credits for their scientific discoveries, but also those research participants' rights who put their lives in danger should be recognized and rewarded too. This is one of the foremost problems of bioresearch. Nevertheless, ethically and morally biotechno-researchers need to be committed to the highest virtuous objectives of humaneness that indicate when disasters occur in experimental cases, they need to mitigate the degree of risks of harm to human subjects. The motivation and humanitarian intentions of voluntary human subjects in bioresearch experiments must be found as Jonas (1974, 119) stated: "the sublime of dedication and ultimate commitment,... the sphere of the holy." Within such a moral context, there are moral reasoning and ethical means and ends.

MORAL REASONING CONCERNING THE MEANS OF HUMAN SUBJECTS

Experimentation of animals as objects in biosciences is not new. There is a long history in performing biological testing on animals. But soon as humans became subjects of experiments for acquisition of bioknowledge then the question of conscience aroused. Conscientiousness is mandating human alertness to respect personal dignity and sacrosanct in civilized world. The major issue in bio-experimental processes is related to separation of individuals from society and misusing individuals as subjects in bioresearch. Then the most serious profound tension arises between individual goodness and common goodness. Such a tension indicates how society and biosciences may infringe the human rights of the individuals in biomedical experiments.

There are some of difficulties hidden in the arguments by the terms of society-individual, and interest-rights in biomoral choices. People are not aimless. Whatever the aim is, they make good and bad choices. People do whatever they intend to do and behave in that manner. What they intend to do is whatever they deliberate on selves and others' reasoning for achieving good and/or evil ends. It is true, in one sense, that an end is last in execution, for it is the last thing to happen. But in another sense the end is first, not in the order of execution, but in the order of intention (Oesterle 1957: 17).

Deliberation is a pragmatic and possible workout of reason. We consider and evaluate reasons for or against doing something. We still need to understand the nature of a choice itself because the act of choice may cause a misunderstanding. Morally, a right choice should be based on goodwill. It should follow the intellectual reasoning for specifying the right ends through the right means. A bioresearcher without intellectual deliberation and good choices cannot succeed at creating an everlasting goodness. Bioresearchers morally need to establish in their character sufficient good intention, goodwill, useful knowledge, and reliable information in order to make good choices and to take good actions. Within such a moral characteristics, there are two important views: (1) eudaemonistic and (2) hedonistic means and ends. Both dimensional characteristics are related to the moral codes of behavior. Therefore, the melioristic global bioethics concentrates on the duel dimensions of human thoughts and behavior namely eudaemonistic and hedonistic means and ends.

EUDAEMONISTIC MEANS AND ENDS

Through eudaemonistic goodness an individual's moral, ethical, and legal ordinations can be characterized by observing conscience, conscientiousness, integrity, dignity, honesty, rightness, discipline, orders, rights, duties, responsibility, accountability, respectfulness, politeness, courage, prudence, truthfulness, trustfulness, fairness, justness, fortitude, patience, goodwill, good faith, magnanimity, perseverance, sincerity, and loyalty. It spells out what are major moral attributions concerning behavior of biotechno scientists and bioresearchers.

What Is Conscience?

An individual possesses a sense of self-love. According to English Philosopher Joseph Butler (1672-1752) self-love is the effective regulative principle that operates when individuals organize their desires to promote their own best interests. When they control their appetites to further proceeding points of the public good, the operative principle is that of benevolence. Yet, Butler tells us, there is no guarantee that these regulative principles of self-love and benevolence will always reinforce and complement one another. Under these circumstances, conflicts between personal and social interests are frequently resolved by a regulative principle of a higher order, namely, the conscience. The term *conscience* is the functioning of reason that at times acts as the arbiter of conflicting interests between self-love and benevolence. It is the commander of our moral obligations to convince us to perform our moral duties (Butler, 1849). Therefore, conscience is the knowledge of right and the self-evidence of conviction within an individual's personal judgmental perception.

Culturally, we have laid down what must seem to be forbidding rules in our civilization. Having moral faith in transcendent potential capability of humans will ever fail a society that does not destroy evildoers; and only such a one is worthy of conscientiousness. Since the elite biotechno scientists are by nature small and they combine attributes of personal aimed objectives with information within the state of absence of external authoritative pressures, they may tend to do whatever they desire. Such a motivational pressure without conscience consequential awareness infringes the societal order of permissibility. Therefore, conscience mandates individual bioresearchers to shift their personal objectives to docility, ambitious-mindedness to compliance, and judgment to trust.

What Is Conscientiousness?

The term *conscientiousness* is a moral cognitive conviction by an individual who controls his/her decisions and actions according to their conscience. It is a dynamic movement agent in an individual's moral mind that manifests the final self-attestment. As indicated in the above definition, conscientiousness is the self-attestment, from which there can be no appeal to any higher moral or ethical principle. It is the supreme ultimate end in an individual's moral character. That is, the state of excellence in the mind and judgment. For example, biotechno scientists should have faith in sanctity of life. Life itself exists not only by human rights, but also by natural faith. This means that respect for *life* is an implicit natural conscientiousness of attestment by all individuals to enlarge the right to live and avoid the right to shrink.

What Is Integrity?

The term *integrity* means soundness of and adherence to the ultimate state of moral character; excellence. Moral and ethical principles mandate people to preserve their honest thoughts and express their intellectual ideas without fear of retaliation. The German philosopher Friedrich Nietzsche (1844-1900) believed that a moral person needs to be independent in thought and strong in conviction, even in the face of group pressure and government authority (Nietzsche, 1917). Martin Heidigger (1889-1927), another German existentialist philosopher expressed his ideal of nobility and thoughts for the importance of resolutive conviction to personal integrity rather than succumbing into socio-political pressures to conform. He believed personal integrity means that one cannot coexist with everyone who is not ethical, so it is incumbent on each person to choose individual lifestyles and commitments carefully.

What Is Dignity?

Dignity is an undemocratic idea, because it is not an essence of majority and minority group's characteristic. It is related to an individual's personal characteristics. The central notion etymologically, both in English and in its Latin root (*dignitas*) is that of worthiness, elevation, honor, and nobility in short, excellence in character. Dignity is closely related to the degree of excellence in relation to the manifestation of self-identity. Dignity means qualitative self-respect to the conformity of excellence in an individual's moral character. It is an honorable worthiness for suitable and sustainable characteristic traits for a person. An individual with a high quality of dignity tries to elevate their moral behavior to the highest standard of morality and ethics. For an individual, self-worthiness is normally extended to the consideration for oneself as an independent dynamic agent. Thus, dignity is the highest honorable behavioral tendency to represent a favorable manifestation of self-identity, based on a comparison of one's own worth comparing with that of others.

Biotechno scientists are particularly relevant examples of group-pressure that can potentially damage individual integrity and dignity (Heidigger, 1962). *Dignity* is closely related to self-consideration in relation to the manifestation of self-identity. Dignity means self-respect gained by the conformity of excellence in an individual's moral character. It is a base for suitable characteristic traits for a person. Individuals with a high quality of integrity try to elevate their moral character to the highest standard of morality and ethics. For an individual self-respect is normally extended to the consideration for oneself as an independent agent. Self-respect is the opposite of self-contempt. Thus, integrity is an ultimate tendency to represent a favorable opinion of self-image according to the highest state of intellectual excellence.

What is exactly the human dignity in bioscientific deliberations? In the strictest sense, human dignity would mean that *life* is something sacred and transcendent. The sacredness of life should not be violated or destroyed by passion and desires of others. By natural law, life should be defended and preserved. Through sanctity of life, it is not something as such but life lived in certain natural way. Nevertheless, this doesn't mean that bioscientists should not try to enhance human life.

What Is Honesty?

The term *honesty* means an individual is a straightforward and trustworthy in dealing with the discovery of truth and expression of the truthful judgments concerning self and others. An honest person does not withhold one's own feelings, ideas, and knowledge relevant to realization and expression of the whole truth. A moral person reveals, by all means and ends, the whole truth, only the truth, and not beyond the truth, while an amoral person reveals only a portion of the truth.

What Is Rightness?

Moral and ethical decisions and actions are nothing less than the full awareness of what one ought to be according to their religious faith and cultural value systems. Thinking about revealing the truth in biosciences is no more than acknowledging that one has taken into account and is willing to be righteously responsible for their effectiveness and efficiency in relationship with other rational findings. Rightness in bioscientific deliberation is a mandated self-conviction for attesting to justness and being decisive to attest the rightful judgment on the basis of three principles as follows:

- **Careful consideration** of the rightful principles needs to be applied. This considers causes, means, ends, subsequent consequences, and such specific concerns as justness.

- The need for prompt rightness of **contributions** to the well being of a society through the value and quality of the usefulness of judgments.

- The need to be committed to carefully viewing the impartial **consequences** of the usefulness of judgments in relation to the intentional and unintended reputation of self, one's own institution, and an industry.

For example, in the forensic expert witnessing and/or hearing, the most important ethical and moral convictions of experts are to be neutral and express the whole truth.

What Is Discipline?

The term *discipline* is an intrinsic precision of one's own mind through behavior to act in accordance to the rules of self-conscience conduct and/or organizational mandated beliefs. It is an orderly behavior in accordance with the maintenance of self-integrity and dignity. Obedience to the intellectual conscientiousness or to the mission (the legitimate reasons for the existence) of a pharmaceutical or biotech corporation is a matter of discipline. There are several personal attributions related directly to disciplinary behavior such as appearance, respect, politeness, punctuality, dependability, efficiency, and cooperation. Although disciplinary actions in organizations are considered as desirable and necessary for orderliness, they raise concerns about fairness, justness, and rightness for the individuals in the way they are treated.

What Is Orderliness?

The term *orderliness* is an extrinsic precision of one's surrounding belongings and/or atmospheric environment. It is a purity of neatness and putting in a sequence of arrangement all things on the basis of necessitated arrangements. Orderly people do not live in a messy and filthy environment. We need to avoid living in a messy condition. Ethical and moral people need to keep their environments clean. Many bioscientists and bioresearchers are observed to be in love with carelessness or by negligence in destroying the experimental hazardous substances. They may destroy species by pollution and by introducing new species that overtake native species (Kempton et al., 1995: 27).

What Are Rights?

Rights are legitimate claims which one person has or can make on another. A right defines a freedom of choice and action. Rights are moral entitlements or privileges that invoke corresponding duties on the part of others. A right to own material objects is a voluntary choice of the use to which those objects will be managed. A right to a specific action, such as free speech, is the freedom to engage in that activity without repression or prosecution. The connection between rights and duties is that if someone has a right to own something, then someone else has a correlative duty to act in certain ways. We have moral rights derived from specific relationships, roles, or circumstances in which we ought to be. For example, as individuals, we have the right to survive and others have the duty to respect it. Rights are divided into two classes: (1) Natural Rights, and (2) Other Rights.

Natural rights are those rights that are created by nature. Natural rights are those entitlements that morally constrain social orders. Natural rights ought to be developed through a mandatory process. Natural rights are self-evidence of coexistence. All men and women view them equally. In modern days, natural rights, through the Charter of the United Nations, are called *human rights*. The other rights are societal agreements and/or entitlements (e.g., parental rights, civil rights, collective bargaining contracts rights, etc.) concerning social privileges for individuals and institutions. For example, Title VII of the Civil Rights Act of 1964 in the United States with the *Equal Employment Opportunity Commission (EECO)* protects employment rights against discrimination. Also, the *Human Development Report of the United Nations* (2000), in terms of human rights, indicates that having access to income and education is an example of competing claims on resources, not rights. In addition, it indicates that the rule of social rights is not only vital to protect the interests of domestic and foreign investors, it is also essential for all domestic citizens, above all the powerless (*Financial Times*, 2000: 12). Or in the United States to have access to medical facilities is viewed as a privilege not as a right. This means that if you are employed by an institution which provides you with health care insurance, you will be able to manage your health and medical care costs. Otherwise you will have difficulty in supporting your medical costs. Also the Act of 1978 prohibits discrimination against pregnant women. The 1967 Age Discrimination in Employment Act extends protection to people 40 years of age and older. The Americans with Disabilities Act (ADA) of 1990 extends protection to the private sector by requiring all companies with more than 15 employees to make reasonable accommodations in order to employ workers with disabilities. Also, HIV infection diseases such as AIDS are considered as a set of disability and the ADA law protects people who have it.

What Are Duties?

Duties are those self-mandatory commitments to conform to natural and societal rights. Duties are what one is morally required to do to self and others. Duties are conscientious determinations of a person either to do or to refrain from performing certain acts. British scholar W. D. Ross (1930: 42) divides duties into seven basic types:

- **Duties of fidelity:** that is, to respect explicit and implicit promises to deal with people, to create expectations, reliance, and trust.
- **Duties of reparation:** that is, for previous wrongful acts.
- **Duties of gratitude:** that is being grateful or thankful for receiving favors.
- **Duties of justice:** that is, by the quality that a person is virtuous in all respects.
- **Duties of beneficence:** that is, to make the condition of others better.
- **Duties of self-improvement:** that is, to drive a person progressively to become what one is capable of becoming.
- **Duties to not injure others:** that is, to avoid vicious decisions and actions.

What Are Responsibilities?

Responsibility is closely related with rights, duties, and obligations. Responsibility is the self-conviction to comply with a formal societal just cause. An individual has a responsibility, in the moral sense, to do those things that are mandated by moral duty. For example, biotechno scientists and bioresearchers have three major moral and ethical responsibilities:

- They are trustees of various scientific discoveries.
- They are powerful agents for the wise execution of scientific principles, policies, and procedures.
- They have the obligation to balance the interests of the bioscientific community and institutions in which they are working in.

These three interrelated responsibilities trusteeship, executive, balancing of interests, and coordination are the main ethical and moral responsibilities of contemporary biotechno scientists.

What Is Accountability?

Accountability is closely related to several other concepts besides duties and responsibilities, obligatory and mandatory commitments, possibilities and capabilities in doing something, and finally making alternative choices for doing right or wrong actions. Accountability means the acceptance of the consequential results of self-conducts, and the willingness to answer to higher authorities what is being done. It is the obligation to give an account of our decisions and actions to higher scientific authorities and/or society. Accountability is conditional. A person needs to be accountable, if causes and consequences can clearly justify reasonability, appropriateness, correctness, and prudence in his/her decisions and actions. Accountability includes liability in intentional and consequential outcomes within the boundary of self-mandated behavior.

There are many attributions attached to accountability such as: praise and pride, blame and condemnation, and shame and remorse. *Liability* for one's actions means that one can rightly pay a compensatory price for the adverse effects of one's own actions on others. There are moral and legal liabilities. For example, the Superintendent of the Corpus Christi School District was found accountable for buying liquor with the school district's money. According to the records, he lost his jobs over a 1995 receipt that included a glass of wine in his lunch, paid with taxpayers' money. Taxpayer's money should be spent for educational purposes, not for personal pleasure (*Laredo Morning Times*, 2000: 10A).

What Is Magnanimity?

Magnanimity means being generous in mind. The word magnanimity is made up of two Latin words: *magna*, means signifying great and *anima*, means signifying the soul. Therefore, the nominal meaning of this value is to be generous in mind. For example, for a bioresearcher, magnanimity means to have deliberation with good reasoning by the demonstration of great prudential efforts, regardless of cost and benefit analysis for disposing dangerous substances. Magnanimity is the breath of qualitative intention and action toward building and maintaining conformity in high qualitative character. In the lab nobody is present when a bioscientists dumps dangerous viruses and leftover of hazardous substances into the drain or garbage cans. It is his/her moral and ethical magnanimity to dispose them scientifically.

What Is Perseverance?

Perseverance is another moral virtue where an individual is persistent to achieve specific legitimate objectives regardless of obstacles and annoyances. A biotechno scientist perseveres in the virtuous sense, if he/she reasonably persists in achieving a difficult action, even though the length of time necessary to complete that action is long and laborious. For example, bioresearchers strategists need to develop the virtue of perseverance in their thoughts and behaviors because they have to wait scientifically to achieve their strategic objectives over a long period of time with continual efforts. They should not be hasty.

What Is Courage?

Courage means the high quality of mind in decisions and actions that enables one withstand facing with difficulty, danger, and pain as the result of standing against unethical and immoral people. In the course of bioscientific deliberation, some scientists need to stand firmly and without fear against unjust and unfair practicing human subject. Courageous people tend to be fearless in expression of their rational reasoning with acceptance of possible retaliatory actions. Courageous decisions and actions are very risky.

What Is Prudence?

Prudence is an intellectual manner of careful consideration when an individual is faced with problems and issues and acting or reacting with care. Prudence is a careful moral obligation toward particular decisions and actions for achieving good-ends through good-means without risk. A biotechno scientist needs to carefully assess the circumstances of a decision or an action in order to understand what should or shouldn't be decided. In addition, bioresearchers need to make sure that a decision or an action should have an assent to suitable scientific means and ends. A bioresearcher needs to avoid inconsistency in his/her intentions and negligence in actions. We should not give credit to a selfish biotechno scientists or biomedical practitioners with good intentions who does the wrong thing. Crisis in biohazardous substances needs courageous people to solve problems. All professionals, paraprofessionals, should know prudent decisions and actions and occupationals and all employees should be expected to act accordingly. However, prudence may be either good or evil.

What Is Truthfulness?

Truthfulness means conformity with causal fact or reality. An individual's moral and ethical conduct is based upon truthfulness, and validity of causes and reasoning in decision- making processes and actions. Sometimes reasoning is based upon sensational and emotional attachment of an individual to pleasure and enjoyment (to enjoy for a logical success or to enjoy with unjust reasoning of failure of others as a sign of revenge), and sometimes it is the result of intellectual deliberation on factual logical reasoning for actuality of existence. To say that a statement is true is to make the claim that it accurately manifests the signs of reality for the factual existence of an object or a state of affairs. The term *validity*, on the other hand, is only our attestment of the existence of reality with the structure of reasoning regardless of just causes.

The truthful ethical decisions and actions in bioexperimental projects and the use of human subject depend on how consistent a bioresearcher is with the ethics of knowledge. In regard of these issues, there are several questions that should be answered as follows:

- Is it true that the concept of scientific thoughts and statements and those of ethics and values belong to different worlds?
- Is it true that the world of scientific thoughts and actions are subject to tests? Is it true that the world of *what* is subject to test, and the world of *what ought to be* subject to no tests?
- Is it true that the power of intellect differs from the power of willingness and from the power of desire?

To know something well through reason is to know something as true. Truthfulness, therefore, is the reasoning of intellect to perceive facts or reality. For example, *CNN.Com* (2005) reports:

> Vioxx was withdrawn in September 2004 after being shown to double the risk of heart attack and stroke in clients taking it for more than 18 month. More than 6,00 lawsuits have been filed against Merk in the United States, alleging Vioxx caused hearth attacks and deaths... In reviewing the diskette that data on cardiovascular events had been deleted from the manuscript before it was submitted (to the New England Journal of Medicine)... The evidence has raised questions about the integrity of data on adverse cardiovascular events in the article and about some of the article's conclusions.

Truthfulness in decision-making processes and actions should be based on three conditions:

- Correctness of the just cause
- Soundness of structural reasoning
- Validity of information and data

What Is Trustfulness?

The term *trustfulness* is the reliance on the dignity, integrity, and confidence in a moral and ethical character. Trust is fragile. It takes a long time to build. It takes a short time to break. It is hard to regain (Sonnenberg, 1993: 22). Recent research by Schindler and Thomas (1993: 563) identified five dimensions that underlay the concept of trust: Integrity, Competence, Consistency, Loyalty, and Openness. They found that importance of these five dimensions is relatively constant:

Integrity > Competence > Loyalty > Consistency > Openness

Moreover, integrity and competence are the most critical characteristics that an individual looks for determining another's trustworthiness. They found that integrity seems to be rated highest in such a magnitude of values because without a perception of the other's moral character and basic honesty, other dimensions of trust were meaningless (Butler and Cantrell, 1984: 19-28).

What Is Fairness?

Fairness is a moral characteristic and ethical obligation of an individual to judge about self and others' behavior free from bias, discrimination, dishonesty, and inappropriate comments. A decision or an action is fair if all involved parties engage in the process freely, without coercion. If all parties have adequate and appreciative knowledge of the relevant aspects of an issue, then the deliberative judgment can be fair. If one of the parties misrepresents the criteria, hides relevant information in some way, or intimidates the other party, then the procedural and consequential result of judgment would be unfair. Fairness is a meaningful word to be considered in the behavior of bioresearchers and biomedical practitioners. When we talk about fairness, we are not talking about equality; we are doing something equitably, reciprocally, and impartially.

What Is Justness?

The proper object of *justness* is right, that which is just. The proper Latin word for right is *jus,* and hence right is only another name for the just. Through an ethical point of view, justness does have three clarifications:

- The first is that the source of justness is natural law. Natural law is a generalized principle for an individual action inclining feelings toward what is good in nature.
- The second point is related to an individual's extrinsic cultural reasoning, which is related to econo-political and sociocultural value systems. These value systems are called rights, in relation to and consequences upon the end-results of goodness.
- The third point is related to an individual's intrinsic cognitive conception concerning human rights. Individuals are concerned about themselves regardless of the consequences for the common good.

Justice is a matter that essentially dissolves serious disputes between parties. Justice is based on an individual's moral rights. Justice is essentially comparative. Justice becomes an issue when parties unevenly compete with each other, when benefits and treatments are not equitably distributed, and when rules and laws are discriminatory administered. The moral right of an individual entitles that person to be justly treated like others. Justness depends on the idea that benefits or penalties should be distributed equitably for all. In other words, the moral rights of some individuals cannot be ignored or sacrificed merely in order to guarantee a somewhat better distribution of benefits for others. If we think that exploitation of less endowed nations by some multinational pharmaceutical corporations in the Third World Countries is unjust, then such an action is immoral and unethical. We then condemn a pharmaceutical corporation that exercises exploitation, even if exploitation makes those citizens economically stronger. The greatest benefits for some economically deprived children in a country cannot justify injustice for all children around the world. Philosophically, standards of justice do not override the moral rights of individuals. There are three types of justness:

- *Distributive Justness:* That is concerned with the fair distribution of benefits and related burdens on all. However, unjustness is unjust.
- *Retributive Justness:* That is concerned with the imposition of punishments, penalties, and fines upon those who do wrong.
- *Compensatory Justness:* That is concerned with the just remedies for those people who lost some rights when others wronged them.

What Is Righteousness?

Righteousness means an individual is suitable to what they are supposed to do, or that a judgment should be suitable to what is in conformity with facts, reasons, standards or principles. From an ethical point of view, any decision or judgment could stay with the right course of action by too little or too much. An obvious instance is found in our daily attachment to special habits, tendencies, or extravagancy such as workaholism, alcoholism, sexism, prejudicism, and others. A biotechno scientist and bioresearcher need to reason correctly when it comes time to expressing causes of judgments and decisions according to a speculative order of knowledge. The right reason is true knowledge of ethical principles.

What Is Fortitude?

Fortitude is a blending behavioral mode of endurance during expected emotional fear and intellectual expression of boldness in making the right decision. People possess different levels of fortitude. These levels are the potential strengths in their minds that enable them to endure adverse events with courageous actions. Fortitude is clearly an admirable intellectual virtue that an individual can create through a high quality in thinking, strong positioning power in choices, and positive attitudes in progressive actions. A biotechno-scientist needs to have the best-known intelligible attitudes toward successful and useful means and ends of self-conduct. Fortitude is not equivalent to courage. Fortitude brings out more accomplishment in intellectual deliberations, whereas courage is sometimes applied to an emotional or sensational action without assurance of the final possibility of positive consequences.

What Is Patience?

Patience is a virtue that moderates behavioral frustration during various hasty decisions and actions. Patience promotes and develops cheerfulness and principally tranquility of the state of the generous mind despite great injuries and other subversive actions. Fortitude is closely related to the extent of endurance and tolerance. Patience in times of miserable situations prevents morale breakdown. Patience mitigates grief and sorrow. Some times a biotechno scientist or a bioresearcher will be exposed to unpleasant situations as a result of failure of his/her error, negligence, carelessness, or bad intention. They need to relieve themselves from such a grief and boldly face with the harsh reality.

They need to be patient because they are behaving as a thoughtful and intellectual people who have the responsibility of leading their discipline. They have to bear unpleasant consequences. In contrast, impatience often promotes selfishness, hastiness, greediness, anguish, fear, frustration, and anger.

What Is Sincerity?

Sincerity denotes to a moral character that possesses a sense of justness free from deceit, hypocrisy, or falseness. A biotechno scientist or bioresearcher needs to be sincere in his/her mind and action. Sometimes people say something but act differently. These people are not judged as sincere people.

What Is Loyalty?

Loyalty means willingness to promote and respect the interest of someone to whom an individual has an obligation or commitment. Loyalty is associated with fidelity. Loyalty is a reciprocal obligation of two parties to each other (e.g., husband and wife; employers and employees). According to the American Idealist, Josiah Royce (1916: 16-17):

> Loyalty is the willingness and practical commitment through-going devotion of a person to a cause. A man is loyal when, first, he has some cause to which he is loyal; secondly, he willingly and thoroughly devotes

himself to this cause; and when, thirdly, he expresses his devotion in some sustained and practical way, by acting steadily in the service of cause.

However, loyalty is not ethical and moral when we notice the loyalty of a thief to another thief. Biologists are celebrating a historic achievement with the announcement of drafting the first human genome *the Book of Life*) that provides our biochemical blueprint in 3 billion genetic letters (*Financial Times*, 2000: 16). Francis Collins and Eric Lander (*CNN.com*, 2004) indicated:

> We humans don't look very impressive in the completion… It is not just the numbers of genes that matters; it really is how nature uses these genes. … In comparison to simpler organisms, humans benefit more from genes that turn out multiple proteins rather than one, and from complex proteins that do more than one job.

Also, Gerald Rubin, another gene expert at the University of California, Berkeley, said: "The result is good a guess as one can make at this point… I think the estimate is unlikely to change very much… So how can human be so complex with relative few genes?" (*CNN.com* 2004). The new estimate is 20,000 to 25,000 genes, a drop from the 30,000 to 40,000 the same group of scientists published in 2001. Since, half of each individual's DNA is inherited from parents, traditionally, a DNA paternity client was an angry mother trying to pin responsibility on her ex-lover to support their children. This action has been changed.

Today, in the field of biotechnology, men are now turning to DNA labs to identify their partners' fidelity. The major moral, ethical, and legal issues are related to the loyalty of a married couple. Through the testing of children's DNA spouses can discover their partners' loyalty. A biologists, professionally, is committed to discover and express the truth. However, through ethical and moral commitments there are two different sides of these issues: (1) according to the deontological theory of ethics bioscientists should be loyal to their profession and tell the discovered truth or (2) according to the utilitarian ethical theory to be loyal to the cohesiveness of a family and not to disclose the truth. In today's liberal societies, male insecurity about their partners' fidelity is creating a massive new client base for DNA experts, fueling an expansion in the testing industry (Adiga, 2000: 16). In different cultures, there are different proponents of both consequences.

What Is the Goodwill?

Choice and deliberation are two major component parts of a *will*. We need to understand the nature of moral obligations, *the goodwill*, in order to make a right choice. An individual can make a choice on the basis of either emotional or intellectual reasoning. Emotional choices can end with pleasure (appropriate sensational and feeling enjoyment) or pain (excessive sensational and emotional deprivation). In contrast, intellectual choices can end up with happiness (appropriate usage of intellect) and avoidance of misery (inappropriate and/or no usage of wisdom). Simple emotional acts of desire are not choices of an individual's will. Emotional desires are acts of tendencies for pleasure. An individual's will is an intellectual satisfactory intention in reasoning. Intellectual choices are not necessarily connected with pleasure or pain, but with happiness and satisfaction. Also, intellectual choices are associated with self-volition, that is, as being very intent on getting what people seek.

What determines the goodness of good will? Kant (1724-1804) answered this by saying that the will is good when it is completely devoted to duty for the sake of duty. As for duty, it is prescribed by the moral imperatives. Thus, the goodwill is reverence for the duty and duty is founded on reason.

What Is the Good Faith?

The *good faith* is considered as reaching to the perfect stage of human moral power. It attains whatever is the good of a power. The good faith differs from the power of willingness and from the power of desire. Both of these powers are appetitive powers. However, abuse of power has always happened, and will always happen. Whereas the faith is a cognitive power, greedy power is an emotional power. The good faith consists of grasping things in a rational and reasonable mode of assurance. To know something is good because it is good to know something as true. For example, in a medical laboratory or pathological test work on a sample, a microbiologist or a pathologist decision to rework an unusual testing result with good faith is considered as moral decision to treat patients with good faith through retesting. Sometimes symptoms or sampling tissues are contaminated, thus it is necessary to retest them. It also makes bioscientists be conscious of doing what is right even with more costs and efforts.

What Is the Good Humor?

Dooley (1941: 37) stated:

> *Humor* is an attitude toward an event, situation, or to a life that makes what otherwise would appear sad and terrible seem insignificant and amusing (or at least tolerable). It rather tends constantly to turn aside suffering to create happiness.

Freud (1960) stated that humor is one of the highest psychic functions enjoying the special favor of thinkers. He describes humor as the vehicle that lets energy that has built up in certain psychic channels be used or discharged in spite of the usual censoring by the superego. This energy may be discharged or converted in a language or behavior that is funny. Good humor is viewed as a brake in a serious situation. It helps to curb expanding energy on feelings. Turning psychic suffering, pain, and pleasure into energy, which is felt as humorous pleasure, is efficient (Buchman, 1980: 1715). Laughing truly takes less energy and time than crying, and we feel better. We can be in pain for extended periods of time but we cannot keep on laughing for long. Freud (1928: 2) states that: "Like jokes and the comic, humor has something liberating, about it; but it is also has something of grandeur and elevation, which is lacking in the other two ways of obtaining pleasure from intellectual activity."

Good humor is different from bad language. In good humor, people consider moral and ethical behavior, while in bad language; people use dirty jokes and unethical or immoral slang.

Grotjahn (1956) spoke of four humorous moral or immoral or ethical and unethical behaviors:

- The *Kidder,* a derivative of the word like a child, is, like a child, in a position of humility and passive endurance. This humor style mocks playfully, yet with an element of cruelty. Usually, women do not kid, as it is socially unacceptable. Instead, they tease.
- The *practical joker* is an eternal adolescent. As a style of humor that employs cruelty, practical joking falls halfway between an intended aggression and its intended witty, verbal, and nonverbal expression.
- The *wit* is a person whose humorous personality style is formed by destiny, not by choice. When angry, he/she uses his/her natural talent as a weapon.
- The *clown* has his origins in his costume and acting funny things out.

Coser (1960) studied humor as a communication facilitator among colleagues. It is known as an equalizing function, which reduces distances between people. Salameh (1983) classifies humor into four levels: (1) destructive humor, (2) minimally helpful humor, (3) very helpful humor, (4) outstanding humorous language.

What Is Serenity?

Serenity means the desire for quality in making peaceful and tranquil discoveries of relationship with goodwill. It is a moral characteristic in which an individual creates an honorable, respectful, and reverent social atmosphere by using good and polite words in communication. Serenity is not only respecting others, it is also related to showing dignity in self-identity.

What Is Politeness?

Politeness means showing good manners and courteous respect toward others in the forms of verbal and written communication, body language, and behavior.

HEDONISTIC MEANS AND ENDS

Sometimes for some people the denominator of goodness is based on their emotional, sensational, pleasurable, and enjoyable ends. These good characteristics are called hedonism. *Hedonism* holds that the basic values of goodness are the differentiation power between pleasure and pain. According to this type of view, everything that people pursue or demand should be directed toward enjoyment or simply as the absence of pain. This view contains selfishness. Just as a healthy body that cannot compromise with the filthy and vicious mind, intrinsic moral goodness cannot work by compromising between vicious and rational intentions. The goodness comes from the healthy mind and the healthy mind comes from the healthy body. If not, then evil ideas and vicious actions are giving rise to the greedy means of appetitive selfishness to win evil ends. Through hedonistic perceptions an individual's behavior may be exposed to evil means and vicious ends such as: cynicism, nepotism, favoritism, cruelty, filthiness, felony, slithery, greediness, heartlessness, falsification, viciousness, revengefulness, cheating, stealing, plagiarism, gossip, rudeness, dishonesty, egoistic, incompetence, offensiveness, reproachful, fraudulence, negligence, deception, harmfulness, harassment, intimidation, influencing, falsification, corruption, scandals, unfairness, unjustness, and wrong doing, exploitation, discrimination, false advertising, and breach the contract. In order to understand in depth these human characteristics, we will define them as following.

What Is Cynicism?

Cynicism is a pessimistic mental characteristic of an individual who doubts or denies the goodness of human motives and who often displays attitudes by sarcasm. It is a bad habit that manifests in a contemptuous mistrust of scientists, politicians, religious, and business leaders, (Olasky, 1985).

What Is Cruelty?

Cruelty means letting nothing stand in one's own way and using any methods and all means and ends to wipe undesirable things out. Cruelty is an extreme degree of selfishness by a person willfully and knowingly causing pain and harm to others. Such an emotional motive is derived from the lack of kindness, gentleness, and compassion.

Many critics of bioresearch with animals believe that simply having the capacity to suffer, known as biosciences, gives nonhuman animals the right to be treated as ends in themselves, rather than simply as means to human ends. For Caplan (1993: 175), the use of animals in bioresearch is a tragic and cruel event even where justified. At least researchers must recognize their moral responsibilities to animal subjects. They should eliminate atrocity and minimizing their suffering.

What Is Filthiness?

In the field of ethics a *filthy* character means having moral impurity, corruption, and obscenity in an individual's mind and action. Usually, those people who do not observe politeness in their daily communications treat other people impolitely. They use vulgar or obscene words, sentences, and metaphoric slang of foul words and languages to offend others.

What Is Felony?

Felony means committing any various vicious actions that, by law, are prohibited. This malicious and treacherous characteristic converts people into savagery. Misdemeanor character is the pure immoral, unethical, and illegal characteristic of a felon who deserves to be severely punished. Unfortunately, there are many examples of this horrible immoral characteristic in today's field of biomedical ethics. For example, recently there was an English physician, Dr. Harold Shipman, who murdered 215 patients in England (*CNN.com* 2002).

What Is Greediness?

Greediness is an excessive and rapacious desire and appetite for accumulation of wealth and power beyond the legitimate share. We can identify greedy businesses from a moral point of view, how they behave through hostile takeovers, junk bonds, and greenmail. Greed is viewed as an infectious psychological disease, not only to motivate the greedy people to acquire soft money, but also, it motivates others to be absorbed into such a trap. Pernicious greed is nonproductive and its only aim is quick acquisition by almost any means of personal gain as their justified ends.

What Is Churning?

Churning is a special greed in which a selfish person pushes other people to use their rights, assets, and/or reputation for achieving his/her own self-interests as ends in them. Eichenwald (1993: C1) indicated in his article entitled "Commissions Are Many, Profits Few," in the stock market, when brokers encourage unnecessarily their clients to buy and/or sell their stocks in order to reap a commission. This action is not based on moral trust, but it is based on greed and selfishness; churning. The brokers' targets in a churning process are to make deals in order to get their commissions regardless of the client's interests. Likewise, Kant would object to churning in the field of medicine. Churning means when a physician uses patients and/or their specimens such as sperm, eggs, ovaries tissues, stem cells, and blood as subjects in a medical experiment without the patients' consent. Even though great social benefit might result, the bioresearchers would intentionally use the patients as a means to the bioresearchers' own goals and thus fail to respect the patient's basic humanity (Shaw, 1996: 61).

What Is Heartlessness?

Human experiences are conveyed into emotional expressions that allow us to center the perspective of other human beings. Personal feelings take shape within a culture and articulate the experiences of a given life into a more or less meaningful whole. *Heartlessness* means unfeeling and unsympathetic ways of judging others with dysfunctional or fragmented feelings. As long as we behave inhumanely, we ignore our moral and ethical commitments to self and others. Such a cold feeling of unjustness and unfairness motivates of heartlessness people to view their business behaviors as a sole milking customers to the last purchase power abilities.

What Is Revengefulness?

Revengefulness refers to a type of punishment or injury inflicted in return for one received. It is a bitter experience to be carried out to injure another person for a wrong doing to one or to those who are felt to be like one. Different cultural beliefs and religious faiths have different ideas concerning revengefulness. Some believe in forgiveness and forgetfulness while others believe in "an eye for an eye." Nevertheless, revengefulness constructs a chain of sequential aggression and ruthlessness.

What Is Rudeness?

Rudeness refers to deliberated roughness in behavior and language (oral, written, body, and sign languages) with harsh intentions to insult others by *words and bodily symbolic signs*. These types of behavior and communications can turn people into enemies.

What Is Viciousness?

Viciousness refers to grossly immoral intention and action to give or to be readily disposed to evil. Such immoral and unethical means and ends characterize a person by faults and defects. Viciousness may be the most hatred characteristic of inhumane behavior.

What Is Falsification?

Falsification is a form of faithlessness. It is a form of deceit that so clearly identifiable that it has its own name, faithlessness. It is a condition for someone being incorrect, untruthful, and treacherous to testify against innocent people.

What Is Deception?

Deception means any various kinds of concealing, acting, or a statement of fraud in a misrepresentation or conversion of a fact. Deception is an attempt to wrongly persuade somebody to buy a defected and outdated medication as non-defected and usable one with a regular price. It exploits patients with ambiguity, concealing the facts, and exaggerating the superficial usefulness of medicine.

What Is Fraud?

Fraud means breaching the confidence to gain some unfair or dishonest advantage over somebody. Fraud is viewed as an evil act. It is unethical, immoral, illegal, and inhumane for someone who makes deceitful statements to gain illegitimate self-interest. Fraud, in the fields of pharmaceutical and medical industries, is a deliberated use of deception to cause the loss of some value to either one of the buyers or sellers' advantages. In any case of buying or selling out dated or defected drugs and supplements or providing medical services, there is an obligation on the part of buyers and sellers to take reasonable care that the exchange is one of equitable values. For example, if a seller morally injures a buyer with deception, then the seller has committed fraud. In such a case, the seller practices fraud by knowing that the product is defective and does not carry any discount in its price accordingly or does not inform the buyer of the defectiveness.

What is Cheating?

Cheating is a deliberate act of violation of moral and ethical principles. In a legal term, it is viewed as a violation of the rules and regulations of the society. It refers to the use of fraud deliberately to hoodwink someone or to obtain an unfair advantage over another. For example, Schwartz (1996: 22) indicated:

> In the 1940s in *Skinner v. Oklahoma* the court addressed a state statute that provided for eugenic sterilization of some third-offense felons. While the Court found that the statute was a violation of the United States Constitution, its reasoning was not based on the uncertainty of the scientific information or the significance of the decision to reproduce; rather, the opinion was grounded on the finding that the statute violated the equal protection clause of the Fourteenth Amendment because it provided for sterilization of third-time offenders who had committed certain listed crimes (generally, blue collar crimes) and excepted those who had committed other crimes (generally, fraud-based white collar crimes) without any rational basis for that distinction.

In the biopharmaceutical industry, for example, a pharmacist may cheat customers by selling short in dosage of formula or in weight. On the other hand, morally, ethically, and legally, if a buyer practices fraud by a known fact that the seller is ignorant of the true value of a product, he/she takes advantage of the fact and does not pay the seller with the appropriate true value. Buyers also may cheat the sellers if they take deliberated advantage of an error in calculation on the part of the seller or if the seller inadvertently gives back more change to buyers than is due to him/her.

What Is Stealing?

Stealing means to take property of others without permission or right, secretly, or by force. Stealing is the vice of taking unjustly what belongs to others. Shoplifting, money laundering, robbery, pick pocketing, and embezzling are vices of unjustly taking money and/or merchandise that are belonged to others. The above injustices are all committed by deed. There are other injustices such as an inappropriate act of copyright, patent, trademarks, and piracy. These are committed by words. Most of the above injustices not only are immoral and unethical, but also they deserve to be exposed to lawsuits and trials in the courtrooms. For example, the so-called Tuskeggee Syphilis Study in which treatment was withheld from poor African-American men who did not know they were part of a long-term research project on the natural course of the disease conducted by the PHS. Such an experiment caused to steal life on more than 600 prisoners.

What Is Usury?

Usury is a vice of charging excessive interest on a loan of money. This meaning of usury is a modern one. In some cultures, by their religious faiths (e.g., Islamic Faith), usury is observed as a sin and prohibited because money is conceived to have only one essential use, to be properly spent. However, today money is employed for investments as capital in order to develop wealth without human efforts. As long as the borrower is taking advantage of the money, therefore the lender has the right to share an appropriate portion of that profit. At the present time, therefore, usury is understood to consist of a charging a rate of interest that is excessive, (e.g., beyond a rate usually determined by law) (Oesterle, 1957: 156).

What Is Egoistic Habit?

An *egoistic* habit pertains to being self-centered and preoccupied with self-desires. It is a habit of valuing only interference to oneself personal interest. In an immoral behavior, an egoistic habit is that people regard their own welfare as the supreme end of action beyond the contextual boundary of the public conscientiousness.

ANALYSIS OF BIOSCIENTIFIC ADVANCEMENTS AND BIOTECHNOLOGICAL CONSEQUENTIAL DEVELOPMENTS

As we indicated in Chapter 7, there are two major cultural beliefs concerning existence: (1) creation and (2) evolution. Creation is a theosophical foundational belief that everything including human beings are created by a super power; God. Therefore, according to this theory, bioscientific deliberations with ethical and moral foundations are viewed as God's blessing inspirations. Biotechno scientists should not interfere in the principles of natural realm of God's will. If they do, they will commit sin and the consequence is eternal misery and curse.

Historically, our ancestors with their moral commitments, ethical responsibilities, and religious faiths perceived that science is the spiritual manifestation of God's image to save people through their wisdom. Humans should respect God's creatures and they have to avoid abusing human subjects in their experiments. According to such a theosophical view, bioscientists should not interfere in changing the path of God's will because if they violate such summon they will be ended up with misery. Therefore, bioscientists in searching for knowledge should not follow too far. In a sense to play the role of creator; God.

From the other point of view, evolution is a kind of biosophical foundation believing that existence of everything is based on a gradual processing change in universe towards two directions: (1) life and (2) death. According to the evolutionary biosophy of social Darwinism all fittest things will survive and continue to grow and all unfitted things including the sickest and weakest will die and perish. Survival is the competitive result of confrontational means and ends of the fittest and the weakest and/or the sickest.

The Twentieth century, science and technology have advanced and developed far beyond what our ancestors dared imagine. Today, biotechno scientists and biomedical practitioners have created a body of wisdom in which it can enable them to cure diseases that used to wipe out the entire population in a limited geographical area. They have found effective methods to prolong life of the terminally ill people and have replaced the damaged organs of those suffering patients from heart, kidney, and liver diseases. Also, today bioscientists created bioweapons and biochemical germs such as Antrax, Boutulism, Plague, Small Pox. Tulacema, VHF, Sulfur B the nerve agent Vx, Mustard Gas, Chlorine, Sarin, H.Syanide, Sudiom Hydroxide, Cyclosarin and others in mass scales which can wipe out the total population.

Within the contextual boundary of such a biotechnological and bioscientific efforts the line between what can be done and what should be done is sometimes very thin. For example, the Promethean scientific innovativeness has accelerated the creed for creation a new possibility to determine the sex of a child within a few days after it has been conceived. Such a bioknowledge has created a fear that it will abort healthy children merely because of their gender-type. Or may soon gene engineering and DNA recumbent can remove an aggressive gene from the genetic makeup of a fetus and replace it with an obedient and emotionless gene or vice versa. Don't you think by placing the awesome power of the Promethean authority in the hands of biotechno scientists within the domain of creation by human beings can conjure up the natural images of humanity? This means that biotechno scientific innovativeness has created two types of bioresearchers: (1) ethical and moral smart biotechno scientists and (2) mad or criminal-minded ones. The smart ones within their conscientious perceptions proceed with care and prudence within three domains of biokowledge: (1) causes, (2) processes, and (3) effects. But the mad or criminal-minded ones proceed with devil intention and irresponsible desire for their experimental objectively consequences (e.g., biological, bacteriological, and biochemical weapons and germs for mass destruction). Therefore, ethically and morally not necessarily legally, biotechno scientists should not do everything that they can do (Bender and Leone, 1994:13).

There are different conflicting causes, processes, and effects between the roles of biomedical practitioners and bioresearchers. In order to understand fundamental differences between the two we will elaborate on (1) clinical observational research, and (2) laboratory experimental bioresearch.

CLINICAL OBSERVATIONAL EXPERIENCES

Generally, bioscientists and biomedical researchers are exposed to two types of observational phenomena and events: (1) experimental and (2) experiential. Experimental observations are highly pre-expected plans with signs of provisional manipulation of data and events. But experimental are those experiences that they get with natural data and events as they pop-up during observations. While in experimental observation, bioscientists and researchers concentrate on preplanned causes, processes, and effects, in experiential observations they are looking at effects as they appear and then they search to discover causes and processes.

There is no doubt that the use of human subject in bioresearch can lead us to better understanding of biological mysteries and ultimately to improve diagnosis, treatment, and prognostic processes of patients' deceases. The reasons for this march of folly are many and included, perhaps most importantly, the lack of complete bioknowledge of human biology and patho-physiology. Traditionally, biomedical practitioners have attempted to understand diseases in order to cure patients' suffering. The clinical research was based on trial and error, through non-randomized clinical observations. Until recently, medical and health developments and progresses depended largely on a very slow pace of process of carefully observing groups of patients through non-randomized therapy. Prognostic outcome was based on non-randomized comparison between previously observed and perceived processes and present evidence of such trials and errors through observations.

Today, a physician's task includes an array of preventive, diagnostic, and therapeutic maneuvers. Such a task has not undergone rigorous assessment. Every therapy adopted by physicians has been based on observational studies and plausible mechanisms. Thus, clinical observation lost its scientific reliability because of non-scientific path of inquiry.

LABORATORY EXPERIMENTAL RESEARCH

Since the traditional clinical research was based on non-randomized studies, they could be obsolete very easily by new evidence of opposing experiences. Thus, physicians have been aware of the fragility of their clinical research outcomes. They have realized that randomized scientific clinical trials may have profound effects on their practices. The importance of the scientific randomized laboratory research can control medical trials and safeguard current and future patients against therapeutic errors. Most biomedical physicians have recognized this fact. Today, traditional clinical observational techniques have been replaced by biotechno scientific randomized experimentations in laboratories by bioscientists, pathologists, medical pharmacologists, and biotechnologists. Within the new domain of biotechno scientific randomized research the first necessity is to use human subjects. To do this, randomized bioresearch strategic projects require getting the consent of human subjects.

Bioethics mandated bioresearchers before obtaining the consent from human subjects; they need to inform experimental participants explicitly the possible potential benefits and risks of harm for them and their rights to withdrawal from the trial at any time. However, as practicing medicine has become highly commercialized and increasingly scientifically oriented, the randomized controlled laboratory experimental research becomes the standardized techniques for mass diagnosis, treatment, and prognosis of human diseases.

The trial and errors of laboratory medical experiments have created moral and ethical dilemmas. Despite the innovative mass diagnosis, treatment, and prognosis, laboratory experimental researchers are required to modify their bioethical commitments to individual participants and be less empathetic to their sampling participants. Randomization of laboratory experimental bioresearch tends to design treatment plans among different control groups that are evenly balanced in both known and unknown prognostic factors. This permits bioresearchers a more reliable treatment effect in groups of patients assigned to experimental and standard therapies. This has created a controversial issue concerning obtaining the consent of human subjects. Whether informed consent is ethically and morally required in all bioresearch trials, it is debatable. In order to make it clear who owns what and why in a laboratory experimental research we need to understand the relationships between property rights and the somatic cells' rights.

INTELLECTUAL PROPERTY RIGHTS AND SOMATIC CELL LINE PATENTS

Commercialization of human body parts, cells, and tissues and practices of scientific medicine have created opportunities for some biomedical practitioners, biotechno-scientists, and biopharmaceutical corporations to make huge profits by patenting innovative discoveries and manufacturing lucrative products such as drugs, diagnostic tests, stem cells, and human proteins. Annas (1994: 35) reported:

> In 1976 John Moore's physician, David W. Golde, (MD) recommended that Moore's spleen be removed as a treatment for hairy-cell leukemia. After surgeons removed the spleen, Golde and others took cells from it and cultured them into an immortal cell line that produced a variety of useful medical products. In 1984 this cell line was patented, and Golde and others reaped substantial profit from it. Moore alleged that he was never informed of any of this and never agreed to it.

There are several ethical, moral, and legal questions concerning the ownership of Moore's body parts including cell line of his spleen:

- Is the Moore's spleen cell line belonged to Moore, or to Dr. Golde and his associates, or to both parties?
- Have Dr. Glode and other surgeons violated the professional codes of ethics by either not obtaining Moore's consent or if they did, they did not inform Moore for researching and patenting his removed spleen for the purpose of creating spleen cell line, marketing it, and making profit from it?

By responding to the above questions and analyzing alternative ethical, moral, and legal issues, we are confronting with different views concerning the ownership rights of Moore's spleen and cell line as a part of his body and ownership of the spleen cell line as the labor efforts of Dr. Golde and his associates as patent-holders.

First, we need to review the property rights of Moore's spleen. Second we need to discuss the issue of Moore's consent. Third, we need to debate on the protection of proprietary rights of patent-holders. Fourth, we need to question the preemptive nature of patents skewing research directions. Fifth, we need to discuss the moral codes of conduct and the ethical codes of professional medicine. Sixth, we need to make it clear, should bioresearchers compromise the independence of scientific research processes. Seventh, how do we justify the scientific neutral bioinformation as a common body of knowledge? Eighth, we need to discuss about the legitimacy of conversion of Moore's spleen into cell line for the purpose of commercialization and profitability. Tenth, we need to examine the ethical and moral consequences of patenting human life.

There are many ethical and moral implications concerning the above issues. Specifically, the transplantable organs and tissues can also be used as viable sources to generate enormous profit. Ethically and morally, it is generally considered that the only options available are to recognize or not recognize property rights in human tissues and cell lines.

Different cultural systems have established property right values attached to the human body cells. This cultural trend has been affirmed regardless of whether the human body was active or not. If it was why Dr. Golde and his associates removed it. If it was active, then how and why the medical team decided to remove it and make a cell line from it. If it was defected, then how come they cultured it and made stem cells to be used for therapeutic treatments. Don't you think in this situation the defected stem cell could cause side effects on other patients in long term?

In some cultures the body is known as a property in its usual recognized sense of the word, yet in others it is as a sort of *quasi* property to which certain individuals may have rights, as they have duties to perform towards it. This property right may be very limited possessor rights. For example, we have to know what is the right of a surrogate mother or sperm donators in regards their body cell and/or material donations. Before analyzing these attributive issues we need to know what are rights, duties, and justice.

In order to understand foundational values concerning human property rights, first we must understand political ideologies, cultural beliefs, and religious faiths. Second, accordingly we must identify those three distinctive levels of human perceptions concerning the values of human beings as properties.

CHAPTER 9

BIOETHICAL DIMENSIONS OF ORGAN AND BODY MATERIAL TRANSPLANTATION

OBJECTIVES OF THIS CHAPTER

When you have read this chapter you will be able to do the following:

- Know how should a limited number of organs be allocated among a large number of potential recipients.
- Know what are the appropriate ways to obtain organs from potential donors.
- Assess how should transplantation therapy be balanced against other forms of medical care.
- Reason why the idea and action of organ transplant could be repugnant.
- Know why organ donation is reaffirmation of an individualized self-altruism.
- Identify what human body parts and materials should ethically be used.
- Know what are the purposes for which they should be used.

- Reason why buying and selling body parts and materials of human beings degrade human integrity and dignity.
- Know what is the subsequent end result of buying and selling somatic parts of human beings.
- Realize why commercialization of human body parts and materials dehumanize human beings.
- Know why the gift of an organ should save another's life.
- Know why commercialization of human body parts and materials converts human beings into commercial commodities for the purpose of economic profitability.
- Reason why human flesh should or shouldn't be subject to marketing.
- Realize what should be the scientific conditions of body parts to be useful for organ transplantation.
- Know why human body parts and materials be taken from alive human beings or animals and/or from corpses.
- Know what are the traditional and contemporary definitions of "death" in scientific communities?
- Know what are arguments concerning human natural and civil rights concerning organ transplantation.
- Know what is the difference between "vegetable life" and "brain death."
- Know what are ethical and moral arguments concerning actual consent, presumed consent, and proxy consent in biomedical experimentations.
- Know what are consequential affects of organ and material transplant over future generations.

PLAN OF THIS CHAPTER

When the practice of buying and selling human parts including kidneys from live vendors first came to light four decades ago, it aroused ethical and moral objections to such inhumane business transactions. Such horror caused bioethicists, theosophists, biosophists, biomedical professionals, and lay people to denounce it, and nearly all countries have now made it illegal (British Transplantation Society Working Party, 1986; The Council of the Transplantation Society, 1985; The World Health Organization – WHO, 1992).

Within the free world of inquiry, some academicians desire to make all possible biotechno scientific possibilities without regulation. In response bioethicists, biosophists, and theosophists say to them "no." Within a civilized community, there are professional principles and standards that they have to abide. In 1977, *Hastings Center* founder Daniel Callahan characterized bioethicists are trying to wrench control from physicians. Callahan said:

> I think the role of (anesthesiologist) Henry Beecher was very important in the mid 60s when he blew the whistle on some bad experiments with human

subjects that did real harm... Beecher in fact said: "Look, we can't trust ourselves any longer." Some of these researchers do bad things. And Congress came along and established the Institutional Review Board Committee because the scientists said: "We don't need review, we are wonderful, we never did harm anybody" and in fact the government said: "We don't believe you anymore. You've got to have some public oversight." ... I suppose the net effect of all this was that (a) you've got a group of people, doctors and others, that are interested in this field; and (b) doctors couldn't keep these issues to themselves much any longer partly because some doctors were blowing the whistle saying: "Hey public, watch, look here, pay attention. There are some things going on here that are not good and that you should know about." This was probably a very small minority group of doctors. But the doctors were long resistant to the idea of any outside coming in," (Tina Stevens, 1991: 10-12).

Human body parts and materials are diverse as their uses, spanning the entire range of human development. Human body parts and materials can come from sex cells, embryos, fetuses, newborns, children, adults, and cadavers. In some cases, such as blood donation, sperm, and eggs, human materials can be removed without harming the donor. In other cases, materials are essential to life and therefore can be removed only before and/or immediately after death.

Organ transplantation procedures for persons with failed heart, liver, lung, and kidney function are the modern efforts of biotechno scientific research and biomedical pragmatic innovativeness. Specifically, children's body parts to be used for organ transplantation are one of the serious unethical and immoral issues that have degraded human dignity and integrity. Weir and Peters (1999: 163) reported:

> M.C. was ten years old when she was diagnosed with acute lymphoblastic leukemia. During two years of chemotherapy, she maintained excellent grades,... Then the leukemia relapsed... Before she received the transplant, at the age of thirteen, she told her parents and others that she did not want to "grow up to be a vegetable," did not want to be supported on "a lot of machines," and "did not want to be a psychological or financial burden on the family." Two months after the transplant, she was diagnosed as having an Epstein Barr virus-associated lymphoproliferative disorder. Despite aggressive treatment efforts in pediatric ICU, her condition did not improve. Four days later the ventilator sustaining her life was withdrawn, at the request of her family and in keeping with her previously expressed wishes.

The logic behind such a decision by children's biological and/or adopted parents to make final decisions on behalf of them to end their lives is based on that parents believe that children are no more than containers of their genes, and their parents have the right to treat them not as individual human beings, but rather as human embryos; entities that can be split and replicated their whim without any consideration of children's choice or welfare.

Historically, humans have had the power to exercise domination over animals for many purposes, including in biomedical research. Also, humans have had the liberty to use animals to study anatomy. Recently, biomedical professionals have used animal organs to be transplanted into human body. American Medical Association believes that research involving animals is absolutely essential to maintaining and improving the health of people in America and worldwide (Smith et al., 1988: 1849).

The theses of this chapter is that, biosciences and biotechnologies come to have a life of their own, not only because of their attributive substances, but also because of certain universal human traits. Biosciences and biotechnologies come into being to serve the purposes of their innovators and users, but ultimately those innovators and users redefine their own objectives in terms of their suitability and efficacy. To examine ethical and moral issues concerning the wonders or dangers of biotechnological breakthroughs is neither necessary nor useful except to acknowledge their humane existence; life and death. Biotechnological breakthroughs are not the main problems in human civilization. They are the relationship of biotechnologies and those who want to use them that is problematic.

In this chapter, we are analyzing ethical and moral issues concerning organ transplantation. In order to discuss such matters we need to answer to the following questions:

- How should a limited number of organs be allocated among a large number of potential recipients?
- What are he appropriate ways to obtain organs from potential donors?
- How should transplantation therapy be balanced against other forms of medical care?
- Why the idea and action of organ transplants could be repugnant?
- Why organ donation is reaffirmation of an individualized self-altruism?
- What human body parts and materials should ethically be used?
- What are the purposes for which they should be used?
- Why buying and selling body parts and materials of human beings degrade human integrity and dignity?
- What is the subsequent end result of buying and selling somatic parts of human beings?
- Why the gift of an organ should save another's life?
- Why commodiousness of organs converts human beings into commercial commodities for the purpose of economic profitability?
- Why human flesh should be subject to market or not to market?
- What should be the scientific conditions of body parts and materials to be useful for organ transplantation?
- Should body parts and materials be taken from alive human beings or animals and/or from corpses?

- What is the traditional and contemporary definition of "death" in scientific communities?

This chapter summarizes ethical and moral arguments concerning human rights. In addition, this chapter provides a variety of perspectives which help us come to ethical and moral terms with many of the critical issues in accepting or rejecting the use of particular definition of "brain death" as a useful criterion for determining death.

INTRODUCTION

Bioethical commitments among biotechno scientists and biomedical practitioners possess specific objective foundations. It is critical to understand the exact nature of bioethical and biomoral foundations. Since practicing medicine is associated with tragic circumstances where all patients die and most suffer acute illnesses before death, physicians are often faced with choices where all rights and duties can be satisfied and surely not all goods realized. Nevertheless, bioethical principles concerning organ transplantation are not objective, but it only works if we think that it is objective. Bioethical principles only work if we believe that everybody believes in them and comply with its causes, processes, and consequences.

In our modern time, biotechno scientists and biomedical practitioners as Stevens (2000: 75) indicated we have been faced with two separated trajectories of modern medicine:

> The first, dating to the 1950s, was the anguish of physicians and patients trapped in the desolate gulf between the promise of medical cure and the reality of therapeutic limitations: in trying to save lives, doctors often prolong dying. The second trajectory, developing especially in the late 1960s, was professional medicine's desire to protect itself from the legal liabilities of conducting medical research – research sometimes dependent upon prolonging dying.

The moral and ethical issues concerning organ transplants mandated biotechno scientists and biomedical practitioners to seek advice from bioethicists, biosophists, and theosophists. Olson (1989: 47) reported:

> The first successful human transplant of a solid organ took place in 1954, when a young man in Boston, Massachusetts, received a kidney from. his identical twin brother. Since then, scientific, technical, and medical advances have made organ transplantation a relatively common procedure. In 1987, some 1,500 Americans received transplanted heart, approximately 1,200 received livers, another 1,200 received bone marrow, some 10,000 received kidneys, and approximately 35,000 received corneas.

Christian Barnard (1922-2001), the pioneering South African surgeon who performed the world's first successful heart transplant in 1967 in the University of Minnesota died on September 3, 2001from a heart attack while he was in holiday in Cyprus. He was 78. Dr. Barnard transplanted the heart of Denise Darwall, an 18-year-old who died in a car accident, into a 53-year-old dentist Louis Waskasky who suffered acute rejection and died of pneumonia after 18 days, leading to criticism of the operation. Dr. Barnard persisted with his work. The next patient lived more than a year and, three years latter, Dr. Barnard performed the first heart-and lung transplant, a new technique that has become standard procedure for heart transplants. Also, he believed xenotranplants (the use of animal organs) would one day address the shortage of human donors. Dr. Barnard was one of the first physicians to use non-white nurses to assist him and transplanted the heart of a white woman into a black man (David Firm, 2001: 4).

Anthropologically, human race has maintained a special respect and concern about the sanctity of alive and dead bodies of human beings. The invasion of an alive body without consent of an individual and/or dismemberment of corpses without consent of next of kin and/or government are viewed as the ugliest characteristics of a barbaric culture. Just in case anyone is hearing the commercial massage about commercialization of human parts and materials for the purpose of organ transplantation and/or permitting or even encouraging their sales and purchases are repugnant. To some people the subject of organ transplant is human flesh; the objective is to kill (a vegetable life or a brain dead) a human being in order to save another life. Isn't it against humanity?

Within materialistic cultures, there are always tendencies toward somatic invasion, cruelty, and exploitation. For example, in October 1999, members of the Diet, the Japanese parliament, called for regulating inhumane demands by debt collection methods of the banking and loan industry. The loan default rate in Japan is extremely low. Nichiei, a Japanese consumer finance company, allegedly asked a loan guarantor to raise money by selling his body parts to be transplanted into patients in order to pay back the loan for Y5.7 million. Japanese, culturally, are ashamed to admit bankruptcy. Eisuke Arai, a 25-year-old collection officer of Nichiei Company's, offered a 62-year-old debtor Y3 million ($29,000) for his kidney and Y1 million for his eye to help him to finance a loan had guaranteed to a now bankrupt company. Arai reportedly said to the debtor: "You have two, don't you? Many of our borrowers have only one kidney... I want you to sell your heart as well, but if you do that you'll die. So I'll bear with you if you sell everything up to that," (Abrahams, 1999: 1).

To sell a tooth, kidney, eye, and other organs that can be planted in the jawbone of or transplanted into the body of another person for gaining momentarily easier livelihood is viewed as self-selling, and/or partial self-murder. However, this is not the case with the amputation of a dead organs or cut off some organs such as hair, nail, and unusual grown cells over and in the body (i.e., excessive grown cells around foot and finger nails, moles, tumors, and cancerous ovaries tissues). Humans have realized that the repugnance of body invasion and/or dismemberment violate the dignity and integrity of the body.

Ethically, humans should not treat their bodies as a mere means to accommodate pleasure and/or livelihood of others, because their bodies are viewed as ends in nature. If they ignore such sanctity, they degrade the humaneness in themselves. Olson (1989: 48) indicated:

> Much has been said and written about the ethical obligations of those who use human materials, but according to Caplan much of current practice can be boiled down to three simple rules: One, don't worry about it unless the source of the material is a person. Two, treat everything with respect. Three, never violate either (a) God's will with respect to these materials or (b), if you don't believe in God, then nature's order.

In order to understand moral and ethical issues concerning organ transplants, first, we need to define:

- What are rights and duties?
- What is life?
- What is death?
- What we mean by living donor?
- What are the means and ends of cadaver donation?
- What is organ swapping?
- What is organ donation as a gift or as a commercial commodity to be able to buy or to sell?

In the following pages we will elaborate on ethical and moral issues of these attributions.

WHAT ARE RIGHTS?

"What are rights?" and "What rights do people have?" are the broad topics of morality, ethics, and law. Broadly defined, a *right* is an individual's attachment to affiliate with, entitled to, and privileged with having possession of something. Also, rights legitimate entitlements that invoke corresponding duties on the part of others. It is an entitlement to act or have others act in a certain way. If something is mine, I have the right to protect it, to keep it, to sell it, to use it, and in rare cases to abandon it. Rights can be defined in terms of moral, ethical, and legal duties either by an individual or by groups. The question of rights can, therefore, be to put in terms of natural as well as societal entitlements.

In terms of natural, what constitute an individual? Morally and ethically, one approach to this problem has been to try to equate the humane sacredness or moral worth of an entity with its stage of development. For instance, a fetus can be seen as having more moral value than a sex cell, and a newborn as having more value than a fetus. Therefore, moral and ethical values concerning the whole developmental levels of processes of the existence of a human being are relatively different. Such a difference makes a distinctive valuable property to be respected among human beings and their societal institutions. Nevertheless, such a valuable distinctiveness allows them to distinguish consciousness and violation.

Naturally, human beings comparing with other animals are entitled to intellect, memory, communication, innovation, liberty, and socialization. This means that all human beings should have the rights to think critically, to remember past experiences, and have the right to express themselves without fear. They have the right to liberty and free association with others and share their innovative ideas and opinions with others without any limitation. Since human beings are purposive agents, they must be entitled to natural rights to liberty. Also, since freedom and liberty are being the necessary conditions for purposive actions, then they should strive for maintaining and enhancing freedom and liberty. The problem is what liberty is. Is it a natural right of entitlement to a maximum or minimum standard of liberty? Both libertarian and fatalism philosophers believe that freedom and liberty depend on the scarcity of resources.

Human beings through their natural rights are individuals of profound self-esteem. They are entitled to the competence of their own body- mind to deal with the problems of existence. They look at the natural habitat and at the world of humanity, wondering:

- What are their natural individual's rights?
- What are their pluralistic societal rights?
- What ought to be done to respect them?
- How can these rights be maintained or preserved?

Nevertheless, the most important natural rights for human beings is the assurance of continuity of their species through natural selection of inbreeding generations to come. On the other hand, pluralistic societal rights are not like natural inherent individual's rights. They are conventional, legal, and contractual rights that people do not sit waiting for to be given or somebody to give them a chance to be entitled to. They make and take their own rights. Pluralistic societal rights are not like natural rights. People set them. Pluralistic societal rights are not set by chances. They are set by choices. People calculate how to safeguard them against those who attempt to bypass or deny them.

INTRINSIC AND EXTRINSIC RIGHTS

As indicated above, entitlements to, attachment to, affiliated with, possession of, and privileged with bestowed rights can be either from natural norms and principles that specify all human beings are permitted or empowered to do something or are entitled to have something to be done for them (e.g., human rights). We need to identify two major domains of moral values: (1) inherent intrinsic values and (2) entitled extrinsic values. Also, we need to realize either the moral worth concerning the existence of an individual is related to his/her inherent intrinsic natural values or it is related to the standing entitlement of extrinsic social values assigned to their identity.

In examining inherent intrinsic and social extrinsic values of the whole body, body parts, and body materials certain values loom large as forming moral and ethical environment in which we can interact with human beings. One of the most important inherent intrinsic values is that the users of human body parts and body materials should not harm donors. It is morally and ethically (may not be legally) wrong to bring about death of someone prematurely (e.g., brain dead) just to get body parts from a donor to benefit someone else. Thus, notions of redemption and transformation of human body, body parts, and body materials are very critical in dealing with human existence. For example, Hindus believe in reincarnation. They believe by reconstitution of their physical body into a spiritual body for eternal blessing and again transforming it into a new body is something quite similar happens when a surgeon takes a kidney from a healthy person and transplants it into another person. This is the major reason in which most body parts are exported from India to all over the world including cadavers to be used in medical schools and/or in bioresearch institutions.

Natural rights primarily have been established in a universal form by precise ordering of just causes for the existence. Human beings do not make them, but human beings are trying to discover them. But human beings through specific institutionalization of their societal reasoning make moral, civil, property, and criminal rights. Natural rights are not limited to a particular jurisdiction. Also, a natural right can be derived either from a cultural value system within or beyond of a political arena (e.g., religious rights or denominations) or from a specific ideological doctrine (e.g., conservative or libertarian belief, or leftist and rightist). Entitlements can also be derived from a system of religious faith independently of any cultural value system or from a particular legal of denominated system. Nevertheless, all rights are attributed to some intentions and actions. The legal rights are limited to the particular jurisdiction within which the legal system is in force. The legal entitlements permit or empower a person to act in a specific way or that requires others to act in certain ways toward that person (Velasquez, 1992: 59). For example, a key consideration in the use of body parts, body materials, and body tissues is that they could be distributed equitably and fairly among needy patients regardless of their wealth, reputation, and power. It is unfair and unjust when people observe that the rich and/or powerful people get access to transplants but the poor don't, or that physicians make immoral and unethical decisions concerning who should live or who should die. It creates a decimating impact on people's willingness to put faith or trust or confidence in the community of biomedical professionals who deal with organ transplants.

Rights inherently have double faces: (1) positive and (2) negative. Also, rights could be perceived as specific attributive entitlements either to positive or negative duties. Positive rights reflect the vital entitlements of all human beings in receiving certain benefits. For example, the rights to be educated, to be diagnosed and treated, to have equal employment opportunity, to have equitable pays or wages and so on are positive rights. Positive rights are rights to obtain privileged opportunities and/or certain kinds of equal treatments. On the other hand negative rights are those entitlements to be free to be holding and practiced through religious beliefs, professional privileges, political ideologies, and cultural customs and traditions without outside interference. Negative rights protect human dignity and integrity without enforcement by governments, or by radical and partisan groups. Negative rights reflect the vital entitlements that all human beings have in being free from outside-interference such as freedom of speech, assembly, religion, and so on.

Correlated with these rights are duties that indicate all human beings should not interfere with others' pursuit of happiness. There are two philosophical schools in relationships of human beings to God, to themselves, to other human beings, and to nature. In sum, there are two schools of philosophies concerning positive and negative rights: (1) Libertarianism, and (2) Fatalism.

LIBERTARIAN PHILOSOPHY OF RIGHTS

Libertarian philosophy of rights emphasizes on all rights as the finality of a human nature. Within this philosophical ideology, libertarians believe that all human beings are the architectures of their own destiny. These rights provide them with autonomy in their free will to pursue their survival objectives; even the right to die. No other forces have any right to interfere in their personal destiny and make any decision on behalf of them, because human beings are free to act according to their will, purposes, and faiths. However, within this idealistic ideology, there are inclusive negative exceptional rights for children, elderly, sick, and insane people. This right needs to be respected by each individual, other people, and as well as the institutions of society.

Moral rights limit the validity of appeals to social benefits and to the numbers of people. If a person has a right to do something, then it is not the right of others to do it to him/her, even though a large number of people might gain much more utility from such interference.

FATALISM PHILOSOPHY OF RIGHTS

Fatalism is a doctrine that people believe in destiny. They believe all events are subject to fate or inevitable pre-determination by God. They accept all things and events, as they are; even illnesses and death. This type of moral doctrine is based on a belief that all things that are existed are subject to the universal order for their own sake with specific universal purposes. They are bound to consider as the chief quality in everything that that is most useful to them. Furthermore, they believe that they are bound to form abstract notions for explanation of the nature of things, such as goodness, badness, order, confusion, beauty, and deformity. Those who understand the mystery for the causes of existence, they firmly believe that there is an eternal cause or order in all things. These mysteries never ever will be revealed to mankind.

FOUNDATIONAL ARGUMENTS FOR RIGHTS

The notion of rights has received a great deal of attention in civilized societies. Various causes of rights have appeared to be pressed for individuals and groups, such as human rights, civil rights, women's rights, consumers' rights, patients' rights, students' rights, academicians' rights, investors' rights, the rights to live, the rights to die, and the rights of unborn children are examples. Where do these rights come from and what gives rise to the above kinds of rights? These are the main issues in this section of our deliberation.

Through history, people have established new forms of cultural, social, political, and economic power, in order to maintain their own identity. Since all of us are human beings, therefore we are living in the state of humanity. Accordingly, there is a claim that all human beings are subject to the same rights. Some advocates believe that just as God created laws of nature that transcend different cultures and religions, so God created laws of morality and ethics which are available to human reasoning.   Therefore, each society functions according to priorities for its social class-stratification. This means the rights of individuals are based on who do you know, but not based on what do you know; connections. One important difference between the societies of the world according to Max Weber (1946) is the recognition of the rights of individuals and groups in relationships to their body, wealth, power, and prestige. First, the rights of individuals are stemmed from one another by the extent to which they have accumulated economic resources, or in other words, their wealth. Second, the rights of individuals rooted in acquisition of power, in which Weber defined it as the ability to exert it to achieve one's own goals and objectives even against the rights and wills of others. The right to have power can be manipulated and be used at-will.

Power may be evil. This is expressed in Lord Acton's celebrated dictum that: "Power tends to corrupt and absolute power corrupts absolutely," (Steiner and Steiner, 1994: 47). Third, the rights of individuals are formulated according to their prestige or reputation, in which Weber defined them as the social esteem, respect, or admiration that a society confers on people. Accordingly, to one degree or another, all people are socially differentiated on the basis of assuming criteria for profession, education, ideology, age, sex, and possession of political and money-power. In addition, according to Morton Fried (1967), societies are classified according to their rights into three types:

- Egalitarian societies who have few or no groups that have greatest access to the greatest volume of wealth, power, or prestige.
- Rank societies who have unequal access to prestige or status but not unequal access to wealth or power. In rank societies, there are a fixed number of high-status societal positions, which only certain individuals because of their skills, wisdom, industriousness, or family linked to power or other personal traits have access to those rights.
- Stratified societies are characterized by considerable inequality in all forms of societal rights; wealth, power, and prestige. As a general rule, the greater the role specialization to be emphasized, the justice system of stratification becomes more complex.

Nevertheless, social scientists, generally, recognize two different types of stratified societies in regard of rights: (1) class, and (2) caste. In class systems, a certain amount of status mobility of both upward and downward variables exists (i.e., American culture). In contrast, societies based on caste rank the entitlements of rights according to birth. They believe, membership in castes is unchangeable. Therefore, in caste systems upward and downward social mobility virtually are nonexistent (i.e., Anglo, Indian, Kuwaitian, and Saudi Arabian cultures; racial supremacy).

All these rights are tightly correlated with duties. A person, a group, and a nation can only exercise their rights to something if sufficient justifications exist. For clarity of this subject matter, it is suffice to analyze the foundational arguments concerning the rights. In this section, we will divide our arguments into two sections: (1) The International Human Rights, and (2) The National Bill of Rights.

Figure 9.1: United Nations Universal Declaration of Human Rights

---

The right to own property alone as well as in association with others.
The right to work, to free choice of employment, to just and favorable conditions of work, and to protection against unemployment.
The right to just and favorable remuneration ensuring for the worker and his family an existence worthy of human dignity.
The right to form and join trade unions.
The right to rest and leisure, including reasonable limitation of working hours and periodic holidays with pay.

Source: Buchholz, R. A. and Rosenthal, S. B. (1998). *Business Ethics: The Pragmatic Path Beyond Principles to Process*. New York: McGraw-Hill Book Company: 30.

INTERNATIONAL ANALYSIS
OF HUMAN RIGHTS

The connection between natural rights and duties is that, generally speaking, if an individual has a right to live, then others have a correlated duty to act in certain ways to respect it. In addition to natural rights, we also have moral and ethical rights such as human rights. Human rights are universal. Everyone has natural rights, just by virtue of being human, not because they live within the boundary of a certain sociocultural or political-legal system.

Figure 9.2: Protection Guarantied By The Bill of Rights

First Amendment: Guarantees the freedom of religion, speech, and press and the rights to assemble peaceably and to petition the government.
Second Amendment: Guarantees the right to keep and bear arms.
Third Amendment: Prohibits, in peacetime, the lodging of soldiers in any house without the owner's consent.
Fourth Amendment: Prohibits unreasonable searches and seizures of persons or property.
Fifth Amendment: Guarantees the rights to indictment by grand jury, to due process of law, and to fair payment by grand jury, to due process of law, and to fair payment when private property is taken for public use, prohibits compulsory self-incrimination and double jeopardy (trial for the same crime twice if the first trial ends in acquittal or conviction).
Sixth Amendment: Guarantees the accused in a criminal case the right to a speedy and public trial by an impartial jury and with counsel. The accused has the right to cross-examine witnesses against him or her and to solicit testimony from witnesses in his or her favor.
Seventh Amendment: Guarantees the right to a trial by jury in a civil case involving at least twenty dollars.*
Eight Amendment: Prohibits excessive bail and fines, as well as cruel and unusual punishment.
Ninth Amendment: Establishes that people have rights in addition to those specified in the Constitution.
Tenth Amendment: Establishes that those powers neither delegated to the federal government nor denied to the states are reserved for the states.

---

* Twenty dollars was forty day's pay for the average person when the Bill of Rights was written.

If the natural right to live a full life is a human right, then everyone, everywhere at all times, has the right to survive. Therefore, human rights are equal rights. Also, human rights are not transferable either by giving or lending them to other people. That is what is meant when human rights such as life, liberty, and the pursuit of happiness are viewed as human rights, nobody should deny it.

Human rights are based on the natural duties, not in the sense that they can be derived from a study of human nature but in the sense that they do not depend on ideological beliefs of religious, racial and/or political-legal systems. A right to self-preservation is an example of one such right. Since happiness is the virtuous finality of human dignity, rights are the valuable finality of humanity. All human beings are entitled to natural rights regardless of their pluralistic and/or collectivistic political or social institutions. A right to self-preservation, both body and mind, is an example of one such right. As previously indicated, an individual can only exercise a right to something, if they can prove that they are entitled to the existence of sufficient justifications, that is, that a right has overriding status.

FOUNDATION OF SOMATIC PROPERTY RIGHTS

Torn between psychosocial sympathy and politico-economical disgust, life and death of an individual are the major ethical and moral issues in a civilized society. The main issue is related how to price life and death. In some cultures, life is very precious for all classes of people regardless of the levels of their wealth. In others, they ban advertising and criminalizing brokering selling body parts, but you can buy or sell them in the black market. Finally, in some cultures legally permitting the sale of body parts, especially from live donors. Therefore, buying and selling and/or not selling body parts and materials have to do with matters of equity, exploitation of the needy and poor people, and abusing or deceiving people for gaining immoral and unethical material rewards; not excluding theft and even murder to obtain somatic valuable parts as commodities.

Within the contextual boundaries of bioethics, rights may be moral and ethical as well as legal. The moral rights are those entitlements in which all inherent characteristics of the world of humanity are shared by all people regardless their gender, color, ethnicity, race, religion, age, political, cultural, social, and economical characteristics. These moral rights are known as goodness, truthfulness, justness, fairness, worthiness, and beauty. Moral rights are important and justifiable claims or entitlements. Moral rights of either kind are tightly correlated with conscience duties.

Legal rights can be put in terms of the entitlements to intellectual properties or material things including human somatic organ properties. Intellectual property rights are similar to liberty rights, copyrights, shop rights, and patent rights. Material rights are similar to ownership of land, buildings, business outlets, investments, and the like. In both intellectual and material entitlements, the following question can be raised in terms of ethical as well as legal production and usage endeavors. Who owns nature and what are legal and ethical attributive rights attached to those ownerships including human body parts and materials?

PHILOSOPHIES OF PROPERTY RIGHTS

John Locke (1632-1704), the British philosopher, whose theory influenced the Christian capitalism, argued that the Christian capitalism ideology has two gospels, the "Bible," and the other one is the "capitalistic state" (Meiklejohn: 1942: 57). There are several issues concerning the "natural rights" and the "state rights." According to Meiklejohn (1942: 83) the trouble is that people confuse "conscience" with "prudence." People are notoriously deceiving themselves and others regarding their own and other's rights. He stated that the individuals who wish to be religious on all days of the week can accept the urges of prudence as the voice of conscience. Another way of living in the Christian-capitalism society is to serve conscience and God on Sundays and be a rugged individualist on other weekdays on the ground that it is not wrong to do what the state does not forbid.

Locke (1924) held that God created the universe and mankind. When God created human beings, He endowed them with eternal, inalienable rights to such things as freedom, equality, and humanity. God has authority over conscience and moral law. But God "did not create the state." Before people created the state, people were living in a "state of nature" in which they were not fully able to enjoy their rights in which God had bestowed upon them. This was because the rights of human beings were violated by the selfish actions of other mighty human beings. Violations and cruelties of people to each other caused people to organize themselves into a sense of the statehood and consequently initiated the social contract.

The social contract dictated by people's moral prudence and maintained them by legal enforcement. Accordingly, human beings become subject to two types of rights: (1) conscience and (2) prudence. Through the moral contract, the citizens of a state become responsible to God in matters of conscience, but in matters of prudence, they found it was wise to keep an armed truce with other states, respecting their contractual rights so that they could respect their own (Weber, 1960: 29).

According to political ideologies, the notion of the state capitalism in each nation possesses its own characteristics. These characteristics establish the foundations of rights for individuals and groups. For example, the American economy is dominated by a relative handful of large corporations and their domestic retail chained stores. These corporations are linked in a variety of ways to each other in order to create the notion of corporate America. The American statehood capitalism ideology has stemmed from the "Christian Capitalism." This religious and econo-political ideology has created two types of capitalism: (1) people's capitalism and (2) family capitalism.

The People Capitalism

The ideological foundation of people's capitalism has stemmed from the constitutional rights. Within such a pluralistic society no one group has overwhelming power over all others and each may have direct or indirect impact over others. The power is diffused, because decentralization of power makes less possible tyranny and exploitation of a few people or groups over others. The American capitalism is permeated by the competitive value of quality that encourages pluralism. The Constitution encourages pluralism in different ways. It guarantees of rights to protect liberty and freedom for individuals and to pursue their interests. In addition, the Constitution diffuses political power through several independent branches of governmental power. Individuals and groups influence in one branch of government, the other branches can diffuse it. The democratic representative people's power has established its own cultural value systems through different groups. These group representatives are political parties, governmental agencies and bureaucrats, social interest groups and lobbyists, managers and executives, scientists and technologists as experts and technocrats, working class people as labor unions, and auditors and researchers as think thank consultants. The people capitalist power imposes immediate close boundaries on the discretionary exercise of social power, because their power will be restricted and shared with the family capitalists.

The Family Capitalism

Most sectors of American economy are dominated by relatively small groups of the "Family Capitalists." These groups are private Federal Reserve System, corporations, commercial banks, investment banks, law firms, family offices, boards of governance, holding companies, medical and pharmaceutical companies, foundations, charitable organizations, philanthropic agencies, and political parties.

Having access to resources from the state of nature needs to be ruled by strength. Nevertheless, without a state, no property can be held on a legal ground. In a state of nature there is no justice for, because there is no legal law except the moral law. However, in the state of nature, there is an ethical shared law that is sustained by the general goodwill. Then the questions are:

- By what right do certain people possess the exclusive claims to the natural resources simply because they were fortunate enough to have been born in the country where the resources existed?
- Do some people have a right to resources and monopolize them?
- Or the natural resources of the world, such as crude oil, are for the benefit of all people not just for the lucky few ones?

The answers require not only pay attention to legal reasoning but also to moral reasoning and arguments. The main issues concerning resources rights are as following:

- Scarcity of resources
- Availability of scientific potential and technological capabilities
- Accessibility to material resources
- Durability of resources
- Efficacy of resources to meet necessary needs
- Flexibility of the state laws
- Suitability of resources for production systems
- Profitability on economical values of resources.
- Cost-benefit analysis of the alternative resources.
- Consistency in continuity of availability of resources

WHAT ARE DUTIES?

It is clear that all rights establish some sorts of duties. Rights would be of little value as an ordering principle of human acts without duties. Let us investigate what is meant by duties in the moral, ethical, and legal senses. Duties are viewed as notions of completeness. Oral and/or written entitlements to any type of rights for an individual establish specific bases for obligatory binding duties for that individual and others in order to put it in practice. When we speak of a duty, we mean an action that we are obligated to undertake or to refrain from regardless of whether in the case we find it in our interest to do so or not. Duty is a constraint on the scope of permissible actions, but not all constraints are duties.

Moral duties are distinct from legal duties, and the necessary conditions of each are distinct too. A necessary condition of the validity of duties is the validity of the procedure by which the moral duty imposing them is enacted to those duties. Duties, to begin with, apply directly only to actions. To make the issue clear, we must say that what is meant is a duty that we would have to discharge by doing what results are found in our rights. Duties are the result of three types of necessities:

The Necessity of the Obligatory Act in Relation to the Necessity of Causes

This duty needs to be done because of the preservation of the rights of self and/or others. Since moral duties are based upon conscience cognitive virtues, they are bound with the intellectual will in the sense that there is a necessary relation between causes and affects. Such a duty will not destroy the liberty for acting or not acting. It demonstrates a necessity for the existence of good or just causes. We are speaking here primarily of moral obligations in relation to natural rights; existence. Since in this textbook, we have defined morality as an individual's desire toward goodness, and then others cannot impose morality or moral obligations on us. We are the only ones who can recognize such a necessity to be imposed on ourselves. If we desire to exist and survive, then we need to understand the real causes for such a being. Therefore, the moral duties at their highest general level state that the form that a cause needs to be rational and the related courses of actions to that cause must have to be moral, to be good not vicious. Consequently, the moral duties spell out the boundary of obligations, but do not spell out the contents of those duties. Therefore, such reasoning is called a formalistic moral approach. In a formalistic moral obligation, the Hegel's dialectic reasoning as thesis and antithesis combined to form a synthesis is used to understand causes, processes, and effects of duties.

The Necessity of the Act in Relation to the Necessity of the Means

This duty must be done as necessarily leading to the achievement of common good. This obligation applies in an analogous manner to humanity. With respect to human rights, asking usually states the question of ethical obligation whether human rights bind us with our conscience. In answering to this question, we must recognize that the human rights are justified through the doctrine of humanity. The finality of the doctrine of humanity is relied on validity of reasoning in defending a logical statement or an action for the goodness of humanity. It is a feature of deductive discourse in which the relation between premises and conclusions is such that if the premises are true (thesis), then the content of pros and cons (antithesis) is rationalized, and consequently the conclusive results (synthesis) could not be false. Since the means of humanity is good, the ends, therefore, should be good too.

It is a fact that sometimes parts of law are not based on moral or ethical, they are based on categorical imperatives. The categorical imperatives provide us with choosing to follow or not, depending on whether we wish to attend the moral and ethical philosophy of humanity and to achieve it or not. Kant provided us with three formulations of categorical imperative:

- For a necessary action to be moral, it must be amenable to being made consistently universal.
- It must respect rational beings as ends in themselves.
- It must form and respect the autonomy of rational beings.

Are these characteristics possible in the realm of humanity? Are these conditions possible in all socio-cultural, psychosocial, and econo-political arguments? The answer in practice is no.

The Necessity of the Act in Relation to the Necessity of the Ends

In responding to this statement specifically, we must recall that the notion of humanity is not the final cause of civil law in all societies. Civil law is either just or unjust. It depends on political ideologies and fiduciary philosophies. If we assume that final ends of law is happiness for all human beings and it is just, then it needs to have the power of binding with conscience. This duty must be done as necessarily leading to the given ends; the power deriving from natural law, and through natural law, and to the eternal law. Then the necessity of the act in relation to the necessity of ends must aim at the common good; humanity.

Institutionalization of Duties

One common way to institutionalize moral, ethical, and legal concepts of duties is to define those obligatory considerations and actions to control conduct of people by dividing duties into four categories: (1) the required, (2) the permissible, (3) the forbidden, and (4) the contractual. These actions widely accepted fourfold classification is used in different societies differently.

- The required actions are duties, and these are the only actions that have moral merit. The required actions must be obeyed under penalty of punishment in a legal term, or under condemnation in an ethical term, or under blaming in a moral sense. The act in question must be one that an agent may intentionally choose to do it regardless of the merit of its moral, ethical, and legal senses.

- The permissible actions are merely all right duties in which an individual I in certain conditions and situations is obligated to do it. For example, if a family member needs an organ to be transplanted other family members morally and ethically can donate their organs to save his/her life. However, the permissible actions associate with risk. Cairncross (1991: 56) indicated:

  Familiar risks are less frightening than the unfamiliar; visible risks less scary than the invisible sort. People clearly feel more frightened by the remote risk of a large catastrophe than by the greater risk of an equivalent number of deaths spread out over a long period.

- The forbidden actions are those wrong actions that an individual is obligated to avoid them. The forbidden actions must be obeyed under penalty of sin, punishment, condemnation, and blaming. This means that those who wish to lead not simply morally adequate, but morally perfect lives, they need to avoid forbidden actions such as deception, stealing, embezzlement, perjury, corruption, fraud, cheating, etc.

- The contractual duties justify obligations by consent to the rule imposing duty on the part of the agent to whom it applies. The point of contractual justification of duty is to address the problems that arise from justifications of a duty is to address the problems that arise from justifying moral principles by appealing to the aggregated benefits of complying with them. The contractual duty denies the legitimacy of duties that require the sacrifice of one person simply for the good of others.

Moral duties do not presuppose the validity of any legal procedure. An agent might find that a legal duty contradicts a moral duty, unless conformity with moral duty is among the criteria of legitimacy of the legal enactments. To say that one has an actual duty to do a certain thing is to suppose that he/she possesses an available option to do it. It must be something that a person is capable of doing and there must not be special circumstances that prevent him/her from exercising that capacity.

WHAT IS LIFE?

We are living in three highly integrated different worlds: (1) materialistic, (2) spiritualistic, and (3) socialistic. The materialistic world spells out the concept of natural somatic earthly life. Such a natural somatic life consists of highly interrelated and integrated organic systems. It possesses the power of living essentially of hard, material atoms. As Nelson (1994: 265) indicated the word *a-tom* is used to say that it is irreducible; it could not be cut any finer. Bioresearchers in molecular biology and biochemistry rapidly have discovered unknown and surprising characteristics of the DNA molecules as the quintessential unit of life. Just as our entire written language is based upon the alphabet, A, B, C, to Z, we know that the units of living matter have a four-lettered alphabet AGTC: A for adenine, G for guanine, T for thiamine, and C for cytosine. Combine with sugar and a phosphate group, these compositions of atoms of carbon, hydrogen, nitrogen, and oxygen produce the 20 amino acids, which in turn are the elements of proteins. Proteins are the main sources of energy; life.

The spiritual world spells out the belief that the essence of life is the soul, the spirit, or the mind. These phenomena are eternal. The somatic manifestations of integrated atoms of life are only transitory appearances. To the present day, biology and biosophy have been pursued within the tension and arguments to connect these two (materialistic and spiritualistic) different domains of life together through biophilia; the innately emotional affiliation of human beings to other living organisms.

The socialistic world is related to individuals to socially live well. To socially live well as a human being is to live life of reason, by which a human being not only engages in the acts of reason itself, but also directs his/her other acts through reason. Hence, a good societal life appears to consist of the activity of reason and good use of reason to direct other acts.

By summing up all above attributions, we need a notion of a full life that is based on some understanding of human needs and possibilities. We should think that living well is not only related to somatic well being, also, it is related to spiritual and social life span as the achievement of a life that sufficiently long to take advantages of natural and civil lives. People differ on what might be a full natural life span. A longer life does not guarantee a better life. No matter how long medicine enables people to live, death at any time is inevitable, because death is the final stage of life. Death guaranties the natural continuity of the balanced between oncoming and ongoing human species.

THE RIGHT TO LIVE AND
THE RIGHT TO DIE

Moral principles and ethical commitments mandate biomedical professionals and paraprofessionals not to violate patients' rights; both natural rights and civil rights. Physicians are morally and legally bound to act consistently within their professional commitments to diagnose and treat patients with reasonable medical practices. The Bill of Patients' Rights says that patients "have the right to appropriate medical ... care based on individual needs ...[which is] limited where the service is not reimbursable (Minnesota Statutes). Respect for patients' autonomous rights and the professional duty of physicians for rendering reasonable treatments are major foundations of medical and health care profession. However, respect for autonomous patients' rights does not empower patients to oblige physicians to prescribe treatments in ways that are fruitless or inappropriate. Physicians are bound to the ethics of "stewardship." They should exercise their professional stewardship to pursue their duties. This stewardship is not aimed at protecting the assets of insurance companies or the sole desires of patients. It should rest on fairness to patients and insurance companies. It is clear that health care insurance companies desire to reduce and/or eliminate their costs by either denying treatments of patients and/or by termination of life of critically ill people, but professionally physicians should act on the best interest of their patients.

Who should live and who should die? This question raises serious ethical and moral problem for humanity. Some people live and die naturally and others live with artificial internal organs and organ transplantation because they are endowed with financial capabilities. According to this scenario, the problem addresses two key issues: (1) financial capabilities and (2) availability of scarce medical resources. Day after day biomedical professionals and insurance companies make judgments and decisions about allocations of medical care to various segments of our population, to various types of hospitalized patients, and to specific individuals. Nevertheless, the effective types of medical scarce resources such as hemodialysis and kidney and heart transplants have compelled us to address the moral and ethical questions that have been concealed in many aspects of our lives.

To live or to die with dignity is a serious questionable argument in the medical community. Nothing in life is simple anymore, not even dying. Theologian Joseph Fletcher (1960: 141) shared with *Harper's* readers the experience of ministers and physicians in dealing with the "heartbreaking struggle over mercy death." Fletcher related several tragic stories of prolonged dying and explained: "The right to die in dignity is a problem raised often by medicine's success than by its failure... Death control, like birth control, is a matter of human dignity." At one time there was no medical need for the physicians to consider the concept of death because the fact of death was sufficient. In addition, life and death were ultimate, self-evident opposites.

Traditionally, life and death seemed so simple in the history of mankind. Today, the attributions to the corresponding behavior of intellectual, emotional, and sensational difficulty of human beings are related to the "right to the natural processes of life and death." In theory, we can see the law, religion, ethics, and morality that might offer mutual support for such a right. The law secures each person's right to live until the life span ends naturally. Religion, while reminds us of the limitations of earthly life as an end in it, also it promises the sacredness of eternal human life. Ethics and morality provide human beings the notion of dignity to continue life to the last moment of the death "simply happens." In such a conclusive moment to cooperate with the notion of death is a natural mandate. However, biotechno scientific devices and biomedical professionals can dramatically extend life span and the process of natural dying increasingly become manageable clinically.

Today, we are exposed to the circumstances of dying and the very timing of death itself. Hill (1996: 200) raised the indispensable questions such as:

> Whose claims on that discretion come first? (2) Whose death is it? We have now come to understand very clearly that when someone is dying, others have central interests that will be affected by the eventual outcome of the process and the manner in which it has been controlled. Consequently, now, with some measure of control over the process of dying, comes presumably a responsibility to exercise that control in a manner that recognizes and protects as reasonably as possible the interests of all those involved.

Biosophically, a physician is a healer. He/she is a professional individual whose decisions and operations are tied to knowledge of the body. He/she uses biotechnological devices to extend patients' lives. Biotechnology is not bioscience. Biotechnology and biosciences are frequently lumped together, but they are distinct. Here are the findings of biosciences become reality by biotechnologies. The actual essence of biosciences is to see what is there about positron functioning emission tomography (PET) scanner, magnetic resonance imaging (MRI), angioplasty, endoscopy, automated chemistry machines, artificial heart, and so on. The foremost affective means and ends that biotechnology has on human life and death we call them wonder and wonderment. No matter how much we know about being human, we will always be human. The wonder is not easily put aside and is quickly reawakened; an innovation leads to a desire for more. The human body is wondrous and so is its psyche. The wonder helps to solve the lively problems of boredom, absence of meaningful life, and loss of prosperous motivation. Wonderment must be reduced to bring the world back into legitimate order. So people have to figure out:

- What these new wondrous biotechnological instruments are?
- How they work and how they ought to work?
- How to control them?

Nevertheless, the community of bioresearchers, bitechno scientists, and biomedical practitioners need to consider both ethical and moral wonder and wonderment how to use biotechnological devices.

WHAT IS DEATH?

The most significant of the tendencies with which biosophy, theosophy, and materialistic philosophy everywhere grapple is the issue of death. Historically, cessation of heartbeat and spontaneous respiration always produced prompt death of the brain, and, similarly destruction of the brain resulted in prompting cessation of respiration and circulation. In this context, it is reasonable that absence of pulse and respiration became the traditional criteria for pronouncement of death. However, bioscientific advancements and biotechnological developments have made it possible to sustain body parts' function in the absence of spontaneous respiratory and cardiac operation. So the death of a person can no longer be equated with the loss of these latter two natural vital functions (Veith, 1981: 171). However, the professional medical authorities added one more cause of death; a neurological one.

Anthropologically, Malinowski (1925: 49-50) in his well-known analysis of primitive life style of savage brings the problem of death into his theory not only of the functions, but also of the origins of religion:

> The savage (and civilized) is intensely afraid of death. Probably, as the result of some deep-seated instincts it is common to man and animals. He does not want to realize it as an end; he cannot face the idea of complete cessation, of annihilation. The idea of spirit and of spiritual existence is near at hand, furnished by such experiences as are discovered and described by Tylor (the founder of anthropology). Grasping at it, man reaches the comforting belief in spiritual continuity and in the life after

death. Yet this belief does not remain unchallenged in the complex, double-edged play of hope and fear that sets in always in the face of death. To the comforting voice of hope, to the intense desire of immortality, to the difficulty, in one's own case, almost the impossibility, of facing annihilation there are opposed powerful and terrible forebodings. The testimony of the senses, the gruesome decomposition of the corpse, the visible disappearance of personality – certain apparently instinctive suggestions of fear and horror seem to threaten man at all stages of culture with some idea of annihilation, with some hidden fears and forebodings. And here into this play of emotional forces, into this supreme dilemma of life and final death, religion steps in, selecting the positive creed, the comforting view, the culturally valuable belief in immortality, in the spirit independent of the body, and in the continuance of life after death. In the various ceremonies at death, in commemoration and communication with the departed, and worship of ancestral ghosts, religion gives body and form to the saving beliefs.

A number of professional medical authorities have argued persuasively that a person whose brain is totally destroyed is in fact dead (Ramsey 1970; and Haring, 1973). Nevertheless, this use of the concept of the brain death has caused controversy among physicians, lawyers, legislators, philosophers, theologians, and ethicists.

Members of the public and members of the professional authority possess two different views concerning death:

- Extension of life through therapeutic procedural techno-scientific methods; (institutionalized medical care: oxygenation, incubations, medication, and surgery) the new way of techno-scientific torturing dying: delirium and unconsciousness.
- Prolong suffering before death. The dilemma is not the result of a specific biomedical and biotechnological procedure and/or operation. It is a predicament rooted in medical profession that measures success by medicine's ability to stall death, even in the face of death's inevitability.

In this regard Leuba (1950: 213) indicated:

And when death speaks to us, what does it say? It does not speak of itself. It does not say: Fear me. It does not say: Wonder at me. It does not say: Understand me. It bids us think rather of life, of the privileges of life, of how great a thing of life can be made. And we thus reflect, we see that there are things that are mightier than death. Honor is mightier than death, for men and women have died to escape dishonor. Justice is mightier than death, for men and women have chosen death rather than countenance or do injustice.

Biomedical and biotechno scientific professionals often determine life or death for their patients. Dr. Williamson (1966: 139) provided a list of contemporary measures contributing to the dilemma of life and death as follows:

> Improved understanding of body physiology and chemistry, potent drugs, remarkably efficient mechanical respirators, pacemakers, and artificial organs, combined with aggressive medical and nursing care, have saved many lives, cured diseases, and solved many medical problems. Yet, paradoxically, this very progress has created other problems.

REDEFINITION OF DEATH AND ORGAN TRANSPLANTATION

The redefinition of death dates back to Dr. James Apple, president of the American Medical Association from 1965 to 1966 when he raised two fundamental professional inquiries concerning redefinition of death:

- Should the physician attempt to restore heart action in the donor patient and then after a period of time turns off the resuscitator?
- If the heart does not continue to beat independently of the machine, should he declare the patient dead and then start the machine again so that there will be some circulation in the organ to be transplanted?

These two major questions caused the medical community along with ethicists, theologians, and lawyers to wonder if we should not have new criteria to determine legal death (Apple, 1968: 102). Within such a contextual professional deliberation, the community of physicians changed the traditional term of "vegetation life" to "brain death" as a new criterion for redefining of heart donor eligibility (Rutstein, 1969: 526).

In *JAMA*'s article (1977: 982) which was entitled to "An Appraisal of Criteria of Cerebral Death," has redefined the new term for death as follows:

> The need for viable organs led surgeons to seek patients with intracranial pathological findings such as head injuries that resulted in a dead brain. However, if the pronouncement of death were delayed until the heart stopped beating, the organs underwent so much deterioration that a successful transplant was jeopardized. Hence, a definition of human death that considered the lack of cerebral function as important as the cessation of cardiac activity was recognized.

According to the new definition of death by American Medical Association, in May 1968 the heart surgeon Dr. Dentin Cooley at Houston's St. Luke's Episcopal Hospital was prepared to remove the heart of thirty-six-year old Clarence Nicks, a welder who had sustained severe brain damage during a brawl the previous month. The controversial ethical, moral, and legal arguments caused many ethicists, theologians, and lawyers to express their objections for such a new definition of death.

Ethicists raised objection and started to argue that as long as any sign of life is present in a patient and all organs have not completely stopped their functioning operations in a patient including putting him/her under artificial respirator that patient is alive. They expressed their vivid opinion that the "professional codes of medical ethics" for physicians mandate them to do everything to save life of a patient till the last moment of a patient's life. Along this line of argument *Stanford Daily* (1993: 1) reported about the essence of death in regard of ethical, moral, and legal bindings. In 1993 Dr. Norman Shumway transplanted the heart of a patient to another patient. The family of a homicide victim offered Dr. Shumway their consent for their victim's heart to be used for transplantation. Stanford Hospital, however, had agreed with the coroner of Santa Clara County that organs of homicide victims should not be used for organ transplantation. Despite this agreement, Stanford Hospital acquired the heart of the victim, and Dr. Shumway proceeded with the surgery. Later on lawyers for the defendant's defense argued that the defendant did not kill the victim because the victim did not die until his heart was removed. They indicated that the heart transplant surgeon caused the death of the victim. The jury agreed.

Lawyers disagreed over 1977 *JAMA*'s article concerning redefinition of "death" by introducing the "brain dead." In Dr. Cooly's patient case, lawyers started to deliberate their views over Nicks's assailant (Dr. Cooley) could be charged with "homicide" if he removed the respirator while the patient's heart was still functioning (*News Week*, 1968: 68). They raised this legal question: Would Nicks have been killed by the barroom brawler or by the surgeons who removed his heart while it was functioning? Also, since Nicks's death would constitute a homicide when he did die, an autopsy would be necessary. If Nicks' heart was removed before pronouncing him dead, then the performance of autopsy would be tainted and the cause of death could medically not be determined. Then, the legal status of the case could be changed from "homicide" to "murder." It was not clear the Nicks's will whether had a wish for donation of his heart for organ transplantation. Nevertheless, Dr. Cooley transplanted Nicks's heart to a patient without objection of the Harris County Medical Examiner Joseph Jachimczyk. Jachimczyk promised Dr. Cooley not to file criminal charges against him. Dr. Cooley completed the heart transplant as an effective innovative medical procedure.

The theological views concerning death go back to 1950s. In 1957, the International Congress of Anesthesiology attendees expressed their ethical concerns by problems in the use of resuscitative measures. Catholic physicians and biotechno scientists sought moral instructions and guidance from Pope Pius XII. Pope Pius XII (1957:1027) responded:

> A physician must not act without authorization from the patient's family, he consulted, and the family was bound to use ordinary, not

"extraordinary" measure to prolong life. According to the Catholic Church's "principle of double effect," one act – specifically, terminating resuscitation – had two effects. The first and desired affect was to end human suffering. The second effect, namely, death, was only the indirect result of a moral act. In such cases, terminating treatment was not only permissible but advisable.

In biomedical and bioscientific community of professional experts there is a distinction between cellular death and organismal death. But in the community of the Western religious traditions; Orthodox Jewish, Roman Catholic Church, and Protestant; the concept of death is based on irreversible "loss of brain function." As Veith, Jonas, Maguire, and Shannon (1981: 178) indicated: "According to M. Feinstein, there is no religious imperative to continue to use a respirator to inflate and deflate the lungs and thus maintain the cellular viability of other organs in an otherwise dead patient." In addition, the traditional Roman Catholic understanding of the moment of real death has been based on the time of departure of the soul from body. Since this separation is not an observable phenomenon, it must be related to physically measurable signs defining apparent death. However, in the Islamic faith, pronouncement of death is based on all possible exhaustive measures including respiratory failure of body and brain organisms. According to a the Islamic faith a doctor is ethically and morally obligated to diagnose and treat patients even if the patient refuses his/her consent or prefers to die. The emphasis is on the physician's responsibility to heal, to offer maximum professional care, more than on the patient's right to be treated. Also, in the Islamic medical profession a doctor's role is viewed with good faith and good will as a healer not as a murder.

In the Islamic faith there is a path of perception that can lead to refreshment of mind and body. That refreshment is related to what is the life that God has bestowed us to live? Moslems believe that God owns one's body and soul. They believe no human being has autonomy and self-determinative ground to have ultimate control over his/her life. It is subject the will of God (*Ensha Allah*). No human being should deprive himself or herself from God's gift of life. Treatment refusal, advance medical directives, passive euthanasia, and suicides are viewed sinful and prohibited, because life possesses infinite value. Therefore, doctors need to go extra miles to save patients with all costs and efforts. It is prohibited to terminate the patient's vegetable life, because Moslems have faith in God for patients to be cured.

Once the realization of brain death with spontaneous movement and responsively and permanently loses the ability to breaths spontaneously occurred professionals believe the loss of signs of life. From a religious point of view, Jewish, Roman Catholic, and Protestant scholars recognize the complete and permanent absence of any brain-related vital bodily function as death. Supporting such a claim, Catholic theologian, Rev. Bernard Haring (1973) supported such a claim: "I feel that the arguments for the equation of the total death of the person with brain death are fully valid." In the same vein, another Roman Catholic interpretation of medical ethics concerning pronouncing death,

Charles J. McFadden (1976: 202) argued that: "Once the fact of brain death has been established, the person is dead, even though heart beat and respiration are continued by mechanical means."

Rothman (1998:14) reported:

> One group of Belgian citizens, Antwerp's Orthodox Jews, have nonetheless announced they will not serve as donors, only as recipients, since they reject the concept of brain death. An intense, unresolved rabbinic debate has been taking place over the ethics of accepting but not giving organs. Should the Jewish community forswear accepting organs? Should Jews ask to be placed at the bottom of the recipient's waiting list? Or should the Jewish community change its position so as to reduce the prospect of fierce hostility or even persecution?

These and other similar questions may cause serious religious objections against organ transplantation. In 1957 controversial issues concerning the new term for redefining death, by biomedical community caused Harvard's brain death committee to be faced with legal concerns in mind. In 1968, The Ad Hoc Committee of the Harvard Medical School established new required neurological examinations to disclose unreceptively, unresponsiveness, absence of spontaneous movements and breathing, absence reflexes, fixed dilated pupils, and persistence of all these findings over a 24-hour period in the absence of intoxicants or hypothermia (*AMA*, 1968: 337). The Committee members cautioned surgeons that patients, designated as donors, should be declared dead before being removed from artificial ventilation because it would provide surgeons with greater legal protection. Within the international biomedical professional codes of ethics there have been serious objections to the new term of brain death. In May 1966 Dr. Clarence Craford had provoked public outcry in Sweden over the "cannibalizing" of human beings for human body spare parts when he suggested that patients be declared dead when flat electroencephalogram indicated irrevocable brain damage (*Time*, 1966: 78). Within the context of biomedical profession such a redefinition of death caused serious moral objections.

Proponents of redefinition of death specifically the brain death argued that since legally declaration of death of a patient is one of the professional responsibilities of physicians, therefore, adoption of the new definition of death by American Medical Association did not require having statutory change in the law in the United States of America. Also, since the law treats the redefinition of death as one of the facts to be determined by physicians, it has not been necessary the legislative body to change the legal status of death.

Humanity commands biomedical practitioners and biotechno scientists to observe ethical and moral commitments with respect to organ transplantation. Through ethical principles and moral convictions, there are serious objections to the new term of brain death. It is a fact that according to the clinical definition of brain death should not provide legitimacy for ending physical life of a patient and provide opportunities for desperately needed organs for transplantation and other useful medical purposes. In addition, the fact that someone would be useful to others if pronounced brain death should not alone be a sufficient reason for considering that person is dead and cannot be the sole basis for changing to the use of brain-oriented criteria. Rather, there must be sound reasons independent of that if society is going to alter its definition of death (Vieth, 1999: 175).

In 1968 at the World Medical Assembly in Sydney, Australia, the question of organ transplant and the definition of brain death proceeded with serious technical arguments. Britain's Dr. Martin Ware related how in four cases in Edinburgh, an electroencephalograph indicated lack of brain activity, yet all four patients recovered. Netherlands physician G. Dekker reported a similar case in which the machine registered no brain activity for four days, after which the patient recovered (*New York Times*, 1968: 25). Even nowadays, there have been cases that patients after several months or years in coma have been recovered. For example, Jessica Diaz, 17 years old gave birth on January 13, 2002. She could hardly see her newborn because of a brain tumor had blinded one eye and obscured vision in the other. Doctors removed a fast-growing tumor a day after she gave birth. Within 10 minutes of surgery, Jessica became comatose – "brain dead," and doctors told her mother, Jessica was likely to die from medullablatoma, particularly virulent brain tumor. But on April 2, 2003, her mother Eva Diaz knocked on the open door of her daughter's room at Tustin Hospital and Medical Center, Orange County, California, and for the first time in a year, her daughter turned her head toward the sound (*CNN.com*, 2003).

WHAT ARE ETHICAL AND MORAL DIMENSIONS OF LIVING DONORS?

In different cultures ownership of the whole body and its parts is a matter of econo-political interpretation. The principle that either God owns one's body or an individual is different in culture to culture. For example, in the reformed Jews and Christianity values of autonomy and self-determination ground the norm that an individual has ultimate control over his/her life, subject only to the limit of not causing harm to others. Also, within a capitalistic society like America, individuals possess ownership of all things that belong to them including their soul and body organs and materials. In most cultures, it is the personal wish of individuals how to value their own bodies. Governments and medical authorities are required to respect their citizens' wishes concerning how to dispose their citizens' bodies after death.

In most democratic societies, individuals stress on respecting the patient's wishes to live or to die. Selectivity of restoring and/or elimination of those whose lives are deemed a burden upon society at large either by the patients' request and/or by the physician decision is a matter of professional discretionary decision. Accordingly, in non-monolithic religious societies buying and selling body parts including sperm, eggs, ovarian tissues, tooth, kidney, cornea, bone marrow, and other parts from a live body are subject to the wishes of body owners, either to be decided by an individual or by the family to do so. There is a serious flaw within such an immersion. That flaw is related to children's body parts to be sold or bought by parents and/or guardians. Ethically and morally, there is a presumption against self-mutilation, even when good can come of it.

WHAT ARE IMPLICATIONS OF CADAVER DONATIONS?

Ethically and morally, there is a beginning presumption that mutilating a corpse defiles its integrity. Also, mutilation of a dead body defiles its sanctity by violating its dignity. The burial ceremonies or freezing of dead bodies reflects honoring and respecting the life of an individual who lived once that body lived. Dead bodies contain four major inherent connections with their relatives (1) to their spouses, (2) to their children, (3) to their relatives who were living with them, and (4) to their offspring generations who will emerge in future.

Multiculturally, there are different sociocultural views concerning the ownership of a dead body. In some cultures like Americans and Europeans who follow either common law, or code law mandate the body of the deceased to next of kin in order to perform last rites for eternal separation of their earthly emotional connectivity. They celebrate through rosaries in order to admit that the earthly life of such a deceased body is over and expecting to join them in future in other world. That is the main reason that spouses like to be buried side by side in a cemetery. Therefore, in such materialistic cultures, the ownership of an individual extends after life and posses specific values. The deep wisdom of such sentiments carries inherent ownership connotations that allow either the next of kin or government to the disposition of remains and to direct the donation of somatic organs after and/or before death.

In the Middle Eastern cultures, people believe that a deceased body belongs to God and relatives or governments do not have any authoritative ownership to dead bodies. They believe that individuals should be buried immediately after death, because a deceased body is a sacrament; a visible sign instituted by God to confer grace or a divine life on those who worthily receive it. Also, in the Middle Eastern cultures, spouses, children, and relatives do not celebrate the death of their relatives, instead they mourn together for separation of the deceased body from familial members. Biotechno-scientists and biomedical professionals must act extraordinary measures to prolong life. Ethically, morally, and professionally, they are in trust by public to perform extraordinary efforts to save lives of their patients, regardless of patients family members authorization.

ANALYSIS OF PATIENTS' CONSENT

How we structure the ethical, moral, and legal dialogues concerning consent depends on how we define consent. We need to analyze the notion of consent most likely to insure that meaningful communication occurs between patients and biomedical practitioners and institutions of medical and heath care systems, including bioresearch centers. Biomedical professionals are expected to use their professional expertise derived from their education, training, experiences, and experimental research assessments to make judgments about what they believe should or should not be done for patients. Acquisition of consent provides professional autonomy for a physician. However, autonomy triggers the duty to secure consent too. Professional autonomy is important, but it is neither the sole nor the primary principle of biomedical practices. Professional autonomy is derivative of and subordinate to the full extent of obligation that a physician shows respect for a patient. Respecting professional autonomy is simply one way of respecting patients. In order to analyze ethical, moral, and legal dimensions of the consent we will discuss them in five major categories: (1) actual consent, (2) presumed consent, (3) proxy consent, (4) informed consent, and (5) conscript consent.

Ethical and Moral Analysis Concerning Actual Consent

By a deliberative logical thought, professional autonomy does not exclude the fate of a patient on the basis of assumed consent. Yet actual consent concerns itself with matters of respecting human dignity, promotional decision-making processes, encouraging professional self-scrutiny, avoidance of deceit and coercion, and above all respecting both natural and civil rights of doctors and patients.

According to intellectual deliberative process of reasoning, the validity of an actual consent on the extent to which certain permissions have been granted by a patient to a physician or to a medical and health care institution depends on both natural and civil laws. Such consent includes respect for the life and careful consideration of professional codes of ethics concerning diagnostic and treatment alternatives. The actual philosophy of consent indicates that the first command is: "Thou shalt not hypothesis or presume consent to terminate a patient's life." Let us see if we can make this complex professional account clear. In the field of biomedical profession, there are familiar and stabilized procedural elements for diagnosis and treatment of patients, and there are unstable elements (the possibility of alternative explanations, the prospect for efficacious treatment, and the patient's ability to cope with therapy). As the nature of consent unfolds, certain cardinal issues emerge (the likely benefit to the patient of one or another diagnosis and treatment plan, the risk of trial and error on the basis of innovative medical procedures and new experiments, and the unexpected failure or successful outcomes to emerge).

Through professional codes of ethics and occupational codes of conduct attending physicians, biotechno scientists, and paramedical personnel play important roles to prolong or shortening the life of patients; depends how they are using the patient's consent. Therefore, the exercise of patient's actual consent depends on cooperation among professional and paramedical staff of a medical unit to use intelligent decisions and actions with the notions of ethical and moral commitments.

Engelhardt, Jr. (1996: 122-124) has presented two major principles concerning consent as follows:

Principle I. The Principle of Permission

Authority for actions involving others in a secular pluralist society is derived from their permission. As a consequence:

Without such permission or consent there is no authority.

•   Actions against such authority are blameworthy in the sense of placing a violator outside the moral community in general, and making licit (but not obligatory) retaliatory, defensive, or punitive force:

o   Implicit consent: individuals, groups, and states have authority to protest the innocent from unconsented to force.

o   Explicit consent: individuals, groups, and states can decide to enforce contracts or create welfare rights.

o   Justification of the principle: the principle of permission expresses the circumstance that authority for resolving moral disputes in a secular, pluralist society can be derived only from the agreement of the participants, since it cannot be derived from rational argument or common belief. Therefore, permission or consent is the origin of authority, and respect the right of participants to consent is the necessary condition for the possibility of a moral community. The principle of permission provides the minimum grammar for secular moral discourse. It is an inescapable as the interest of persons in blaming and praising with justification and resolving issues with moral authority.

o   Motivation for obeying the principle is tied to interests in acting in a way i) that is justifiable to peaceable persons generally, and ii) that will not justify the use of defensive or punitive force against oneself.

o   Public policy implications: the principle of permission provides moral grounding for public policies aimed at defending the innocent.

o   Maxim: Do not do to others that which they would not have done unto them, and do for them that which one has contracted to do.

o   The principle of permission grounds what can be termed the morality of autonomy as mutual respect?

Principle II: The Principle of Beneficence

The goal of moral action is the achievement of goods and the avoidance of harms. In a secular pluralist society, however, no particular account or ordering of goods and harms can be established as canonical. As a result, within the bounds of respecting autonomy, no particular content-full môral vision can be established over competing senses (at least within a peaceable secular pluralist society). Still, a commitment to beneficence characterizes the undertaking of morality, because without a commitment to beneficence the moral life has no content. As a consequence:

• On the one hand, there is no general content-full principle of beneficence to which one can appeal.

• On the other hand, actions without regard to concerns of beneficence are blameworthy in the sense of placing violators outside the context of any particular content-full moral community. Such actions place individuals beyond claims to beneficence. In particular, malevolence is a rejection of the bonds of beneficence. Insofar as one rejects only particular rules of beneficence, grounded in a particular view of the good life, one loses only one's own claims to beneficence within that particular moral community; in either case, petitions for mercy (charity) can still have standing. Actions against beneficence constitute moral impropriety. They are against the content proper to the moral life:

o Implicit contract: content for fashioning a community with a common view of the proper account or ordering of goods and harms acquires principle of beneficence.

o Explicit contract: content for duties of beneficence can be derived as well as from explicit agreements. In this case, as in the previous case, the content of a duty of beneficence is grounded in the principle of permission.

o Justification of the principle: the principle of beneficence reflects the circumstances that moral concerns encompass the pursuit of goods and avoidance of harms. Since such disputes can be resolved in secular pluralistic societies only by an appeal to the principle of permission, the principle of permission is conceptually prior to the principle of beneficence. One can know when one is violating the morality of mutual respect, even when one cannot know, because of its lack on content, whether one is violating the principle of beneficence. However, recognition of the principle of beneficence provides the minimal characterization of the content required for moral concerns.

o Motivation for obeying the principle is tied to interests in acting in a way: I) that is justifiable to beneficent persons generally, and ii) that will not justify one in being characterized as an unsympathetic individual who may be excluded from a particular or any community's beneficence.

o Public policy implications: the principle of beneficence provides the moral grounding for reusable welfare rights drown from common holdings.

o Maxim: Do to others their good.

o The principle of beneficence grounds what can be termed the morality of welfare and social sympathies?

Ethical and Moral Analysis Concerning Presumed Consent

Imposing on patients' consequences they have not assumed is a form of coercion. Respect for human dignity requires truth telling. Patients are entitled to know what are wrong with them. Patients need medical information to make choices; especially when no medical options exist. Specifically, those patients who are expected to die, they need to know what are presumed options ahead of them; to plan a funeral, say farewell to their beloved ones, and simply to realize their life time is drawing to a close. Younger (1988: 2094) indicated: "Patients are value systems, not organ systems, and consent serves a personal purpose even when it is medically useless."

The idea of presuming that organ donors would consent to the use of their alternative organs and body such as kidney, eye, and body materials, including blood, sperm, eggs, bone marrow, tissues, cells, and genes for life saving transplantation is now receiving serious attention. In order to see why it is necessary to both moral and ethical logic behind presumed consent and the alternatives available, we need to examine diversified views concerning this issue.

One of the major issues in the field of biomedical and biotechno sciences concerning acquisition of a consent is related to emergency medical help that must be supplied at once to avoid loss of life, mutilation, or compromise of bodily or psychological function. The problem is related to two major factors: (1) time and (2) immediate diagnosis and treatment. In these circumstances, biomedical practitioners and paramedical staff face with presumption of the consent. The degree and level of medical aids depend on the severity and acute conditions of the patients. Sometimes physicians and paramedical staff will be required to take a general range of actions where the reasonable presumption will be that persons about to be presumed already to have consented. It is in these situations and circumstances that negative or intrinsic rights and duties are stronger than positive or extrinsic rights and duties. These negative or intrinsic rights and duties will be subject to the physician's conscience. General negative rights and duties based on a physician's conscience are subject to professional arbitrary decisions and actions which are not subject to prior agreements, understanding, and/or consent of a severed injured patient.

Although in our modern civilizations neither the living individuals nor the next of kin technically owns the body parts and body materials, to some extent they can be thought of having quasi-property rights. Nevertheless, professional alternatives are based upon justifications of a set of moral and ethical rules.

Ethical and Moral Dimensions of Proxy Consent

Human organ and material transplantations embrace any of several epithelium, sperm or eggs, or early conception such that genetic changes become permanently encoded in the sex cells of the resulting generational adult. Germ cell alterations such as stem cell, cell line, and mixed germ line by virtue of their intergenerational consequences can create potential ethical and moral controversies. In theory, only changes directed at the germ line can produce heritable changes. However, in practice, some cell alterations also become transmissible. More serious ethical objections apply to intentional germ line interventions because of the uncertainty of using a person solely as a viable source for creating uncertain genetic change in his/her descendants. It is also morally and ethically objectionable to use the promise of future benefit to conduct experiment on fetuses or embryos for whom other biotechnologies exist to achieve the end of being free of major genetic defect.

The proxy consent can affect not only someone as a recipient of organ transplantation and/or somatic material alteration; also it will affect the offspring and future descendants of the treated individual. Since future descendants by the time of transplantation or alteration are not existed, then the rational adequacy and acceptability of proxy consent become questionable. Therefore, future uncertainty of both somatically and germinal transplantation and/or alteration as potential cure for an individual may cause a major heredity disorder (e.g., Huntington's chorea or retinoblastoma) for future generations. To discover whether or not such genetic material changes are in fact beneficial to the recipients and on coming generations it requires bioresearchers to conduct comprehensive strategic experiments to prove that some certainty what the future holds and can faithfully convey those probabilities in a discussion of informed consent by proxy. Since somatic and germinal transplantations and/or alterations may subject at least to one or probably more generations of future persons to the experimentation before the phenotype effects of germinal changes can be tested, the proxy consent is subject to careful consideration. Therefore, proxy consent can be considered as one of the major moral and ethical flaws in biotechnology and biosciences.

Ethical, Moral, and Legal Analysis of Informed Consent

The concept of informed consent is based on econo-political theories of individualistic self-determination in Western civilization. It is the product of the Patient Self-Determination Act, a federal law that went into effect in 1991 in the United States. It requires physicians and medical and health care institutions to comprehensively explain and advice patients about their rights to accept or refuse medical treatments. Also, it provides opportunities for patients to advance treatments with possible medical choices or to deny them.

Informed consent is one of the best-known legal terms, and arguably, one of the best-known routine concepts in modern biotechno-scientific and biomedical practices. Although much of the ethical and moral issues concerning actual, presumed, and proxy consents have traditional roots, the idea of informed consent is relatively new. Until the mid-twentieth century most medical ethical issues were viewed as physicians and medical institutions' professional responsibility to act autonomously, but not to inform or consult with patients either practicing medicine, and/or conducting bioresearch (e.g., Tuskegee Syphilis Bioresearch Project).

The legal term of informed consent came to medical practices through the judiciary system. As Levine (1999: 2) indicated:

> The earliest influential decision was *Shloendorff v. New York Hospital* (1914), in which the court ruled that a patient's right to self-determination obligated a physician to obtain consent. This case laid the basis for further litigation. The most influential series of decisions occurred in the 1950s and 1960s, when rulings went beyond the litigation to obtain consent to include an explicit duty to disclose information relevant to the patient who is making a decision about consent. The term *informed consent* first appeared in *Salgo v. Leland Stanford, Jr., University Board of Trustees* (1957).

The informed consent has been initiated for broadening access to the actual processes of professional decision-making and practices of medicine by patients from legal standpoint. In the legal arena, informed consent has been used to develop minimal standards for doctor-patient interactions and clinical decision-making processes. The most important argument for involving patients in medical decision making processes is based on the philosophy of patients' rights to how and why diagnosis and treatments including therapy should be conducted. Nevertheless, physicians and patients typically assume of informed consent as a legal requirement for a signed piece of paper, rather than a process of normative communication between physicians and patients. Nevertheless, informed consent is viewed as a recitation of risks and benefit analysis to prevent further legal actions against physicians.

Informed consent contains a series of interrelated professional tasks. First, patients and attending physicians must address the agreed real medical diagnostic issues that will be the focus of their attention. Whereas physicians typically focus on biotechno scientific medical methods and procedures, patients typically view the problems within the contextual boundaries of possible recovery of their health and socio-economic implications. Second, informed consents provide treatment and therapeutic plans with affordability of physical, psychological, and financial demands. Third, informed consents should provide comprehensive risk assessments and the possible level of healing achievement through availability of alternative treatment plans and objectives. Fourth, choosing the best suitable treatment strategy in order to achieve therapeutic objectives. Fifth, physicians must have assurance that their patients can understand the required diagnostic, treatment, and prognostic information.

Moral and Ethical Problems With Conscript Consent

There must be a distinction between voluntary and compulsory consents in biomedical services. The call for volunteers with the socio-cultural and econo-political pressures can cause a sort of conscripting. There are many social issues in which individuals do not wish to have any desire to consider them in their private lives. Nevertheless, since individuals are socially interacting with others, they are under pressure to comply with those societal rules and regulations. In such cases some soliciting issues emerge and may infringe individuals' natural rights and civil rights. Then the conscripting consent becomes a non-negotiable minimum requirement for further medical actions. For example, if patients do not sign the medical consent for receiving treatment in a hospital, then they will not be admitted. However, granting soliciting consent to a hospital is a part of medical procedure in which forces patients to give away their rights in return to receive medical services. In such a situation, there is a question: who may conscript and who may be conscripted?

The major medical problem between a patient and a hospital concerning a conscript consent is related to creation of a safety net for hospitals, attending physician, and biomedical researchers concerning their medical research projects and careers. In regard of such issues Jonas (1981: 248) indicated:

> The ineradicable dialectic of this situation – delicate incompatibility problems – calls for particular controls by research community and by public authority that we need not discuss. Then can mitigate, but not eliminate the problem. We have to live with the ambiguity, the treacherous impurity of everything human.

CHAPTER 10

INTELLECTUAL CONTRIBUTIONS AND ACADEMIC INTEGRITY

OBJECTIVES OF THIS CHAPTER

When you have read this chapter you should be able to do the following:

- Develop conceptual skills of ethical and moral principles for effective examination of integrity in bioresearch processes.
- Establish a foundation for analyzing the honorable professional responsibilities of biotechno scientists and their institutions to honest verifiable methods in designing, proposing, performing, evaluating, and publishing bioresearch intellectual contributions.

- Develop comprehensive understanding of the codes of moral conduct and the professional codes of ethics in bioscientific research.
- Understand difference between the utopian and the dystopian views of humanity.
- Know how to convert human weaknesses into strengths.
- Understand the historical progressive trends of biosciences in civilized societies.
- See the integration of sciences, scientists, and society as a holistic multi- dimensional entity for the welfare of the human race.
- Be familiar with cultural philosophies, biosophy, and theosophy concerning gene engineering, cloning, and fertility activities.
- Realize what academic honesty and integrity are in bioscientific research activities.
- Develop a sense of reliable academic knowledge and behavioral norms in laboratories.
- Know what the major attributes of innovative bioresearch are.
- Know what academic professional mandated principles in bioresearch centers are.
- Be able to develop a common body of knowledge for bioethical and biomoral reasoning for biotechno scientists and biomedical practitioners.
- Know what the differences are between Classical and Rogerian analytical reasoning.
- Recognize four types of reasoning: inductive, deductive, analogous, and holistic.
- Understand the traditional academic expectations concerning publish or perish.
- Know how to compete intellectually in academic institutions.
- Know the effects of intellectual contributions through authorship and publications.
- Develop a comprehensive ethical responsibility in the presentation of professional research papers at professional conferences.
- Establish a holistic academic accountability for using public resources.

PLAN OF THIS CHAPTER

Bioknowledge advancement and biotechnological developmental progress depend upon a free exchange of ideas and experimental information through a vast and growing global multicultural professional networking of communication. Such a vital professional mission for academicians is crucial to prevent fraudulent claims and cover up abuses of human subjects. Perspectives on bioresearch practical priorities and biotechno scientists' integrity sometimes manifest conflicting ethical and moral consequences. An examination of empirical bioresearch studies on the behavior of scientists yielded few significant insights. Globally, existing bioscientific research activities, specifically in the area of the human subject, are not adequate to support conclusions about the relative effectiveness of various alternatives for fostering honesty and integrity in bioresearch processes. Although some countries in recent years have developed and adopted formal bioresearch guidelines to foster bioethical practices, global scientific experience with ethical bioresearch guidelines is limited. The most crucial barriers in obtaining biodata are related to politico-economic misconduct. Data on secret bioresearch projects and confidential national scientific reports are not available. For example, because of the secrecy surrounding development of biological and biochemical weapons of mass destruction and/or defensive bioweapon mass destructive experimental programs in some countries are not available. Only some few governmental authorities and organizations know what would be the end results of such horrible crimes against humanity.

In this chapter, our plan is to discuss an ethical and moral framework for effective examination of the integrity of bioresearch processes and honorable professional responsibilities of biotechno scientists and their institutions in relation to honest and verifiable methods in designing, proposing, performing, evaluating, and publishing bioresearch activities. It should be noted that the term bioresearch integrity is sometimes thought to be synonymous with integrity of biosciences, but the terms of reference are different. Whereas, bioresearch integrity has been seen as the code of moral conduct for a social enterprise that involves individuals and institutions, the integrity of biosciences is related to a professional codes of ethics in information, composed of current viable and reliable biotechno scientific methodologies, theories, paradigm, and observations in developing, assessing, certifying, and communicating research results.

At the beginning of this chapter, we will analyze the codes of moral conduct and professional codes of ethics. While violation of the codes of moral conduct is an amorphous term, it covers a spectrum of both significant intentional forms of bad-faith and trivial forms of bad-faith and bad-will in behavior by biotechno scientists. Both bad-faith and bad-will by biotechno scientists are commonly referred to fraud. The moral interpretation of the term *fraud* denotes to an intentional deception and conscious damage to human subjects by bioresearchers. On the other hand, violation of the professional codes of ethics is sometimes referred to as inexcusable ignorance and undeniable negligence. Ignorance is the lack of adequate professional knowledge and information. Negligence is a deliberated carelessness not following expected universal standards of the professional codes of ethics.

INTRODUCTION

Traditionally, to the academic community of researchers, scholars, and scientists the important thing has been not only a creed which expects that they should believe in honesty, modesty, and humility and be faithful to observable codes of ethics in their behavior and intellectual contributions, but also that they should be faithful to the goodness and wisdom of their vision-mission derivatives by attending to the pragmatic courses of constructive actions; not destructive biological and biochemical mass destruction. They should accept that the moral obligations are honorable in their mind and are as unbreakable as that of accuracy and integrity in their behavior. Such a pledge applies to all incumbents including governments, industries, and bioacademicians.

The historical idealistic world of humanity is often traced back to the Greek *eutopia – Platonists*. Can we find an ideal human society? The answer is "no." Can we search for it? The answer is yes. Utopia exists nowhere, except in the human mind. Nevertheless, the utopian genre is old. It is old as the human race. It is a phenomenon that premises a presupposed excellent idealistic human life and nature. Rousseauists are convinced that humanity is naturally good, or at least the journey to perfectibility is promising. Opponents to Rousseauists are Hobbesians who believe that humanity and nature have double characteristics: (1) good and bad, (2) perfect and imperfect, (3) faithful and faithless, (4) graceful and ungraceful, and (5) consistent and inconsistent. Accordingly, humanity possesses two opposite extreme zones:

- On the right, are those who think and behave as if human life, as it should be, is pretty good and life is *utopia*. People should enjoy and appreciate it.
- On the left, are those who think that humans already inhabit the worst of all possibilities and life is *dystopia*. People should suffer in order for tyrants and vicious people to enjoy their lives. Which group will take power in a society? Those who have conspired against humanity or those who are altruistic? For example, in the 1995 Tokyo subway attack on passengers, one of the followers of the Aum Shinrikyo cult Asahara; a partially sighted yoga tutor whose real name was Chizuo Matsumoto released Sarin gas during the peak of rush hour and killed 12 people and caused thousands of others to become sick. There are many passengers who are still suffering with headaches, breathing problems and dizziness. Finally, on February 26, 2004, the former Japanese doomsday cult leader was been found guilty and sentenced to death for masterminding the 1995 nerve gas attack. Sarin gas is extremely toxic. It affects the nervous system when inhaled as a gas or

absorbed through skin. It suffocates victims immediately by paralyzing the muscles around the lungs. A single drop can kill a person in few minutes (*CNN.com*, 2004).

Nevertheless, in between the utopian and dystopian zones of real life, there are remarkable capabilities in which humanity can find dubious processes and consequences because of its strengths and weaknesses. The only serious weakness of humanity that is seeded in its inherent characteristic is ignorance. How can we convert weaknesses into strengths by bioethics? Perhaps we can search for possibilities through the human's flourishing intellectual mind to convert natural defective genes to smart genes through genetic engineering or through social, moral, and ethical reforms. Is this possible? That is a complex question.

Genetic engineering is remodeling and restructuring human psychosomatic characteristics. Within the contextual biological and ecological processes of such a conversion, we should not try to let the ends justify the means; to exterminate rival genes that can threaten the new genes. Biotechno scientists, bioresearchers, and biomedical practitioners all as academicians have created promising possibilities through enhancing germ cells and stem cells to cure chronic illnesses and deformities. How about social deviations and psychological deformities? Is it the task of biotechno scientists to do so? The answer could be no, because it is the task of bioethicists who criticize all ugly and unpleasant contents within the contexts of real life.

Bioscientific discoveries are the result of relentless efforts of academicians who have individualized a common characteristic or connection among natural genes and proteins and kinesthetic intelligence that were deemed dissimilar or unrelated before. Academicians have created new set of terms in their research endeavors such as:

- Basic bioresearch to serve humans, animals, and plants with scientific methodological novelty.
- Cure bioresearch to find innovative diagnostic and treatment procedures to fight against diseases.
- Targeted bioresearch to apply promotional bio-discoveries and enhance human and animal lives.
- Mission-oriented bioresearch to serve strategic defensive biological and microbiological problem solving.
- Disease-oriented bioresearch to fight against human made diseases and germs.

- Programmatic bioresearch to experiment with new pharmaceutical products and by-products; relevant bioresearch to find ecologically and environmentally related solutions.
- Commission-initiated bioresearch to come out with national innovative and technovative solutions and policies.
- Contract-supported bioresearch to fulfill focused task oriented research projects for utilizing bioscientific supports towards profitability of their sponsors; biopharmaceuticals and/or governments.
- Payoff bioresearch to find quick fix solutions for the biopharmaceutical industry for financially accelerated profit-making purposes.

Nevertheless, in all types of bioresearch, academicians are subject to academic honesty and integrity. This is the theme of this chapter.

PROGRESS IN BIORESEARCH: PAST, PRESENT, AND FUTURE

Biotechno scientific innovativeness and concluding validity of bioresearch end results could be viewed as social enterprises in which involvements of different parties and institutions engaged in initiating competitive ideas, developing scientific procedures, conducting pragmatic experimental research, concluding viable discoveries, filing copyrights and/or patents, and publishing in well known professional journals. Through such a systematic process, bioresearchers and authors focus on the integrity of their efforts to find remedies for deceases. Within the contextual societal boundary of the publishing process there are four major critical issues:

- The innovative integrity of the bioscientific research proposals.
- Questionable operational research processes and applications of biotechno scientific methodologies.
- Peer and/or expert evaluation of journal articles, research papers, conference proceeding papers, and scientific reports.
- Assessment, analysis, and evaluation of bioresearchers' ethical, moral, and legal conduct.

We can claim that many scientific innovative research proposals are the result of individualizing a common socio-medical characteristic or connection between somatic causes, processes, and effects of deceases that were deemed dissimilar or unrelated before. One of the major issues in bioresearch is recognition of the merit of diseases concerning the continuity of human life.

Culturally and scientifically, we need to review acute diseases from the standpoint of social justice. Every year many women die because of diseases. We can claim that justice in diagnosis and treatment of the two genders are not equal. Unnecessary risks to health are not shared equally by gender. Bioethicists argue that gender disease is an important issue to be considered in funding bioresearch projects. Gender disease is a term that draws attention to culturally constructed meanings of masculinity and femininity, which are social elaborations upon human biological sexual differences.

Any research proposal should be oriented toward the needs of the users. In many instances the causes, processes, and effects of creativity consist of discovering an interrelatedness between one system or field of knowledge and another on one hand, and dissimilarities between deductive, inductive, and analogous concepts on the other hand. One of the most important examples of this type is that of Darwin. Arieti (1993: 23) indicated:

> In 1838 Darwin happened to read the book written by Malthus 40 years before, *Essay on the Principle of Population.* Malthus had advanced the idea that Rousseau's optimistic views about humanity are unsound because (1) the natural tendency of population is to increase faster than the means of subsistence; and (2) this fact increases results in a struggle for existence. Darwin, abstracting from all the observations that he made in the Galapagos Islands, had the vision that productive competition between members of the same species is similar to the Malthusian competition found in human society. Thus Darwin applied principles formulated in relation to human society to the origin of life in general.

Nevertheless, we are committed ethically and morally to presume science, scientists, and society (3Ss) as a synthetic holistic multidimensional phenomenon that can create a healthy competitive environment in academia.

It is very difficult to assess the historical process of the natural and artificial world as presented to us at the time of birth. The world is initially strange to us as unlabeled place with mysteries. The numbers of natural events or objects are numerous and their positive and negative contributions and impacts on other elements, including humans, are unknown. This has made bioscientists search for the ways of discovering the key elements of life.

Even with all of the progressive bioresearch discoveries and innovations, our understanding of the natural life is still limited. For many years bioscientists and biotechnologists have wondered how to understand the way nature functions. In recent years the roles of science in general, and biosciences specifically, have become extremely manipulative to such an extent that they are trying to outwit and overturn nature. Nevertheless, we are optimistic that the results of biotechno scientific research will enrich human life and promise to eradicate diseases and enhance human somatic development. Within such a progressive trend in biosciences, the danger in production of bio-weapons of mass destruction (BWMD) including biochemical and biological weapons is frightening.

By nature, governmental bureaucratic authorities are not qualified to conduct research in biology and medicine. They can manipulate biotechnologists' mind to justify their ambitious ends through bioresearch means. If governmental bureaucratic authorities' mindset and operations are autocratic then the process and consequences of bioresearch becomes catastrophic. This is related to the dark side of human nature that converts bioscientists into some of the groups of smart criminals. Specifically, in culturally militarized societies, interest groups provide monetary rewards for bioscientific and biotechnological end-results into inhumane processes. They convert human spiritual nature into viciousness.

Historically, professional bioscientists searched generation by generation for more blessings and desirable innovative life enhancement. There is a crucial question:

What might happen if the coming generations grow up only in a pre-designed eugenic culture, where they come to think and proceed their lives as a mere process of pre-revolutionized creatures?

The answer would be based upon the consequential uncertainty of trial and error. Are they able to ignore the mystery of the process of natural evolution as they did in the cloning process of Dolly the sheep? In the bio-methodological process of Dolly the sheep, bioresearchers asserted utilitarian (consequential) bioethics rather than deontological (causality) bioethics.

From another point of view, gene engineering is advancement in science and a risky technological development that structures genes for wholesale and/or retail sale in the world's gene banks. It is an international legal mandate for the biotech industry to patent genetically human embryos and fetuses as well as human genes, cell lines, germ lines, and tissues. This can cause potential ethical and moral arguments concerning patenting all separate parts of eugenic products except the whole process of human cloning. The main ethical and moral reasoning for not having potentially patentable whole human beings is constitutional law and human rights forbidding any type of slavery. Nevertheless, the debate over the life patent is one of the most important legal, ethical, and moral issues ever to face civilization. The life patent targets the core concept of our religious and political beliefs about the very nature of life on Earth. The debate over life patents is the issue of whether it is to be conceived of as having intrinsic family moral values or mere utility of legal material values. In the event that, in the free market economy, producers do have the right to own and freely allocate their products, the main problem will be of ownership in eugenic production system in reference to human ownership (slavery). As long as nations are subject to the charter of the United Nations, biotech corporations and/or governments cannot patent their whole products; cloned human beings.

Historically, in responding to patented life, the lifelong slavery arguments finally came to end in the Ninetieth century with abolitionists who argued that every human being has intrinsic value and cannot be made the personal commercial property of another human being. Some nations believe that genetic materials are facts of nature and therefore must be considered as a discovery and not as an innovation. However, holders of Promethean biosophical beliefs state that creation of cloned humans by the biotech industry and gene engineering is an innovative reproduction system that can create fabricated cloned humans with specific characteristics and valuable genes. By such a claim, eventually cloned humans will not be free of commercialization values including ownership and trademarks and they will be subject to profits from selling their organs in biotech retail stores. If this happens, then humanity will lose its integrity and dignity.

Agribusinesses, biopharmaceutical, and biotech corporations are already seeking patents on superior plants, animals, and chemical genotypes that can be replicated and mass-produced for use chemical factories, for organ transplantation and for meat consumption. Some biotech industry leaders hope to create brand-name identification for their cloned plants and animals by spending large sums of money on marketing their version of Dolly the sheep.

The biotech Group (Geron) bought Dolly's cloning technology, specifically in embryo, from a Scottish company for $28 million. The U.S. Biotech Group aimed to clone a patient's cells to produce specialized tissues for transplantation. Geron, a U. S. Corporation based in California, bought cloning technology from Roslin-Bio-Med, a private company which set up a newly sophisticated system in biotechnology to commercialize cloning research in the public sector, at the Roslin Institute in Edinburgh, Scotland. British bioscientists at the Roslin-Bio-Med Institute believe that "biosciences are global activities which should have freedom to pursue their biotech scientific objectives." Nevertheless the acquisition of the Roslin Bio-Med corporation offered Geron a strong lead in the biotechnologies needed to grow specialized cells; eventually whole organs for transplantation (Cookson, 1999: 10).

In the decade of 1990s, the number of domestic and international alliances grew by more than 25 percent annually (Black and Ernest, 1995: 97). Peter Drucker made a comment that the greatest change in the way scientists, corporations, and nations are conducting their activities is in the accelerating growth of scientific relationships based not on ownership but on partnership (Drucker, 1995: 12). Alliances provide networking societies with a unique opportunity to leverage their strategic focus, flexibility, and innovativeness. Eugenic-networking societies in the third millennium will create potential opportunities to acquire and exchange knowledge and information associated with their partner's skill and capabilities. Rifkin (1998: 37) indicated:

> Global chemical and pharmaceutical giants are moving quickly to consolidate their control over the world's remaining germ plasma reserves... Just a century ago, hundreds of millions of farmers, scattered across the planet, controlled their own seed stocks, trading them freely among neighbors and friends. Today, much of the seed stock has been brought up, engineered, and patented by global companies and kept in·the form of intellectual property.

In addition, chemical companies are buying seed companies. They hope to own the green gold of the biotech century (Fowler and Mooney, 1990:123).

Promethean biotechno scientific innovativeness without consideration of the natural evolutionary process may end up with catastrophes. Revolutionary biotechno scientific efforts need to synthesize both natural and artificial genetic engineering and therapy, intrinsic and extrinsic utility of gene values, and reduction of natural and artificial harmful factors for the purpose of ethically objectionable status of species. The ability to discover innovativeness in biomedical therapy and to reinvent new species is an important phase of gene proliferation because it allows the organism to seek out suitable environments and resources and to avoid unsuitable ones.

ACADEMIC MORAL AND ETHICAL PHILOSOPHIES

For a few years, one thing that caught our attention was the interest in ethical behavior within the contextual boundaries of medicine, education, business, and above all biosciences. By reviewing academic philosophies of teaching and research, we may find crossroads of thoughts and behavior through the realm of academic highways of choices and forces. Academic highways of thought point out two directions: (1) scientific deliberated instruction and (2) virtuous alternative solutions to be free from forced deceptive decisions or manipulative actions. In crossroads of academic thought and communication, academicians are capable of free choices and actions whether or not they are accorded the right to such consequences. Nevertheless, when academicians are caught between choices and forces at a deceptive and manipulative crossroad, they are more exposed to possibility of getting lost.

The foremost ethical inquiry concerning the nature of academic responsibilities is related to the academic philosophy of our institutions of higher learning. Consequential ethicists believe that academicians should be treated equally. That is what justice and fairness demand. This philosophy is based on the standardization of academia and professions, regardless of differences among constituencies. Professional authorities must make equity in their fair judgmental alternative objectives. They should believe that equal treatment simply means to provide the same facilities for all constituencies regardless of their relevant differences. They view academic achievement as a base on an honest competition. For example, when students receive A's because they have proven that they have reached a higher level of achievement than D students. Equity, justness, and fairness demand a reward system in competitive achievement and those differences that make a difference (Strike and Soltis, 1992: 57).

On the other hand, deontological ethicists believe that academicians should be treated differently according to their related differences. At this level individuality is a matter of meritocracy. Individuality is viewed as the notion of purposive being. No matter how much academicians are alike, they are individuals because they are different by physical and mental traits, and social position. They deserve to be treated differently. This does not mean that academicians are essentially different creatures and naturally they should be treated unequally. We must presume that academicians should be treated equitably unless some relevant differences exist. This does not mean to taking away of academic resources and opportunities from those capable researchers to give them to those groups, who are lazy and do not deserve them. Therefore, accordingly we need to identify the needs of academicians and provide them with appropriate resources for their effective intellectual contributions.

WHAT IS ACADEMIC HONESTY?

The term *honesty* means an individual is straightforward and trustworthy in dealing with the discovery of truth and the expression of the truthful judgments concerning self and others. An honest person does not withhold one's own feelings, ideas, and knowledge relevant to realization and expression of the whole truth. A *moral* person reveals, by all means and ends, the whole truth, only the truth, and not beyond the truth, while an *amoral* person reveals only a portion of the truth. An honest individual possesses two moral and ethical characteristics: (1) integrity and (2) dignity.

The term *integrity* means soundness of and adherence to the ultimate state of moral character; excellence. Moral and ethical principles mandate people to preserve their honest thoughts and express their intellectual ideas without fear of retaliation. The philosopher Friedrich Nietzsche (1844-1900) expressed his opinion that a moral person needs to be independent in thoughts and strong in convictions, even in the face of group pressure and government authority (Nietzsche, 1917, 1924). Martin Heidigger (1889-1927), another existentialist philosopher, expressed his ideal of nobility and thoughts for the importance of resolutive conviction in relation to personal integrity rather than succumbing into socio-political pressures to conform. He believed personal integrity means that one cannot coexist with everyone who is not ethical, so it is incumbent on each person to choose individual lifestyles and commitments carefully.

The term *dignity* is closely related to self-consideration in relation to the maintenance and manifestation of self-identity. Dignity means self-respect gained by the conformity to excellence in an individual's moral character. It is a base for suitable characteristic traits for a person. Individuals with a high quality of integrity try to elevate their moral character to the highest standard of morality and ethics. For an individual, self-respect is normally extended to the consideration for oneself as an independent agent. Self-respect is the opposite of self-contempt. Thus, integrity is an "ultimate" tendency to represent a favorable intellectual optimistic opinion of self-image according to the highest state of excellence.

THE ROOTS OF HONOR AND INTEGRITY IN BIOACADEMIA

The values of humanity appreciate the worth of dignity of each human being. They recognize the supreme importance of an individual's integrity that exists within the process of ethical and moral socialization. They promote the notion of excellence in character and enhancement in behavior. In stating these propositions, we need to explain more precisely what we mean by an act of honorable choice. We need to distinguish choice from forced decisions and actions, because the character of an academician depends more upon what he/she chooses than upon any other type of act he/she performs. Furthermore, we know from our experience that we deliberately attribute freedom to our choices and acts in proportion, as we are able to choose one type of behavior or thing rather than other.

Since people live in a very complex social cluster, let us begin by stating what we mean by academic values of moral and ethical socialization. The values of moral and ethical socialization motivate academicians to pursue the truth. While, on one hand, every deliberated social decision is voluntary, on the other hand, not every act is strictly a free act or an act of choice. A choice refers to one specific kind of deliberated act performed and controlled by will. We mean any academic value of ethical and moral socialization is under control of the individual's will. Nevertheless, to think of will in terms of freedom of will in academia is not an act of free-will, because we are influenced by socio-cultural codes of moral behavior and econo-political codes of conducts.

In the field of academic ethics, essential to the values of humanity, moral and ethical socialization is the protection of free choice in research. Along such a desirable academic objective, bioresearchers need to be concerned with sound moral character and the well-being behavior of themselves and of their intellectual contributions. For example, *CNN.com* (2005) reported:

> South Korean's most renowned stem-cell scientist (Professor Hwang Woo-suk, a veterinarian)... speaks publicly about media reports that he wanted a landmark study retracted because key parts were fabricated... Professor Hwang admitted to fabrication. Roh told media nine of the 11 stem cell-lines – batches – that were part of the tailored stem-cell study paper were fabricated and the authenticity of other two was questionable... In the disputed study, Hwang's team reported they had used a cloning method called somatic cell nuclear transfer to create lines of genetically identical stem cells from nine different patients, most with a rare neurological disease... Other stem-cell experts have said they are worried by the controversy. Human cloning is itself controversial, with opponents saying it is unethical to experiment on human embryos.

Nevertheless, Glass (1993: 43) stated:

> It has been said that science has no ethical basis that it is no more than a cold, impersonal way of arriving at the objective truth about natural phenomena... Human values have themselves evolved. Man arose after some two billions of years of organic evolution, during which species after species originated, flourished, and fell, or occasionally became the progenitors of species that were new and better adapted, on the basis of evolutionary scheme of values. Fitness, like it or not, in the long run meant simply the contribution of each trait and its underlying genes to survive.

Therefore, what makes biosciences and biotechnologies ethical and moral are academicians and biomedical practitioners.

It is said never fall in love with bioscienctific hypotheses, because love may make you blind. All bioethicists, bioscientists, biotechnologists, bioresearchers, and biomedical practitioners should shape their professions with honesty and integrity through their intellectual contributions. In the community of academicians, lying, distortion, fabrication of data, and dishonesty are condemned. Unfortunately, deliberate deceptions or carelessness and negligence in some biopharmaceutical and biomedical entities seem to be universally accepted and sometimes even promoted through false advertisements and propaganda. We do not claim that all bioscientistists, biotechnologists, bioresearchers and biomedical practitioners are careless and/or ignorant. Nevertheless, those who are deprived of adequate ethical and moral standards clearly may violate human rights and their professional codes of ethics and codes of moral conduct. What we need is to analyze bioacademic responsibilities and duties within a broad intellectual deliberation in order for the truth to be prevailed.

CODE OF ETHICS IN THE EDUCATION PROFESSION: ADOPTED BY THE 1975 NATIONAL EDUCATION ASSOCIATION REPRESENTATIVE ASSEMBLY

PREAMBLE:

The educator, believing in the worth and dignity of each human being, recognizes the supreme importance of the pursuit of truth, devotion to excellence, and the nurture of democratic principles. Essential to these goals is the protection of the freedom to learn and to teach and the guarantee of equal educational opportunity for all. The educator accepts the responsibility to adhere to the highest ethical standards.

The educator recognizes the magnitude of the responsibility inherent in the teaching process. The desire for the respect and confidence of one's colleagues, of students, of parents, and of the members of the community provides the incentive to attain and maintain the highest possible degree of ethical conduct. The Code of Ethics of the Education Profession indicates the aspiration of all educators and provides standards by which to judge conduct.

The remedies specified by the NEA and/or its affiliates for violation of any provision of this Code shall be exclusive and no such provision shall be enforceable in any form other than one specifically designated by the NEA or its affiliates.

PRINCIPLE I: Commitment to the Student

The educator strives to help each student realize his or her potential as a worthy and effective member of society. The educator therefore works to stimulate the spirit of inquiry, the acquisition of knowledge and understanding, and the thoughtful formulation of worthy goals.

In fulfillment of the obligation to the student, the educator:

Shall not unreasonably restrain the student from independent action in the pursuit of learning.

Shall not unreasonably deny the student access to varying points of view.

Shall not deliberately suppress or distort subject matter relevant to the student's progress.

Shall make reasonable effort to protect the student from conditions harmful to learning or to health and safety.

Shall not intentionally expose the student to embarrassment or disparagement.

Shall not on the basis of race, color, creed, sex, national origin, marital status, political or religious beliefs, family, social or cultural background, or sexual orientation, unfairly:

Exclude any student from participation in any program,
Deny benefits to any student,
Grant any advantage to any student.

Shall not use professional relationships with students for private advantage.

Shall not disclose information about students obtained in the course of professional service, unless disclosure serve a compelling professional purpose or is required by law.

PRINCIPLE II: Commitment to the Profession

The public with a trust and responsibility requiring the highest ideals of professional service vests the education profession.

In the belief that the quality of the services of the education profession directly influences the nation and its citizens, the educator shall exert every effort to raise professional standards, to promote a climate that encourages the exercise of professional judgment, to achieve conditions which attract persons worthy of the trust to careers in education, and to assist in preventing the practice of the profession by unqualified persons.

In fulfillment of the obligations to the profession, the educator:

Shall not in an application for a professional position deliberately make a false statement or fail to disclose a material fact related to competency and qualifications.

Shall not misrepresent his/her professional qualifications.

Shall not assist entry into the profession of a person known to be unqualified in respect to character, education, or other relevant attribute.

Shall not knowingly make a false statement concerning the qualifications of a candidate for a professional position.

Shall not assist a noneducator in the unauthorized practice of teaching.

Shall not disclose information about colleagues obtained in the course of professional service unless disclosure serves a compelling professional purpose or is required by law.

Shall not knowingly make false or malicious statements about a colleague.

Shall not disclose information about students obtained in the course of professional service, unless disclosure serves a compelling professional purpose or is required by law.

RELIABLE ACADEMIC KNOWLEDGE
AND BEHAVIORAL ORDINATIONS

The growing interdependence of socially, politically, economically, and legally diverse countries has caused academic systems to reexamine a variety of their existing policies. Among these revisions are strategic management philosophies, strategic academic alliances, cooperative academic partnerships, service positions, total quality education (TQE), quality enhancement planning and performance (QEPP), and ethical-legal conduct. These revisions mandate academic institutions to create a new mission on the basis of both domestic and global perspectives, with ever-increasing awareness of multiculturalization and multiethicalizaion of academic visions. It seems clear that the dynamic forces of environmental academia of today is the subject of much criticism in light of varying unethical decisions and immoral conducts concerning the pressure to publish. Although many academic institutions recognize the need to establish a sound competition, they nevertheless tend to view the real world from academic ethical and moral perspectives. There are several questions that address academia's mission concerning research. These questions are:

- Why is there so much pressure to publish?
- Is there sufficient pressure to publish or perish in all institutions of higher learning?
- Why are the issues of "publish or perish" so complicated?
- Are publications the real products of intellectual deliberations and contributors and/or authors?
- Does the public expect new knowledge and ideas?
- How do academicians know which intellectual contributive results represent advances in academic socialization?
- If journal articles, proceedings papers, and professional conference presentations and show cases are refereed either by peers and/or experts, do they represent real professional impartiality in promoting professional knowledge?
- Should academicians evaluate their intellectual contributions on the basis of the quality of ideas or the quantity of published articles and proceeding papers?
- Should promotion and tenure granting committees meet in secret in a democratic institution such as a college or university and their views to be open to the public?
- Are there systematic sufficient and comprehensive criteria as expected standards of academic performances for evaluating faculty

performance? If not, why are academic merit systems so critical for the reputation of faculty members and their affiliated institutions?

- Are there implicit rather than explicit pressures to publish in an academic institution for specific research fields in a discipline rather than in others?
- How do we know what decision or an action is right?
- What we must do to make educational services right?

To make the right decisions and take the right actions, we need to probe the real nature of intellectuality within the contextual boundaries of ethical, moral, and legal reasoning of ethicism, elitism, liberalism, and pragmatism. Our initial concern is to state precisely what kind of decision, action, and behavior or knowledge is ethical, moral, and legal. Do we believe that academic moral education is a compromised agreement between faculty members and their institutions? These and other similar questions raise some doubts that some academic institutions are not moving alongside of ethical and moral convictions. They are concerned about educational amorality.

BIOETHICAL ATTRIBUTIONS OF INNOVATIVE RESEARCH

We are defining and analyzing value ethics of the socio-cultural and politico-economical implications of bioresearch concerning innovativeness, patents, copyrights, and shop rights. Despite the apparent lack of ethics in an oligopolistically competitive biopharmaceutical industry, the current state of bioresearch offers unparallel opportunities for ethical systems to influence the relationship between academicians and market-based development of biotechno-scientific discoveries. Ethical considerations between bioresearchers and bioethicists can establish reflective wisdom on the issues of justice, patents, copyrights, and shop rights.

One of the major discoveries in the field of biotechno sciences is the emergence of new capabilities offered by recombinant genetics. It is the ability to cure diseases and to modify our own genetic structure. Bioresearchers for the first time have discovered how to alter the very concept of what innovativeness means. This is true because the current objectives of bioresearchers are to find solutions for curing human diseases and extending enriched life. Pharmacologists and biomedical experts work hand-in-hand with physiologists to perform the work that results in drugs to cure diseases.

Philosophers, biosophers, and bioethicists have been concerned about past, present, and future since the day of Plato. In his classic utopian book, *The*

Republic, Plato vividly expressed his vision about future and the kind of philosophy necessary to sustain it. Biosophists and bioscientists have been intimately connected with the future state of life and their scientific institutions. They have expressed their scientific deliberations with preferred logical outcomes. Questions like "what ought they to do?" or, "what objectives ought the colleges and universities to have?" are related to a future time. Thus, it is safe to say that the first and the most dynamic branches of knowledge of the future have been, are, and will be, biosophically oriented within the context of bioethics. In this endeavor, we will examine alternative concepts of the futuristic ideas by questioning why and what shall we call the study of the future? While at first glance these exhibit to be academic questions, they really bear careful scrutiny about logic, innovation, discoveries, and generalization. Historically, the research of the future has been called prospectivism, futurism, and futurology.

In today's bioresearch endeavor, some professional biomedical practitioners, specifically in the field of fertility clinics, have converted their altruistic medical profession into profit-making entities as brokerage centers to buy and sell human stem cell, genes, eggs, sperm, and body tissues and parts. For example, *FOX NEWS. COM* (2006) reported:

> A presidential advisory committee on bioethics said in an interim report on Hwang's research that he had used 2,221 human eggs donated by 119 women, and that 62 of the women were paid for it. Hwang had earlier said he used only a small number of eggs... Lee said Hwang is believed to have coerced junior researchers in his lab into donating their eggs for the research, a practice widely considered unethical. Las month, Soul National University said Hwang's team fabricated data in papers published in 2004 and 2005 that purported to show they created stem cells from the world's first cloned human embryos. *The Journal of Science* retracted both papers. Hwang publicly apologized for faking data, but claimed fellow researchers deceived him. He said some of the stem cells at his lab had been maliciously switched...

Some bioresearchers have changed their professional practical diagnostic and treatment procedures into biobusiness by researching, finding, and matching human body parts and materials between donors and receivers. Such a biotechno scientific option allows people as customers to order their prospective children. We must ethically and morally pay attention to this new path of fertilization of the sanctity of natural genes, sperm, and eggs by not ignoring what eugenic cybertechnology offers to mothers and fathers and to the traditional way we have defined and practiced the notion of family.

In bioresearch fertility clinics, children are assumed as commodities to be valued on the basis of demand and supply in the biomarketplace. Parenting is viewed as mass nurturing foster cares laboratories and hospitals are viewed as human body shops. In addition, cybernetic eugenic enterprises, in the foster-care markets, are sorting sperm and egg banks by worth of genes. Also, the cybernetic eugenic enterprises, through bioresearch innovative processes, promise to eradicate natural and human mistakes in child bearing. Nevertheless, the concept of bio-progressive innovativeness forces humans to be exposed to the question of "what makes for worth" in our society. The end result derives us to the competitive innovativeness to convert families, biotechno scientists, biomedical practitioners, and biopharmaceutical corporations actively seeking "the very best genes money can buy." Besides commercialization of genes, the packages of patented human life come with body materials such as semen, blood, and milk. Every biomarket possesses its own cultural value system and has invested capital with different expected outcomes as profits every time. Nevertheless, bio-profitability depends heavily on bioresearch activities. Rothman (1999: A52) indicated:

> The market has long affected sperm banks, too, with ads for sperm donors aimed at medical students through 1970s, but shifting to business students in the 1980s. Surely that change reflected the increasing status of business executives in our culture.

Ethically and morally, to what direction societies are moving provide sufficient ground to examine the integrity and dignity of human beings.

BIOACADEMIC PROFESSIONAL MANDATES

Academic intellectual vision-mission mandates grow out of a set of deliberated challenges through the dynamic argument of intellectual reasoning. They require constructive preliminary professional informative planning processes. Stating and listing reasons for believing in specific paths of scientific delineations for the purpose of professionalism is most likely to be effective in life problem solving with innovative views. Bioresearchers now must wisely respond to a number of questions:

- Where and how should we begin our intellectual analytical reasoning?
- In what biosophical and scientific ground and order should we build our hypothetical premises point by point on how we intend to plan our research?
- How can we most efficiently and effectively respond to opposing arguable reasoning?
- How should we conclude our predictable reliable causes-effects?

The answer to those questions will vary from one research project to another. Bioacademicians not only should have the scientific empirical reasoning, but also they should develop their skills in writing journal articles and conference proceedings papers. They should pay attention to the notion that experimental scientific mechanisms cannot be separated from all other works when they are designing, planning, organizing, and implementing their research projects.

If a group of bioresearchers are planning to design a basic research project, which may not require following the principles of classical arrangements, they need to generate novel ideas that are suitable for their research plans. Or if they begin by generating creative ideas with applying concrete viable disciplinary and/or interdisciplinary principles, then they must decide what types of scientific methodological procedures will be suitable for their ideas to be considered and implemented in the scientific practical endeavor in order to provide adequate ground for further academic communication. These steps do not happen in isolation or in linear progression in which it is impossible to revisit an earlier part of experimental work. When generating novel ideas, they may find that a tentative outline for their arrangement is beginning to emerge.

Any scientific argument concerning proving or disproving a hypothetical assumption needs to be persuasive. Nevertheless, the purpose of any persuasion varies from one occasion to another. Biotechno scientists and bioresearchers may express themselves in writing and/or by oral presentations of their analysis to persuade other people to accept the legitimacy and viability of their scientific positions. They may be invited by other bioscientists to exchange their reasoning or to undertake a specific action. Or they may to write and present refutable papers in order to encourage conflicting scientific parties to accept scientifically a compromise. In any case, they need to utilize their intellectual abilities with suitable purposes and methodological arguable analysis. Within contextual boundaries of bioresearch methodological procedures, there are two major types of analytical arrangements: (1) classical and (2) Rogerian.

Classical Analytical Reasoning – CAR

The theories of classical analytical reasoning emphasize upon the importance of scientific persuasion concerning assertion of a novel scientific procedure with purposive objectives. Because these theories have been historically developed at a time when most scientific arguments were oral an audience could easily understand the reasoning processes and conclusions. If orators follow essentially the same formulated traditional analytical arrangements, audiences will be able to follow long, complex analytical reasoning because the main components are easily recognizable. Classical analytical reasoning composes as follows:

- *Introduction*: State the issues that the presenters hope to tackle. By presenting issues as major problems which need solutions through reviewing possible variable alternatives and choosing the best.
- *Executive Summary*: Presenters state as accurately and neutrally as possible the briefing description of their distinctive dimensions of their presentations.
- *Statement of the Self Interest*: Presenters may provide their scientific interests. They may be different from audiences' views that do not share their views.
- *Benefits*: Presenters: may start their reasoning to respect causes and effects of analytical solutions. Then, they may generalize their statements as new evidence of solutions and add them into the body of literature.
- *Alternative Views*: Views of previous scientific relevant reasoning with which presenters disagree. By doing this, presenters provide an opportunity for the audience who think differently from presenters to review literature with a fair and deep understanding. Presenters show that they understand there are situations in which these views are valid. In other words, they are offering a kind of concession.
- *Statement of Issues*: Presenters need to summarize their own scientific views differently.
- *Understanding Others*: Presenters are not conceding that other views are always right, but they recognize that there are conditions under which presenters would share their comprehensive views of their opponents.
- *Analytical Assessments*: Having won the attention of the audience concerning opponent's scientific views.
- *Statement of Points of View*: Presenters scientifically explain their syllogistic reasoning to validate their findings.
- *Presenters' Views*: Presenters generate an interest for hearing further analytical scientific reasoning of others. Now that the audience has discovered the presenters' scientific fair considerations, they will be prepared to listen fairly to presenters' innovative views.
- *Using Analytical Reasoning*: Analytical statements of presenters' views could be perceived as a final view in problem solving.
- *Logical Reasoning*: Presenters may apply four types of types of logical reasoning: (1) Inductive, (2) Deductive, (3) Analogous, and (4) Holistic.
- *Statement of the Context*: The statement of context describes situations in which presenters conducted their research. They hope for the audience to honor their views. By persuading audience concerning

presenters' scientific position, they will provide them with merit in a specific context or contexts. This will increase the likelihood that opponents will agree with presenters, at least in part.

- *Conclusive Results*: Presenters conclude their analytical reasoning by appealing to audience to challenge their findings and/or to assert their views concerning problem solving.

Rogerian Analytical Reasoning – RAR

Although Classical Analytical Reasoning (CAR) composes of fifteen parts., Rogerian Analytical Reasoning (RAR) needs not to be limited to those types of scientific segmentation. According to the RAR, presenters need to look at complexity of the issues, the extent to which scientific professional authorities are divided about them, and the points of reasoning in which presenters want to analyze.

Rogerian Analytical Reasoning summarizes all scientific procedures and freely emphasizes on any part of analysis that can be expanded. RAR is effective in situations where presenters address their reasoning to a scientific community who are divided as to the result of different values or perceptions. RAR emphasizes more on methodological procedures, random sampling, conclusive quantitative assessments, and holistic evidential conclusions. RAR makes presenters as a kind of scientific negotiators that may allow professional authorities to move forward even though some differences remain. For example, one of the crucial ethical and moral issues in biotechno scientific deliberations is related to bioethics in cloning.

FOUR TYPES OF LOGICAL REASONING

In both classical and Rogerian analytical reasoning, there are four types of conclusive methods which researchers may use them in their reasoning. These are:

- Inductive Logical Reasoning
- Deductive Logical Reasoning
- Analogous Logical Reasoning
- Holistic Logical Reasoning

Inductive Logical Reasoning

When bioresearchers use induction, they can draw general conclusions based on specific experimental evidence in advance. Their pragmatic scientific reasoning rests on a methodological foundation of procedural details that they have been accumulated for their reasoning support. This type of reasoning is based upon predictable judgments concerning conclusive results. For example, when we listen to the weather forecast before leaving our house, we hear the range of cold, mild, or warm temperatures. If the sun is shining, the temperature is higher and the weather is warmer and if it is cloudy the temperature is cooler. By this type of reasoning, we have not proven that the day will be pleasant and/or unpleasant. We have concluded that it will be within a certain range of temperatures. This is a kind of reasoning that we can do in inductive logical reasoning. Therefore, in inductive logical reasoning we arrive at a conclusion that seems likely to be true. Ultimate and positive proof is usually beyond reaching at the time of judgment.

Inductive logical reasoning is especially important in bioscientific experimentation. Bioresearchers may have specific logical reasoning that they hope to prove in the future. But to work toward proving them needs hundreds or thousands of experiments to be conducted to generalize their hypothetical assumptions. In practice, they may need periodically to adjust environmental conditions to the establishment of creation of specific processes and gather enough data to justify their conclusive generalized results. Bioresearch metrical variables sometimes reach to a point where they seem incontestable. Biologists, pharmacologists, physiologist, pathologists, immunologists, oncologists, biochemists, and biophysicists are usually aware of inductive reasoning. They believe in inductive reasoning unless new discoveries can come under challenge. So again, bioresearchers go back to their experiments and keep working on their projects, hopefully truthful mindset evidence will be emerging. This is the beautiful side of bioresearch that motivates bioresearchers to continue their experiments.

Deductive Logical Reasoning

Deductive logical reasoning is based on proven fundamental truthful values, or rights rather than specific pieces of new evidence. In deductive logical reasoning, evidence is of secondary importance. Such a logical reasoning argument will be based upon declaration of conceptual values or beliefs that will prepare the way for the reasoning. In deductive logical reasoning we first, must create a foundational right, value, or belief from which we wish to deduce our premise. What we mean by a premise?

A *premise* is the most effective attribute when we think about values. Those values are viewed as foundations for building our reasoning. A good premise should satisfy three requirements:

- Your audience should accept those pragmatic values as fundamental beliefs in their disciplines. This indicates that you and your audience possess a common ground for pursuing your reasoning.
- You need to structure a scientific mechanism to prepare the way for your reasoning so that you will follow on the same path of experimental reasoning mechanism on top of those values and beliefs.
- You need to conclude with a careful consideration to frame a good premise within the domain of your scientific reasoning by illustrating the expected results of your hypothesis.

Also, the premise is viewed as an underlying assumption that must be agreed on point-by-point and step-by-step to present your reasoning. In deductive reasoning, there are two strategies to be used in order to prove your rational reasoning:

- In advance, if you know tentatively what the conclusion your deductive reasoning is expected to reach, we first mention our conclusion and then we analyze variables till to reach to that conclusion. For example, making sexless babies by biotechno scientific methods in fertility clinics as cloning can violate the continuity of human somatic connectivity. This means that instead of the newborn being delivered through the body of a mother, he/she can be born from a tube (e.g., the Baby M who is 28 years old now). Such an innovative system may alienate dignity and integrity of natural child bearing.
- If you do not know the concrete conclusion in advance, first you start to build your reasoning step by step and then to get to a final conclusive result. For example, in eugenic gene engineering and cloning we are violating the natural endowment of a pair system for fertility. We will convert it into multiple systems of combination of eggs and sperm. The strategic end result may cause natural disaster; such as the result of such a gene engineering process whereby brothers and sisters unknowingly may marry each other. Not only this will be against natural selection, also it will be against the integrity of humanity. Therefore, in deductive reasoning, there are some laden ethical values that must be considered in your reasoning.

You should already know how to build or formulate your premise. Your premise is an outline of logical reasoning. Then for scientific reasoning to prove your points, you need to follow the pattern of what is called syllogism. Syllogism contains three parts of reasoning in which the conclusion rests on two premises:

- The first is called the major premise because it is the point at which you begin to analyze truthful reasoning to reach to your conclusion.
- The second is called minor premise. Here is a simple example of a bioethical syllogism:

  o *Major premise*: John is a by-product of sexless fertility clinic through gene engineering from enhanced and manipulated sperm A, B,
  o *Minor premise*: Elizabeth is a by-product of sexless fertility clinic through the same bioengineered eggs that John was created.
  o *Conclusion*: Therefore, John is brother of Elizabeth and they should not marry each other, because they share the same eggs.

- If the major and minor premise are both true, then the conclusion reached is true. Note that the major premise and the minor premise share a term in common (the eggs). It should be indicated that through ethical, moral, and legal mandates of humanity, that marriage between brothers and sisters is a taboo. In addition, all offspring of John and Elizabeth through generation by generation will carry the same heredity of mutual genes. What is the strategic prediction of such deductive reasoning in the above syllogism? It is creation of Promethean classes of human species. Thus, a syllogism such as the one just cited may seem very simple. Since we accept the major and minor premises, then we will have to accept the conclusion.

Within contextual boundaries of deductive reasoning, there is another type of analysis. That is enthymeme. An enthymeme is a syllogistic reasoning which has lost its major premise. Enthymeme usually results in deductive understanding when the major premise is obvious. What is obvious to someone trying to convince us with an enthymeme is not necessarily obvious to those that who are trying to understand it. For example:

- *The minor premise*: John and Elizabeth are products of a sexless baby making process through eugenic shared gene engineering by a combination and manipulated specific known of eggs.
- *Conclusion*: Both John and Elizabeth's offspring are viewed through heredity as cousins. Therefore, ethically, morally, legally their offspring should not marry each other (not necessarily in the Islamic and Judaism cultures).

Analogous Logical Reasoning

Comparative experimental data assessment is a scientific tool for conducting examining procedures on different groups with a control group. In an analogous logical reasoning you must first be sure that the comparative procedural factors you are comparing have several characteristics in common with others and that these similarities are relevant to the conclusion you intend to draw. If a drug is causing depression in chimpanzees, you could reason that the affect of that drug can cause a similar problem for human beings. The validity of your conclusive result would depend on the degree to which chimps are analogous to humans, and then you would need to conceive with care and demonstrate that there are important similarities between the two species.

The analogous logical reasoning is based on speculation. We need to be careful of using analogous reasoning in proving some final conclusions because it is often misused. A type of reasoning from analogy that reaches a strong conclusion could be fallacious. Therefore, bioresearchers need to be careful in their animal experimental experiences not to use analogous logical reasoning if they find that the analogy itself is inappropriate.

Holistic Logical Reasoning

Although all three inductive, deductive, and analogous logical reasoning methods suggest concrete judgmental assessments, they also have their limitations. Within the contextual boundaries of biosciences, bioresearchers should not bound by a predetermined biomedical procedure and regard the syllogism, in particular, as unnecessarily rigid. They need to generalize their logical reasoning with combined inductive, deductive, and analogous reasoning to get to an effective result. We should indicate that logical experimental reasoning is concerned with probability more often than certainty. Accordingly, we need to be concerned with three factorial types of analytical reasoning in order to holistically generalize our bioresearch conclusions. Those are: (1) hypothesis, (2) data, and (3) warrant.

- *Hypothesis*: Hypothesis is defined as the equivalent of the conclusive result or whatever it is a bioresearcher wants to try to prove.
- *Data*: The gathered defined and quantified information or experimental evidence a bioresearcher offers in support of the hypotheses.
- *Warrant*: A general conclusive, viable, and reliable statement that establishes a trustworthy relationship between the data and the hypothesis. The holistic warrant should be explicit, especially when bioresearchers believe that the warrant is effective in repetitive similar conditional and situational circumstances.

THE WARRANT OF PUBLISH OR PERISH IN ACADEMIA

One of the crucial issues of today's academia is related to the notion of publish or perish. Because of such an overwhelming pressure, faculty members feel that they have to seriously do something about it. This has caused some faculty members to have access to some biodata and in rare cases to use them fraudulently in their papers without indication of the original sources and/or acknowledgment of the consent of the source of references. There are serious questions concerning biodata:

Should bioresearchers share their data by the time of journal article publication? Are there any exceptional circumstances that permit bioresearchers not to share their biodata with other scientists?

According to the academic codes of ethics if a research plan is a part of a faculty's professional intellectual contribution, then biodata should be an integral part of a research plan and its data-sharing plan should be accessible by other bioresearchers. Bioresearchers should record and maintain their experimental data and keep them for certain period of time in case other researchers need to have access to them. Bioresearchers are required to provide other researchers their data after publication of results. In return, it should be noted that subsequent analysis of biodata by other researchers should explicitly acknowledge the efforts of original bioresearchers and provide recognition for the intellectual contributions of the original bioresearcher(s).

It is an academic rule in scientific experimental disciplines that all procedures, step-by-step and point-by-point should be recorded and the data of several control groups should be recorded and kept. It is the scientific rule that laboratory technicians should make their own notes concerning experiments as a second source of viability of experimental procedures and accuracy of data. Of course technicians are prohibited from disclosing procedures and data to others without oral permission and/or written consent of the principal researcher. In addition, departments of pure sciences such as biology, physiology, pharmacology, chemistry, physics, and the like should maintain the records of purchase orders for experimental packages, sets, and animals used in the experiments, and biochemical substances. Records of purchased substances, materials, and animals will be used as a part of an academic defense concerning validity of performance of some experiments.

It is the professional expectation journal editors that submissions should contain either actual data or secret keys to provide reviewers the actual data for their judgments. It is unethical that some bioresearchers might exploit the peer review process and without providing the actual biodata misrepresent their work as peer reviewed articles. Such an action can cause fraud in bioacademia. Academic fraud not only will expose the first author of an article and/or a proceedings paper to academic dishonesty, but also, all other coauthors as well as in some cases their academic institutions will be exposed to such allegations. Kennedy (1986: 26) stated:

> Science relies very heavily on the capacity to replicate experiments; it is the only way at all to correct fraud. Although we referee journal articles, evaluate the logic of propositions, and check arithmetic, we cannot decide, merely from reading a report, that a result is right – only that it is not wrong in some obvious way. Accordingly, we require that scientific communications include enough detail about the way an experiment was done so that a competent investigator in the field can do it in exactly the same way. This is an exciting requirement; it compels the release of all relevant information about methods and techniques. Secret ingredients, magic sauces, and your own special glassware are fine in cookery or in product development, but in fundamental science they are out.

In addition to the principal researchers, there are others such as graduate students who are working on their Ph.D. dissertations, postdoctoral fellows, and clinical fellows who are working in labs for the enhancement and up dating of their knowledge. Some of these graduate students, postdoctoral, and clinical fellows may end up in academic medicine and/or in biotechno scientific research, and others go to industries. They need to observe academic honesty and integrity. In relation to academic dishonesty, for example, Petersdof (1993: 95) indicated:

> A young faculty member about to be appointed in a clinical department was discovered to have submitted several papers containing fraudulent data to several reputable journals... He had done superbly in medical school and was excellently trained; during his fellowship he wrote over 30 papers. When he was proposed for his initial faculty appointment, he had authored in excess of 100 papers... In assembling the proposal for this

man's academic appointment, a senior member of the department reviewed some of these publications. The data of several control groups were the same in several papers: normally, different experiments should have different controls... When the young investigator was confronted with the doubts, he denied all allegations, but was unable to marshal proof that allegations were false. His letter of resignation from the faculty followed shortly thereafter.

COMPETITIVE INTELLECTUAL CONTRIBUTIONS

The intellectual knowledge-based view of the academia holds that each academician has unique know-how knowledge and competence in a specialized field of science and skills in application of specific technology. Also, each institution of higher learning and research possesses specific capabilities in advancement of knowledge and technological development to seek to improve its academic performance by concentrating on those scientific research projects that best fit its competencies. High caliber researchers and large, diversified interdisciplinary research universities are constantly realigning their intellectual contributions to focus on their academic strengths. Yet despite constant changes in the science and technology the basic moral and ethical inquiries remains the same.

- What does it mean to exploit human life as raw material in research in order to discover new therapeutic medicine?
- What are the likely future of techno-scientific possibilities and ethical problems that our present experimental research projects are creating willy-nilly? What ought the moral and ethical boundaries for academicians to be, whether they spend governmental and/or private funds in research?
- What does it mean to blur the line between cooperative procreation and competitive Promethean evolution?
- What are the final objectives of, and what are proper limits to, the project of human genome?
- Do we know how to control where this project is taking us, so as to reap the benefits without losing human dignity and integrity? If so, how?

We need to know and realize that it is more at stake in revolutionary Promethean biological advancement than just saving life or avoiding pain and suffering.

Competitive intellectual contributions have always had ethos that called for effective communication among scholars. It is a professional tradition that academicians feel some pressure to publish their research results. Publishing articles and presenting conference research papers advance scientific knowledge. It is through publications that science and technology can advance, develop, and flourish.

Scientific research viability should be evaluated through peers and experts in the field before they are published. Such a refereed processing of publications allows other scientists, scholars, and researchers to further their research and use them as bases for scientific synergistic usage. The validity of the content of an article and/or a conference research paper is based upon application of those ideas in practice. In addition, scientific articles and research papers represent in depth qualification of scientists, scholars, and researchers; in many cases they are the primary factors to be applied for professional merit pays, promotion, tenure, and post-tenure review (PTR). In addition, intellectual contributions of faculty members facilitate conducting more systematic research projects and discovering new information about the relation of publications to professional advancement.

INTELLECTUAL CONTRIBUTIONS THROUGH AUTHORSHIP AND PUBLICATIONS

What makes bioacademic contributing authors distinguish in community of scholars are their professional ethical and moral commitments to conduct truthful research projects and write their cognitive observational conclusions as journal articles, research papers, books, and reports? Clearly, some journal articles, research papers, books, and reports include the names of those individuals who really contributed their knowledge and efforts for advancing human civilization. Meanwhile, on a very rare occasion, there are some academic free riders that are looking for taking advantage of the good faith and goodwill of the principal author(s) and desire to include their own names in those manuscripts for enjoying illegitimate personal gain. Such a fraudulent claim in publication can cause a matter of deep academic deception and dishonesty.

There are several ethical principles concerning intellectual contributions. These principles warrant biotechno scientists, bioresearchers, and biomedical practitioners as authors. The main concern is related to the emergence of intellectual ideas in the forms of scientific hypotheses. The immediate questions can be raised as following:

- Should the source of a working bioresearch hypothesis be given authorship credit?
- What about affiliated and/or those academicians who facilitated either the experimental set up procedures or cooperated in conducting research projects? What about those professional mentors who refine bioresearchers' thoughts and facilitated the research funding, provided laboratory space, equipment, and relentless efforts to reexamine the validity of the experimental conclusive results?
- Should professors, mentors, advisors, and/or peers who made some vital contributions for processing data to be listed in the final product of a scientific work or should be appreciated by naming them in the acknowledgment?

In order to answer to the above questions, we need to consider specific principles in the following pages. The first principle is related to the scientists' personal integrity. In science, truthful declaration is a crucial type of professional ethical and moral conviction. Scientists are expected to be praiseworthy authorities because rationally they should be disassociated with ignorance, carelessness, deception, fabrication, dishonesty, and fraud. One of the most important dimensions of scientific progress is related to the intellectual innovativeness and creativity through expression of valid inferences established to imaginative hypothetical formulation of elegant experiments designed and conducted and/or procedural methods developed in a research project. Nevertheless, among scientists, the notion of innovativeness and creativity creates professional credibility through specific qualitative rewards via publishing a first-class article. Also, innovative scientific ideas establish professional status, respect for colleagues, academic reputation, expertise power, and monetary income for their viable intellectual contributions. Such rewards may sometimes count for more than self-respect and the joy of discovery. In addition, in scientific deliberated contributive endeavor, there always is intensive competition. Therefore, fraud in stealing and/or plagiarizing scientific ideas may distort academic honesty. We must therefore be attentive to observe professional codes of professional ethics and codes of moral conduct.

The second principle is related to ethical and moral commitments of authors to disclose real repeated experimental data, procedures, and conclusions. The immediate question can be raised as following:

How can these data be validated through scientific methodological procedures and their relative proclivity of scientific sufficiency in concluding either direct observational results and/or deductive ones?

Statistical testing validation procedures sometimes can be deceptive (e. g., the calculating of p values: *post hoc* hypothesis). It is usually recognized that t-tests, chi-square tests, and other statistical tests be carried out before data should be examined. Statistical tests usually are used in discovering the validity of probability of hypothetical occurrences. Also, statistical tests are used in non-probability ways to discover rough measures of the size of an effect rather than to test hypotheses.

The third principle is related to the selectivity of report findings and the repeated reported findings as supporting evidence in a study in multiple fragments. These types of issues can obscure critical aspects of an experiment. Such an obscured dimension of a research project can mislead the evidential values of the collected data.

The fourth principle is related to the originality of scientific ideas and experimental procedural processes. In scientific deliberative analysis, the innovative mindset of bioresearchers fosters biotechno scientists to grow intellectually. They know that being innovative doesn't only mean much more than just expanding and/or accelerating the progress of a line of research. It is a new way of critical thinking that drives every aspect of a successful and dynamic progress of thoughts and ideas towards more accomplishment. Scientific innovativeness is not based upon imitation. It is a new way toward discovering original thoughts and ideas. Research oriented innovativeness is a type of scientific mindset to present new ideas, adapt new procedural methods, and invent new biotechno devices. Therefore, the originality of an innovative research proposal is a novel way of focused thinking beyond the present domain of a research entity to be directed towards the future.

The fifth principle is related to the analytical breadth and power of quality of the scientific experimental procedures, processes, and conclusions. The concept of qualitative research power is defined in terms of scientific random selectivity of the data, scientific validity of multi-variance of the scope of the experiment and variability of scientific results in which they are inherent in specified combination of classes of data through structuring; by sample size, by statistical models, and by both observational and cognitive deductive, inductive, analogous, and holistic judgments.

The sixth principle is related to the professional ethical obligations of journal articles. Scientific journal articles should be of excellent quality, original in content, and provide all previous related literature in a reproducible fashion. In addition, comprehensive heuristic writings concerning minutiae of methods are of the highest importance. Bernard (1927) indicated that the greatest scientific truths are rooted in details of experimental investigation that form, as it were, the soil in which these truths develop. Within the contextual boundaries of this principle, causal inspections, reduction, relational, reactional processes, and consequential new compounds and/or conditions should be perfectly described.

Nevertheless, in heuristic experimental reports, a very detailed comprehensive scientific reasoning for new compounds and or procedures should describe their identities and effective results. Since some highly respected scientific journals urge authors to shorten their articles, authors must have a great care to avoid elimination of important details.

The seventh principle urges authors of journal articles to have professional tolerance for receiving criticism and disagreements from experts concerning the content and context of their articles. They need to be open-minded people. Also, they need to be exposed to critical examination and the testing of their results by other researchers in the field. Since biotechno scientific experiments are based upon trial and error, authors of journal articles are ethically obligated in case they have published some articles that have some mistakes or errors, which should be publicly acknowledged. Wise (1946: 1299) indicated:

> The research worker should not permit himself (herself) to become embittered or involved in useless polemics... It simply means that his (her) criticism must be objective and that they must not descend to the plane of personalities. He (she) must show that he (she) is dealing with a set of data, not with an enemy.

The eighth principle indicates to authors of journal articles and proceedings papers professional ethical obligations concerning intellectual property copyright, shop right, and patent considerations in their works. In general terms, scientific article authorship copyrights belong to the original writers. However, since some professional associations, universities, colleges, research centers, and private publishing companies will publish scientific articles, the copyright issues carry duel ethical and legal considerations. Up to 1968, the decision to try to publish or reveal a researcher's intellectual property copyrights had been the sole right of the scientists. Nevertheless, the appearance of the legislative copyrights and patents changed such a right and extended it to financial sponsors of research projects. Now, with researchers receiving financial support from others, the final decision is tending to fall on the provider of the funds. Monetary profit sharing is one of the solutions for arrangement of contractual agreements between authors and publishers with an agreeable percentage of royalty for both parties.

The ninth principle is related to ethical and moral publicity issues. Since the works of scientists are viewed as professional, scientists are obligated to serve beyond selves. There are three types of scientists' perception concerning professional publicity. Those are as following:

- Some scientists aggressively oppose general publicity and popularization of their works because of their professional codes of ethics.
- Some scientists seek publicity in order for their peers to recognize and appreciate their professional works because they believe that they have the ethical and moral rights to appreciate their professional hardworking on the basis of the codes of moral conduct.
- Others seek publicity beyond their ethical and moral rights and even condone or support erroneous and misleading publicity.

With consideration of the above behavioral attitudes of scientists, authors and writers, there are serious questionable issues at stake: Do scientists owe the public a duty to inform them about their discoveries and the significance of their discoveries? Of course, all scientists are entitled to inform the public how they have sacrificed their efforts for promotion of knowledge and human welfare. Nevertheless, scientists by all means and ends should avoid chicanery and excessive or misleading publicity.

The tenth principle is related to ethical and moral issues concerning joint venture academic partnership among a group of researchers. There are several issues such as scientific seniority, merit, efforts, expertise, and originality of research ideas that should be considered. To many researchers and institutions of higher learning, the order of the authors for journal articles, proceedings papers, and scientific reports has significance. It recognizes academic credit weight for their efforts and contributions. Such weight and efforts are considered during promotion, tenure, and post-tenure review processes.

Academic meritocracy is a critical issue that is not only related to professional ethical and moral obligations, but also related to cultural etiquette. In different cultures implementation of such etiquette is different. For example, in Asian and Middle Eastern cultures traditional etiquette is based on seniority, while in European and American cultures it is based upon the level of contributions for producing the final product. Therefore, there are three different concepts concerning the order of authorship as following:

Senior Authorship: This type of arrangement is based on academic cultural administrative rank system. The one who has the most academic interest, experience, and reputation should be named first as a mentor, the one who has the most contributive efforts second as a principal researcher, the one who has furnished the original idea third, the one who has provided the technical skill in writing an article, paper, or report fourth, and the one who has assisted any of the aforementioned researchers the last.

Merit Authorship: This type of arrangement is based on the merit of academic leadership efforts of researchers from the beginning to the final product. Merit authorship is bound to actual efforts of authors who have sustained substantial, continuous, and of a high level of contribution. It should be indicated that research in biosciences requires relentless efforts in conducting experimental tests in laboratories. Therefore, according to this system, the one who has done most of laboratory work should be first, the one who has written the article, paper and report second, the one who has furnished the original idea third, the one who has played the roles of mentors and provided technical, administrative, and financial support last.

Scholastic Authorship: One of the controversial issues in bioresearch activities is related to the works of graduate students in laboratories. They assist researchers by setting up technical experimental equipment, collecting related data, and analyzing test results. Should their efforts be recognized and appreciated by including their names in the authorship of articles, papers, and reports? Or should the directing professor treat graduate students as laboratory assistants? Or should the senior author of an article, paper, or report promote senior graduate students, especially Ph.D. candidates, and appreciate their help by including their names in authorship? The concrete ethical answer to the above questions is that senior professors should not expect to obtain free academic rides from their graduate students. In addition, senior faculty members should safeguard the academic integrity and graduate students' rights by not permitting abuse of their efforts. In some countries, it is unethical and immoral for faculty members to expect graduate students to include their names in their research papers as the second or third author, unless after the date of their graduation. The rationale for such an academic ethical and moral tradition is that students work as laboratory staff by receiving salary to work in a laboratory, also professors receive a salary and incentives to teach, advise, and prepare students as new generation of scholars in their field. Therefore, Ph.D. students should have entitlements of their scholastic hardworking efforts.

In summary, as we have pointed out, violation of the professional codes of ethics on the part of scientists results in academic dishonesty. Such deliberated violations can cause a faculty member to be exposed to academic indecency for discharge. We suggest that each institution of higher learning and research center should establish definite professional codes of ethics and codes of moral conduct in order to safeguard profound and favorable effects for science, society, and the scientists.

INTELLECTUAL CONTRIBUTIONS THROUGH PROFESSIONAL CONFERENCE PRESENTATIONS

Every year many professional experts get together to exchange their research findings in academic conferences around the world. Within the contextual boundaries of bioethics, we need to analyze the effects of these gatherings. There are certain points of view that presenters should follow. These are as following:

- Presenters should provide new formatted and organized scientific information related to the theme of the conference.
- Presenters should provide comprehensive accurate data with supporting prior literature in the field and have concise analytical arguments concerning hypothetical assumptions to be accepted or rejected.
- Presenters should provide the audience with very well defined objectives of their research alongside scientific tools, research methodologies, and comprehensive statistical data in order to prove accuracy of their findings.
- Presenters should avoid providing the audience irrelevant information that may be misleading.
- Presenters should avoid application of untried procedures and/or individualized speculative results beyond their biodata.
- Presenters should illustrate a balanced comprehensive menu for their presentations within the appropriate time-line of the conference.
- Presenters should avoid redundancy, oversight, and/or exaggeration in conducting their experimental hypothetical testing.
- Presenters should show professional tolerance for being criticized by peers and/or experts. They should not only appreciate criticism, but also welcome scientific suggestions and recommendations for the enhancement of their articles.
- Presenters should be ready to hear new comments concerning their work and should be ready to obtain new insights from experts in the field that will be helpful for revising their research papers.

REFERENCES

Chapter 1

Albert, E. M., Denise, T. C., and Peterfreund, S. P. (1984). *Great Traditions in Ethics*. Belmont, California: Wadsworth Publishing Company: 203, 223, and 231.

Ayer, A. J. (1950). *Language, Truth, and Logic*. New York: Dover Publications: 107-108.

Baillar III, J. C. (1993). "Science, Statistics, and Deception." In Bulger, R. E., Heitman, E., and Reiser, S. J. (Eds.). *The Ethical Dimensions of the Biological Sciences*. Cambridge: Cambridge University Press: 104.

Barlow, T. (2001). "Some Eminent Scientists Have Taken Part in Very Unethical Research." *Financial Times*. (Weekend, July 14-15): 11.

Barlow, T. (2001). "Religious Repression; Western Style." *Financial Times*. (Weekend, December 8 and 9): 11.

Barrett, M. (1991). *The Politics of Truth: From Marx to Foucault*. Stanford, CA: Stanford University Press: 194.

Beauchamp, T. L. and Childress, J. F. (1994). *Principles of Biomedical Ethics*. 4th Edition. New York: Oxford University Press.

Beecher, H. (1966). "Abuses in Human Experimentation." *New England Journal of Medicine*. Vol. 74: 1354-1360.

Berelson, B., and Steiner, G. A. (1964). *Human Behavior*. New York: Harcourt, Brace and World: 87.

Berenheim, R. E. (1987). *Corporate Ethics*. New York: The Conference Board, Inc.

Berg, B. L. (1995). *Quantitative Research Methods For the Social Sciences, Second Edition*, Boston: Allyn and Bacon: 5.

Berman, B. J. (1993). "Only Glancing Blow Roger Penrose and Critique of Artificial Intelligence." *Science as Culture*. Vol. 3, Part 3, No. 16: 404-426.

Billingham, J. (1982). *Life in the Universe*. Cambridge, Mass: The MIT Press.

Bowe, C. (1999). "Biotech Companies Plan to Milk Herds of Cloned Cows for Human Drug Needs." *Financial Times*. (Wednesday October 13): 6.

Brooks, L. J. (1989). "Corporate Codes of Ethics." *Journal of Business Ethics*. Vol. 8: 117.

Brown, D. R., Qin, K., Herms, J.W., Madlung, A., Mason, J. Strome, R. Fraser, P.E., Kruck, T., von Bohlen, A., Schulz-Schaeffer, W., Giese, A., Westaway, D., and Kretzschmar, H. (1997). "The Cellular Prion Protein Binds Copper in Vivo." *Nature*. (December, 18-25), Vol. 390, No. 6661: 684-7.

Bull, J. P. (1959). "The Historical Development of Clinical Therapeutic Trials." *Journal of Chronicle Diseases*. Vol. 10: 218.

Burns, C. (1977). "Richard Cabot and Reformation in American Medical Ethics." *Bulletin of the History of Medicine*. Vol. 51: 353-368, Quote on 368.

Cabot, R. (1919). "A Study of Mistaken Diagnosis." *Journal of the American Medical Association*. Vol. 55: 1343-1350.

Cabot (1919). *Social Work: Essays on the Meeting Ground of Doctor and Social Worker*. Boston/New York: Houghton-Mifflin Company.

Cassirer, E. (1956). *An Essay on Man*. New York: Doubleday: 43.

Clark, D. C. (1997). "Social Issues and Genetic Studies: A Case Study Using Advocacy Group." *Journal of College Science Teaching*. Vol. 27: 17.

CNN.com (2003). <wysiwyg://3/http://www.cnn.com/2003/HEALTH/02 /06/biotech.pigs.ap/index.html>

Cookson, C. (2000). "BSE Could Have Happened Anywhere." *Financial Times*. (November 4 & 5, II Weekend FT): 11.

Corbett, E. P. J. (1991). *The Elements of Reasoning*. New York: Macmillan Publishing Company: 32.

Darwin, C.R., (1958). *The Autobiography of Charles Darwin 1809-1882 With Original Omissions Restored*. London: Collins: 120.

Dinsmore, J. H., Manhart, C., Raineri, R. Jacoby, D.B., Moore, A., and Diacrin Inc. (2000). "No Evidence for Infection of Human Cells With Porcine Endogenous Retrovirus (PERV After Exposure to Porcine Fetal Neuronal Cells." *Transplantation*. November 15, Vol. 70, No. 9: 1382-9.

Dobzhansky, T. (1967). "Changing Man." *Science*. Vol. 155: 409.

Drane, J. (1972). "A Philosophy of Man and Higher Education." *Main Currents in Modern Thought*. Vol. 29: 99.

Drucker P. (1980). *Managing in Turbulent Times*. New York: Harper & Row: 191.

Edmondson, G., Carey, J., and J. O. C. Hamilton (1996). "Science and Technology, Biotech, Europe's Ace Gene Hunter, Can Daniel Cohen's Startup Outrun U. S. Rivals?" *Business Week*. (September 30): 86 and 88.

Edwards, F. (1999). "How Biotechnology Is Transforming What We Believe and How We Live?" *The Humanist*. (September/October), Vol. 59, No. 5: 24.

Eisenberg, L. (1973). "On the Humanizing of Human Nature." *Impact of Science on Society*. Vol. 23: 214.

Ferraro, G. P. (1994). *The Cultural Dimension of International Business*. Second Edition, Englewood Cliffs, New Jersey: Prentice Hall: 21.

Financial Times (2000). "The Book of Life." (Monday June 26): 16.

Fisher, L. M. (1996). "Genetic Institute in Deal to Share Biochemical Library." *New York Times*. (September 26): D1, D4.

Flowers, E. B. (1998). "The Ethics of Economics of Patenting the Human Genome." *Journal of Business Ethics*. Vol. 17, No. 15: 1737-1745.

Fluehr-Lobban, C. (2000). "How Anthropology Should Respond to an Ethical Crisis?" *The Chronicle of Higher Education*. Section 2, October 6, 2000: B24.

Fox, M. W. (1990). *Inhumane Society: The American Way of Animal Exploitation*. New York: St. Martin's Press.

Fox, M. W. (2001). *Bringing Life to Ethics*. New York: State University of New York Press: 29.

Free Inquiry in Creative Sociology. "A Reexamination of Triangulation and Objectivity in Qualitative Nursing Research." Vol. 21, No. 1: 65-72.

Gardener, H. (1993). *Frames of Mind: The Theory of Multiple Intelligence*. New York: Basic Books: xvii.

Gates, D. (2000). "Fundamentalism 101: Why That Old-Time Religion Is Thoroughly Modern." *Business Week*. (March 20).

George, N. (2000). "Ethical Practices May Have Prevented Outbreak in Sweden." *Financial Times*. (Thursday November 30): 2.

Gert, B., Culver, C. M., and Clouser, K. D. (1997). *Bioethics: A Return to Fundamentals*. Oxford: Oxford University Press: 2.

Gregory, M. S. (1984). "Science and Humanities: Toward a New Worldview." In D. H. Brock and A. Harward (1984). *The Culture of Biomedicine: Studies in Science and Culture*. Vol. 1, Newark: NJ: University of Delaware Press: 11-33.

Griffith, V. (2001). "Searching for the Real Staff of Life." *Financial Times*. (Wednesday February 21): 11.

Griffith, V. (2001). "Forever Young." *Financial Times*. (Weekend, August 25-2): 11.

Harvey, F. (2001). "A Miniature World of Tubes, Balls, and Locusts." *Financial Times*. (Monday April 23): 16.

Heilbroner (1974). *The Human Prospect*. New York: W. W. Norton.

Heller, J. (1972). "Syphilis Victims in US Study Went Untreated for 40 Years." *New York Times*. (July 26): A1, A8.

Higgins, J. M. (1994). *The Management Challenge*. New York: Second Edition. Macmillan Publishing Company: 61.

Hildyard, N. and Sexton, S. (2000). "No Patents on Life." *Forum for Applied Research and Public Policy*. Knoxville, TN: Spring, Vol. 1591: 69-74.

Hosmer, L. T. (1987). *The Ethics of Management*. Homewood, Illinois: Irwin: 82.

Jones, W. H. S. (1924). *The Doctor's Oath: An Essay in the History of Medicine*. Cambridge: The University Press.

Jonsen, A. R. (1998). *The Birth of Bioethics*. New York/Oxford; Oxford University Press: 12 and 125.

Jonsen, A. R. (1991). "American Moralism and the Origin of Bioethics in the United States." *Journal of Medicine and Philosophy*. Vol. 16: 114.

Jonsen, A. R. (1993). "The Birth of Bioethics." *Hastings Center Report*, # 23, November/December Edition.

Juengst, E. T. (1997). "Can Enhancement be Distinguished From Prevention in Genetic Medicine?" *The Journal of Medicine and Philosophy*. Vol. 22: 125.

Kaplan, A. (1964). *The Conduct of Inquiry*. Chandler Publishing: 206.

Lane, R. E. (1962). *Political Ideology: Why the American Common Man Beliefs What He Does*. New York: Free Press: 3, 15.

Leake, C. D. (1927). *Perceival's Medical Ethics.* 18.

Leake, C. D. (1928). "How is Medical Ethics to Be Taught?" *Bulletin of the Association of American Medical Colleges.* Vol. 3: 343.

Lui, H., Farr-Jones, S., Ulyanov, N.B., Llinas, M., Marqusee, S. Groth, D., Cohen, F.E., Prusiner, S.B., and James, T. L. (1997). "Solution Structure of Syrian Hamster Prion Protein rPrP." *Biochemistry.* Vol. 38: 5362-5377.

Madison, J. (1961). "Federalist 51." In *The Federalist Papers.* In Alexander Hamilton, James Madison, and John Jay (Eds.). New York: New American Library: 320-325.

Mahnaimi, U. and Colvin, M. (1998). "Israel Planning Ethnic Bomb as Sadam Caves in." *The London Times.* Sunday Edition. (November 15).

Malik, S. (2000). "Cracking the Genetic Code; What's Next After Genetic Decoding? Will We Be Able to Control Our Feelings and Desires? Will We Control Every Aspect of Our Lives?" *Time.* (July 24): 15.

Marger, M. N. (1985). *Race and Ethnic Relations: American and Global Perspectives.* Belmont, California: Wadsworth Publishing Company: 16.

Meilaender, G. C. (1995). *Body, Soul, and Bioethics.* Notre Dame: University of Notre Dame Press: 2.

Michael, M., Grimyer, A. and Turner, J. (1997). "Teaching Biology: Identify in the Context of Ignorance and Knowledge Ability." *Public Understanding of Science.* Vol. 6: 1-17.

Mill, J. S. (1897). *Utilitarianism.* London: Longmans.

Morrison, S. (2000). "Mad Cow Panic Blights Farmer of Water Buffalo." *Financial Times.* Weekends December 9-10: 3.

Mullins, W. A. (1972). "On the Concept of Ideologies in Political Science." *American Political Science Review.* Vol. 66: 498-511.

Munson, R. (1983). *Intervention and Reflection: Basic Issues in Medical Ethics.* Belmont, California: Wadsworth Publishing Company: 239-24, 246, and 378.

Murray, G. (1970). *Five Stages of Greek Religion.* New York: Doubleday.

Olby, R. C. (1966). *The Origins of Mendelism.* New York: Shocken Books.

Pauly, P. C. and Harris, D.A. (1998). "Copper Stimulates Endocytosis of the Prion Protein." *Journal of Biological Chemistry.* (December 11, 1998), Vol. 273, No. 50: 33107-10.

Percival, T. (1803). *Medical Ethics: Or, a Code of Institute and Precepts, Adapted to the Professional Conduct of physicians and Surgeons.* London: S. Russell. In Leake, C. (1927), (Ed.). *Perceival's Medical Ethics.* Williams and Wilkins.

Pilling, D. (1999). "Researchers Weigh the Risk of Animal-to-Human Transplants." *Financial Times.* (Friday August 20): 3.

Porter, V. R. (1971). *Bioethics, Bridge to the Future.* Englewood Cliffs: Prentice Hall.

Poter, V. R. and Poter, L. (1995). "Global Bioethics: Converting Sustainable Development to Global Survival." *Medicine and Global Survival.* Vol. 2: 185-90.

Prusiner, S. B. (1997). "Molecular Biological, Genetic, and Protein Structural Studies of Prion Disease." *Noble Foundation.* Stockholm, Sweden. Reprinted in (1998) *Proceedings: National Academy of Science*, U.S.A. Vol. 95: 13363-13383.

Rawls, J. (1971). "Justice as Reciprocity." *From John Stuart Mill, Utilitarianism.* S. Gorovitz (Ed.), New York: Bobbs-Merrill.

Reuters (2001). "U.S. Quarantines Texas Cattle Over Mad Cow Rules." *Netscape*: <wysiwyg://6/http:// dailynews.netscape.com...able'n&cat' 50100&id"200101251849000210734>.

Rothman, B. K. (1999). "The Potential Cost of the Best Genes Money Can Buy." *The Chronicle of Higher Education.* June 11: A52.

Rothman, D. (1991). *Strangers at the Bedside: A History of How Law and Bioethics Transformed Medical Decision Making.* New York: Basic Books: 3.

Rubenstein, E. C., Anderson, C. J. D., & Hall, W. B. (1996). "Drama Drive a DNA Fingerprinting." *Lab Exercise.* Vol. 26: 103-106.

Schoen, E. J., Margaret, M. H., and Falchek, J. S. (2000). "An Examination of the Legal and Ethical Public Policy Considering Underlying DES Market Share Liability." *Journal of Business Ethics.* Vol. 24, No. 2: 141-163.

Sidel, V.W. (1971). "New Technologies and the Practice of Medicine." *Human Aspects of Biomedical Innovation.* Cambridge, Mass.: Harvard University Press: 147.

Skinner, B. F. (1953). *Science and Human Behavior.* New York: Free Press. Spooner, 2001: <http://news.cnet.com/news/0-1003-200-5744137.html>.

Sproul, L. S. (1981) "Beliefs in Organizations" in P. C. Nystrom and W. H. Starbuck (Eds). *Handbook of Organizational Design.* New York: Oxford University Press: 204.

Steiner, G. A. and Steiner, J. F. (2003). *Business, Government, and Society.* Tenth Edition. McGraw-Hill-Irwin: 199.

Stockel, J., Safar, J., Wallace, A.C., Cohen, F. E., and Prusiner, S. B. (1998). "Prion Protein Selectively Binds Copper (II) Ions." *Biochemistry.* May 19, Vol. 37, No. 20: 7185-93.

Supattapone, S. Bosque, P., Muramoto, T., White, H., Aagaard, C., Peretz, D., Nguyen, H., O.B., Heinrich, C., Torchia, M. Safar, J., Cohen, F.E., DeArmond, S.J., Prusiner, S.B., and Scott, M. (1999). "Prion Prottein of 106 Residues Creates an Artificial Transmisssion Barrier for Prion Replication in Transgenic Mice." *Cell.* Vol. 96: 869-878.

Tatum, E. (1966). "The Possibility of Manipulating Genetic Change." in J. D. Roslansly (Ed.). *Genetics and Future of Man.* New York: Appleton-Century-Crofts: 55-60.

Taviss, I. (1971). "Problems in the Social Control of Biomedical Science and Technology." In E. Mendelsohn, J. P. Swazey, and I. Taviss (Eds.). *Human*

Aspects of Biomedical Innovation. Cambridge, Mass: Harvard University Press: 3-45.

Terpstra, V. and David, K. (1991). *The Cultural Environment of International Business.* Cincinnati: South-Western Publishing Co.: 106.

Tofler R. L. (1970). *Future Shock.* New York: Random House.

Trosko, J. E. (1984). "Scientific Views of Human Nature: Implications for the Ethics of Technological Intervention." In D. H. Brock and A. Harward (1984). *The Culture of Biomedicine: Studies in Science and Culture.* Volume 1. Newark: NJ: University of Delaware Press: 70-76.

Viles, J.H., Cohen, F.E., Prusiner, S.B., Goodin, D.B., Wright, P.E., and Dyson, H.J. (1999). "Copper Binding to the Prion Protein: Structural Implications of Four Identical Cooperative Binding Sites." *Proceeding: National Academy of Science*, USA. Vol. 96: 2042-2047.

Watson, J. and Crick, F. (1953). "The Molecular Structure of Nucleic Acids." *Nature.* Vol. 4356: 737.

Weber, D. O. (2000). "The Bionic Century: More and More Doctors Will Be Replacing Worn-Out Organs With or Manufactured Body Part." *Health Forum Journal.* (May-June Edition): 16-19.

White, R. (1970). In Weber, D. O. (2000). "The Bionic Century: More and More Doctors Will be Replacing Worn- out Organs With or Manufactured Body Part." *Health Forum Journal:* 16.

Wilson, E. O. and Kellert, S. R. (1993). *The Biophilia Hypothesis.* Washington: Island Press.

Wrong, M. (2000). "EU to Prop up French Beef Market." *Financial Times.* (Thursday November 16): 6.

Chapter 2

ABC.com (2002). <wysiwyg://4/http://Abcnews.go.com/section/us/ DailyNews/doctor021115.html>.

Ahmed, M. M. (1999). "Cultural and Contextual Aspects in Business Ethics: Three Controversies and One Dilemma." *Journal of Transnational Management Development.* Vol. 4, No. 1: 111-129.

Albert, E. M., Denise, T. C., and Peterfreund, S. P. (1984). *Great Traditions in Ethics.* Belmont, California: Wadsworth Publishing Company: 1-7 and 128.

Barton, L. (1995). *Ethics: The Enemy in the Workplace.* Cincinnati, Ohio: South-Western College Publishing: 109.

Benn, S. (1967). "Power." In Paul Edwards (Ed.). *The Encyclopedia of Philosophy.* New York: The Free Press, Vol. 6: 424-427.

Council on Ethical and Judicial Affairs (1998). "Code of Medical Ethics: Current Opinions." *American Medical Association.* Chicago, Illinois: Annotations prepared by the Southern Illinois University Schools of Medicine and Law: 61 and 164.

De George, R. 1995. *Business Ethics*. Englewood Cliffs, New Jersey: Prentice Hall: 5, 19, 87 and 256.

De Mente, B. L. (1989). *Chinese Etiquette & Ethics in Business: A Penetrating Analysis of the Morals and Values that Shape the Chinese Business Personality*. Chicago, Illinois: NTC Publishing Group: 27-28.

Emerson, R. M. (1962). "Power-Dependent Relations." *American Sociological Review*. Vol. 27, (February): 31-41.

Findlay, S. (2002). "Do Ads Really Drive Pharmaceutical Sales?" *Marketing Health Services*, Vol. 22, No. 1: 20-25.

Flecher, G. J. O., and Ward, C. (1988). "Attribution Theory and Processes: A Cross-Cultural Perspective." In Bond, M. H. (Ed.), *The Cross-Cultural Challenge to Social Psychology*. Newbury Park, CA, Sage: 230-244.

Frankena, W. K. (1963). *Ethics*. Englewood Cliffs, NJ: Prentice-Hall, Inc.: 6.

French, W. A. and Granrose, J. (1995). *Practical Business Ethics*. Englewood Cliffs, New Jersey: Prentice Hall: 9.

French, J. R. P. and Raven, B. (1959). *Studies in Social Power*. Ann Arbor: Institute for Social Research.

Halbert, T. and Ingulli, E. (2000). *Law and Ethics in the Business Environment*. Canada: West Legal Studies: 19 and 40.

Hemingway, E. (1932). *Death in the Afternoon*. New York: Charles Scibner"s Sons: 4.

Hobbes, T. (1839). *Leviathan and Philosophical Rudiments*. From *The English Works of Thomas Hobbes*. Vol. II, III, Sir William Molesworth (Ed.). London: John Bohn.

Hook, S. (1946). *Education for Modern Man*. New York: Dial Press. <*JAMA,* http://jama.ama-assn.org/issues/v287n3/ffull/joc11123.html.>.

Jansen, E. and Von Glinow, M. A. (1985). "Ethical Ambivalence and Organizational Reward Systems." *Academy of Management Review*. Vol. 10, No. 4: 814-822.

Kant, I. (1969). *Foundation of the Metaphysics of Morals*. Reprinted. Translated by Lewis White Beck. Indianapolis: Bobbs-Merrill Educational Publishing, (Originally Published in 1785).

Kant, I. (1984). *Duty and Reason*. In Albert, E.M. and Denise, T. C. (Eds.), *Great Traditions in Ethics*. Belmont, California: Wadsworth Publishing Company: 199-218.

Latif, D. A. (2001). "The Relationship Between Pharmacists Tenure in the Community Setting and Moral Reasoning." *Journal of Business Ethics*. Vol. 31, No. 2: 131-141.

Lilla, M. T. (1981). "Ethos, Ethics, and Public Service." *The Public Interest*. 3-11.

Newton, L.H. and Schmidt, D. P. (1996). *Wake Up Calls: Classic Cases in Business Ethics*. United States of America: Wadsworth Publishing Company: 3.

Oesterle, J. A. (1957). *Ethics: The Introduction to Moral Science*. Englewood, New Jersey: Prentice Hall, Inc.: 5, 20, and 201.

Parhizgar, K. D. and Jesswein, K. R. (1998). "Ethical and Economical Affordability of Developing Nations's Repayment of International Debt." In Baker, J. C. (1998). *Selected International Investment Portfolios*. Great Britain: Pergamon Publishing Co.: 141.

Parhizgar, K. D. (2002). *Multicultural Behavior and Global Business Environments*. New York: Haworth Press: 297.

Park, J. and Barron, R. W. (1977). "Can Morality be Taught?" In Stiles, L. J. and Johnson, B. D. (Eds). (1977). *Morality Examined: Guidelines for Teachers*. Princeton, NJ: Princeton Book Company Publishers: 3-23.

Paul, R. W. and Elder, L. (2002). *Critical Thinking*. Upper Saddle River, NJ: Prentice Hall: 48.

Shaw, W. H. (1996). *Business Ethics*. Second Edition, Belmont, California: Wadsworth Publishing Company: 4 and 12.

Steiner, G. A. and Steiner, J. F. (1988). *Business, Government, and Society*. New York: Random House Division: 592.

The Oxford English Dictionary (1963). Oxford, Britain: At the Clarendon Press, 287, 312-314: 554, and 656.

Trevino, L. K. and Nelson, K. (1995). *Managing Business Ethics: Straight Talk About How To Do It Right*. New York: John Wiley & Son, Inc.: 52.

Walton, C. C. "Overview." In Walton, C. C. (Ed.), (1977). *The Ethics of Corporate Conduct*. Englewood Cliffs, New Jersey: Prentice-Hall, Inc.: 6.

Whately, R. (1859). *Paley's Moral Philosophy: With Annotations*. London: John W. Parker & Son: 68-90.

Yinger, J. M. (1970). *The Scientific Study of Religion*. London: The Macmillan Company: 45.

Chapter 3

Adler, N. (1986). *International Dimensions of Organizational Behavior*. Boston, Mass.: Kent Publishing Company: 12 and 13.

Aquinas, T. (1945). *Basic Writings of St. Thomas Aquinas*. Vol. II, A. C. Pegis (Ed.). New York: Random House, Article V: 356-357.

Bentham, J. (1823). *An Introduction to the Principles of Morals and Legislation*. 2nd Ed.: Ch. XII, Part 2.

De George, R. T. (1995). *Business Ethics. Fourth Edition*. Englewood Cliffs, New Jersey: Prentice Hall: 63.

Dupuios, A. M. (1985). *Philosophy of Education in Historical Perspective*. Lanham, MD: Rand McNally and Company: 10.

Freud, S. (1949). *An Outline of Psycho-Analysis*. New York: Norton.

Geertz, C. (1970). "The Impact of the Concept of Culture on the Concept of Man." In Hammel, E. A. and Simmonson, W. S. (Ed.). *Man Makes Sense*. Boston: Little Brown: 47.

Herbart, J. (1806). *General Principles of Pedagogy Deduced from the Aims of Education.* (Tr. By A. F. Lange With Annotations by C. De Garmo) London: Macmillan: 1913.

Hobbes, T. (1839) *Leviathan and Philosophical Rudiments.* London: Sir William Molesworth, (Ed.): Part I, Chapter 13, Paragraph 13, Chapter 14, Paragraph 3, and Chapter 15, Paragraph 10.

Kant, I. (1898). *Fundamental Principles of Metaphysics of Morals.* Tr. T. K. Abbott, From *Kant"s Critique of Practical Reason and Other Works on the Theory of Ethics.* London: Longmans, Green: 10 and 539.

Kluckhohn, F. R. and Strodtbeck, F. L. (1961). *Variation· Value Orientations.* Evanston, IL: Row, Peterson, and Company: 11.

Locke, J. (1924). *An Essay Concerning Human Understanding.* (Abr. and Ed. by): A. S. Pringle-Pattison. Oxford: Clarendon Press.

Locke, J. (1693). *Some Thoughts Concerning Education.* Marshal, K. P. (1999). "Has Technology Introduced New Ethical Problems?" *Journal of Business Ethics.* Vol. 19: 81-90.

Marshal, L. (1997). "Facilitating Knowledge Management and Knowledge Sharing." *Online.* Vol. 21, No. 5: 92-98.

Montague, W. P. (1930). *Beliefs Unbound: A Promethean Religion for the Modern World.* New Haven, Conn.: Yale University Press: 44.

Moran, R. T. and Harris, P. R. (1982). *Managing Cultural Synergy.* Volume 2. Houston: Gulf Publishing Company: 19.

Natcher (1999). <http://planning. cancer.gov/whealth/DES/chapter1.html)>. Parhizgar, K. D. (2002). *Multicultural Behavior and Global Business Environments.* New York: Haworth Press: 124 and 221-254.

Parhizgar, K .D., and Lunce, S. E. (1994). "Genealogical Approaches to Ethical Implications of Informational Assimilative Integrated Discovery Systems (AIDS) in Business." In Beardwell, I. (Ed.), *Contemporary Developments in Human Resource Management.* Montpellier, France: An International Publication of the Scientific Committee of the Montpellier Graduate Business School, Editions ESKA: 55-60.

Plato, (1892). *The Dialogues of Plato.* Vols. I, II, and III. Translated by B. Jowett. 3rd Edition. New York: Oxford University Press: 26.

Reid, T. (1764). *Inquiry into the Human Mind on the Principles of Common Sense.*

Smith, E. D. and Pham, C. (1998). "Doing Business in Vietnam: A Cultural Guide." In Maidment, F. (Ed.). *International Business 98/99.* Seventh Edition. Guilford, Connecticut: Dushkin/McGraw-Hill: 174.

Spencer, H. (1888). *Education, Intellectual, Moral, and Physical.* New York: D. Appleton.

Watson, Jr., T. J. (1963). *A Business and Its Beliefs: The Ideas That Helped Build IBM.* New York: McGraw-Hill Book Company, Inc.: 36.

Chapter 4

American National Commission for the Protection of Human Subjects of Biomedical and Behavioral Research (1978). *The Belmont Report: Ethical Guidelines for the Protection of Human Subjects of Research.* DHEW Publication No. (OS) 78-00. Washington, D. C.: Department of Health, Education, and Welfare.

Aristotle (1925). *Nichomachean Ethics.* Translated by W. D. Ross. *Works of Aristotle.* Vol. IX, W. D. Ross, (Ed.). Oxford: Clarendon Press.

Bentham, J. (1838). Edited by J. Bowring. *The Works of Jeremy Bentham.* London: Simpkin, Marshall, Vol. 1: 16, Note.

Bentham, J. (1970). *Introduction to the Principles and Morals of Legislation.* London, England: Athlone Press.

Butler, J. (1949). *Five Sermons.* New York: Liberal Arts Press: 45.

Callahan, D. (1984). "Morality and Contemporary Culture: The President's Commission and Beyond." *Cardoza Law Review.* Vol. 6: 348.

Carroll, A. B. and Buchholtz, A. K. (2003). *Business and Society: Ethics and Stakeholder Management.* United States: Thomson, South-Western: 167.

Childress, J. F. (1994). "Principles-Oriented Bioethics: An Analysis and Assessment From Within." In Dubose, E. R., Hamel, R. P., and O'Connell, L. J. (Eds.). *Matter of Principles? Ferment in U.S. Bioethics.* Valley Forge, Pennsylvania, Trinity Press International: 72-98.

Churchill (1989). "Reviving Distinctive Medical Ethics." *Hastings Center Report,* Vol.19, (May/June): 30.

Epicures, (1866). *The Work of Epictetus.* Translated by T. W. Higginson, Boston, Mass.: Little, Brown.

Fox, M. W. (2001). *Bringing Life to Ethics.* New York: New York University of New York Press: 12.

Frankena, W. K. (1973). *Ethics.* Second Edition. Englewood Cliffs, New Jersey: Prentice-Hall, Inc.: 109.

Hosmer, L. R. T. (1987). *The Ethics of Management.* Homewood, Illinois: Irwin: 12 and 98.

Jonas, H. (1984). *The Imperative of Responsibility: In Search of an Ethics for the Technological Age.* Chicago: University of Chicago Press: 43.

Johnson and Johnson Web Site: <http://www.jni.com/who_is_jnj/cr_usa. html> .

Kass, L. R. (1985). *Toward More Natural Science: Biology and Human Affairs.* New York: The Free Press: 72 and 102.

Kass, L. R. (1989). "Neither For Love Nor Money: Why Doctors Must Not Kill." *The Public Interest.* Vol. 9: 41.

Koller, P. (2002) "Human Genome Technology From the Viewpoint of Efficiency and Justice." In Cosimo Marco Mazzoni (Ed.). *Ethics and Law in Biological Research.* The Hague: Martinus Nijhoff Publishers: 9-20.

Leob, J. M., Hendee, W. R., Smith, S. J., and Schwarz, M. R. (1989). "Human V. Animal Rights: In Defense of Animal Rights." *Journal of the American Medical Association.* Vol. 262, No. 19, (November 17): 2719-2720.

McCollum, K. (1998). "Founder of Utilitarianism Is Present in Spirit at 250th Birthday Teleconference." *The Chronicle of Higher Education.* February 27: A28.

McKenny, G. P. (1997). *To Relieve the Human Condition: Bioethics, Technology, and the Body.* New York: The State University of New York Press: 54.

Mill, J. S. (1897). *Utilitarianism.* London: Longmans, Green.

Moore, G. E. (1948). *Principa Ethica.* New York: Cambridge University Press: vii.

Moore, G. E. (1922). *Philosophical Studies.* London: Kegan Paul, Trench, Trubner: 273.

Moreno, J. D. (1995). *Deciding Together: Bioethics and Moral Consensus.* New York: Oxford University Press: 47.

Moros, D. (1996). "Taking Duties Seriously: Medical Experimentation, Animal Rights, and Moral Incoherence." In David C. Thomasma and Thomasine Kushner (Eds.). *Birth and Death: Science and Bioethics.* Cambridge, Britain: Cambridge University Press: 313-324.

Multinational Monitor. (1996). Vol. 17; No. 6: <http:multinationalmonitor. org/hyper/mm0696.01.html>.

Plato. *Apology, Cerrito, Republic I-II.* Great Books Foundation (Regency): 343.

Plato. *The Republic. Everyman's Library (Dutton).*

Ross, W. D. (1930). *The Right and the Good.* New York: Oxford University Press: 41-42.

Sartre, J. P. (1947). *Existentialism.* New York: Philosophical Library: 27.

Shaw, W. H. (1996). *Business Ethics.* Second Edition. New York: Wadsworth Publishing Company: 11.

White, Jr., L. (1967). "The Historical Roots of Our Ecological Crisis." *Science.* Vol. 155, (March 10): 1203-1207.

Chapter 5

Bayles, M. D. (1987). "The Values of Life." In D. VanDeVeer and T. Regan (Eds.). Philadelphia: Temple University Press: 265-289.

Caplan, A. L., Englehardt Jr., H. T., and McCartney, J. J. (Eds), (1981). *Concepts of Health and Disease: Interdisciplinary Perspectives. Reading.* Mass.: Addison-Wesley: 83.

Carr, D. (2000). *Professionalism and Ethics in Teaching.* London/New York: Routledge, Taylor and Francis Group: 23.

Dawnie, R. S. (1974). *Roles and Values: An Introduction to Social Ethics.* London: Methuen.

De George, R. (1995). *Business Ethics.* Englewood Cliffs, New Jersey: Prentice Hall: 115, and 454-468.

Douglas, J. D. (1978). "Major Tactics of Investigative Research." In Charles H. Swanson, (Ed.). *Focus: Unexplored Deviance.* Guilford, Conn.: Dushkin: 206-221.

DuBose, E. R., Hamel, R. P., and O'Connell, L. J. (1994). *A Matter of Principles? Ferment in U.S. Bioethics.* Valley Forge, Pennsylvania: Trinity Press International: 102.

Gert, B., Culver, C. M. and Clouser, K. D. (1977). *Bioethics: A Return To Fundamentals.* New York/Oxford; Oxford University Press: 98.

Greenwood, E. (1962). "Attributes of a Profession. In Nosow, S. and Form, W. H. (Eds.). *Man, Work, and Society.* New York: Basic Books, 206.

Guterman, L. (2001). "An Armful of Eggs: Ovarian Transplants Could Restore Lost Fertility." *The Chronicle of Higher Education.* January 26: A19.

Moreno, J. D. (1995). *Deciding Together: Bioethics and Moral Consensus.* New York: Oxford University Press: 4.

Oktay, K. (2001). In Guterman, L. "An Armful of Eggs: Ovarian Transplants Could Restore Lost Fertility." *The Chronicle of Higher Education.* January 26: A19.

Parhizgar, K. D. (2002). *Multicultural Behavior and Global Business Environments.* New York: Haworth Press: 126.

Parks, S. D. (1993). "Young Adults, Mentoring Communities, and the Conditions of Moral Choice." In Andrew Garrod (Ed.). *Approaches to Moral Development: New Research and Emerging Themes.* New York: Teachers College Press, Columbia University: 217.

Schein, E. H. (1966). "The Problem of Moral Education for Business Manager." *Industrial Management Review.* Vol. 8: 311.

Schwartz, M. (2001). "The Nature of Relationship Between Corporate Codes of Ethics and Behavior." *Journal of Business Ethics.* Vol. 32: 247-256.

Thompson, V. G. (1961). *Modern Organization.* New York: Knopf: 170.

Wilson, F. A. and Neuhauser, D. (1976) *Health Services in the United States.* Cambridge, Mass.: Balinger Publishing Company: 52.

Chapter 6

Albert, S. and Whetten, D. (1985). "Organizational Identity." In L. L. Cummings and B. M. Staw (Eds.). *Research in Organizational Behavior.* Greenwich, Conn.: JAI Press: 263-295.

Arieti, S. (1993). "Science." In Bulger, R. E., Heitman, E., and Resier, S. J. (Eds.). *The Ethical Dimensions of the Biological Sciences.* Cambridge: Cambridge University Press: 19.

Awadudi, A. A. (1989). *Towards Understanding Islam. Jamaica.* New York: The Message Publications: 121.

Ball, D. A., and McCulloch, Jr., W. H. (1988). *International Business: Introduction and Essentials.* Third Edition. Homewood, IL: Irwin: 269.

Barinagg, M. (1989). "Making Transgenetic Mice: Is It Really That Easy?" *Science.* Vol. 245: 590-591.

Beals, R. L. and Hijer, H. (1959). *An Introduction to Anthropology.* New York: Macmillan: 9.

Behdad, S. (1989). "Property Rights in Contemporary Islamic Economic Thought: A Critical Perspective." *Review of Social Economy.* Vol. 47, No. 2: 185-211.

Benjamin, M. (1995). "The Value of Consensus." In Bulger, R. E., Bobby, E. M., and Fineberg, H. v. (Eds.). *Society's Choices: Social and Ethical Decision Making in Biomedicine.* Washington D.C.: National Academy Press: 249 and 251.

Berelson, B. and Steiner, G. A. (1964). *Human Behavior.* New York: Harcourt, Brace, and World, 16-17.

Blackler, F. (1995) "Knowledge, Knowledge Work and Organizations: An Overview and Interpretation." *Organization Studies.* Vol. 16, No.6: 1021-1046.

Buchholz, R. A. and Rosenthal, S. B. (1998). *Business Ethics.* Upper Saddle River, NJ: Prentice Hall: 60.

Collins, H. (1993). "The Structure of Knowledge." *Social Research.* Vol. 60: 95-116.

Carroll, A. B. (1979). "Three Dimensional Conceptual Model of Corporate Performance." *Academy of Management Review.* (October Issue): 499.

Comroe, Jr., J. H. and Dripps, R. D. (1993). "Scientific Basis for the Support of Biomedical Science." In Bulger, R. E., Heitman, E., and Reiser, S. J. (1993). *The Ethiocal Dimensions of the Biological Science.* Canada: Cambridge University Press: 28.

Dalton, M. (1964). "Preconceptions and Methods in Men Who Manage." In Hammond, P. (Ed.). *Sociologists at Work.* New York: Basic Books: 50-95.

Darwin, C. R. (1982). The Autobiography of Charles Darwin 1809-1882 With Original Omission Restored (1958). London: Collins.

De George, R. T. (1990). *Business Ethics.* Fourth Edition. Englewood Cliffs, New Jersey: Prentice Hall, Inc.: 119.

Denzin, N. K. (1978). *The Research Act: A Theoretical Introduction to Sociological Methods.* 2nd Edition. New York: McGraw-Hill.

Dewey, J. (1929). *The Quest for Certainty.* New York: Mint Balch.

Drucker, P. (1993). *Post-Capitalist Society.* Oxford: Butterworth Heineman: 5.

Financial Times (2001). "The Danger of Knowing Too Much." Weekend May 12/May 13: 11.

Flack, J. (1997). "Contingent Knowledge and Technology Development." Technology Development. *Technology Analysis for Strategic Management.* Vol. 9, No. 4: 383-397.

Fox, M. W. (2001). *Bringing Life to Ethics: Global Bioethics for a Human Society.* New York: State University of New York Press: 71.

Freud, Z. (1856-1939). "Re-Examining Freud." *Psychology Today.*

September 1989: 48-52.

Garvin, D. A. (1998). "Building a Learning Organization." *Harvard Business Review on Knowledge Management.* Boston, Mass.: President and Fellows of Harvard College: 47.

Gold, J. (2000). "Ex-Penny Stock Mogul Arrested on Fraud Charges." *San Antonio Express News.* Wednesday August 2: 2E.

Hall, W. (2000). "Banks Agree Money Laundering Rules." *Financial Times.* Tuesday October 31: 10.

Hammer, R. W., Pursel, V. G., Rexroot, C. E., Jr., et al., (1986). "Genetic Engineering of Mammalian Embryos." *Journal of Animal Science.* Vol. 63: 269-278.

Harvey, C. and Allard, M. J. (1995). *Understanding Diversity: Readings, Cases, and Exercises.* New York: Harper Collins College Publishers: 11.

Keller, S. R. and Wilson, E. O. (1993). *The Biophilia Hypothesis.* Washington: Island Press: 12.

Lundvall, B. A. (1996). "The Social Dimension of the Learning Economy." *Department of Business Studies.* Aalborg University, Denmark.

Luthans, F. (1985). *Organizational Behavior.* New York: McGraw-Hill: 30-39.

Meyes, B. T. and Allen, R. W. (1977). "Toward a Definition of Organizational Politics." *Academy of Management Review.* Vol. 2, No. 4: 672-678.

Miller, J., David, A., and Quintas, P. (1997). "Trans-Organizational Innovation: A Framework for Research." *Technology Analysis of Strategic Management.* Vol. 9, No. 4: 399-418.

Morgan, C., and King, R. (1966). *Introduction to Psychology.* 3rd Ed., New York: McGraw-Hill: 22.

Palmer, J. D. (1989). "Three Paradigms for Diversity Challenge Leaders." *OD Practitioner.* Vol. 21: 15-18.

Parhizgar, K. D. (2002). *Multicultural Behavior and Global Business Environments.* New York: Haworth Press: 125.

Parhizgar, K. D., and Lunce, S. E. (1996). "Implications of Employees" Informational Integrated Discovery Systems." In Beardwell, I. (Ed.). *Contemporary Developments in Human Resource Management.* Montpelier: France: An International Publication of the Scientific Committee of the Montpelier Graduate Business School, Editions ESKA: 393-403.

Parhizgar, K. D. (1996). "Cross-Cultural Implications of the Popular Cultural Damping in the International Movie Market." In Lemaster, J., and Islam, M.M., *Southwest Review of International Business Research, Proceedings of the 1996 Academy of International Business, Southwest Regional Meeting*: 309.

Parhizgar, K. D. (1994). "Affordability and Solvency Implications of Privatization of Government-Owned Industries in the Third World Countries." *Journal of Business and Society.* Vol. 7, No. 1: 110.

Reichenbaqch, H. (1951). *The Rise of Scientific Philosophy.* Berkeley: University of California Press.

Rifkin, J., et al., (1983). "Theological Letter Concerning the Moral Arguments Against Genetic Engineering of Human Germ Line Cell." Reported in C. Norman. "Cleric Urge Ban on Cell." *Science*. Vol. 220: 1360-1361.

Sibley, W. M. (1953). "The Rational Versus the Reasonableness." *Philosophy Review*. Vol. 62: 554-560.

Steidlmeier, P. (1993). "The Moral Legitimacy of Intellectual Property Claims: American Business and Developing Country Perspectives." *Journal of Business Ethics*. Vol. 12, No. 2: 157.

Taylor, G. R. (1969). *The Biological Time Bomb*. New York: Mentor Books: 205.

Terpstra, V. and David, K. (1991). *The Cultural Environment of International Business*. Third Edition. Cincinnati. Ohio: College Division South-Western Publishing Co.: 136.

The Oxford English Dictionary (1989). Second Edition. Prepared by Simpson, J. A. and Weiner, E. S. C. Oxford: Clardon Press.

Turner, M. (2003). "UN Vote Postpones Decision on Banning Human Cloning." <http://news.ft.com/servlet/ContentServer?pagename'FT.com/StoryFT/FullStory&c'Story&cid'1066565...11/6/2003>.

Van Raden, P. M. and Freeman, A. E. (1985). "Potential Genetic Gains From Producing Bulls With Only Sire as Parents." *Journal of Dairy Science*. Vol. 68: 1425-1431.

Weber, C. O. (1960). *Basic Philosophies of Education*. New York: Rinehart and Winston: 13-14.

Wundt, W. (1879). In Luthans, F. (1985) *Organizational Behavior*. New York: McGraw-Hill: 36.

Zack, M. H. (1999). "Managing Codified Knowledge." *Sloan Management Review*. Vol. 40, No. 4: 45-58.

Zadeh, L. A. (1965). "Fuzzy Sets." *Information Control*. Vol. 8: 338-353.

Chapter 7

Aeschylus. *Prometheus Bound*. Lines 250ff.

Beauchamp, T. and Childress, J. (1989). *Principles of Biomedical Ethics*. New York: Oxford University Press: 7 and 394.

Berg, P., Baltimore, D., Brenner, S., Roblin III, R. O., and Singer, M. F. (1993). "Summary Statement of the Asilomar Conference on Recombination DNA Molecules." In Bulger, R. E., Heitman, E., and Reiser, S. J. (Eds.). *The Ethical Dimensions of the Biological Sciences*. (1993). Cambridge: Cambridge University Press: 263.

Burkhardt, R. W., Jr., (1977). *The Spirit of System: Lamarck and Evolutionary Biology*. Boston: Harvard University press.

Callahan (1989). "Morality and Contemporary Culture: The President's Commission and Beyond." *Cardoza Law Review*. Vol. 6: 348.

Campbell, N.A. (1993). *Biology*. Redwood City, California: The Benjamin/Cummings Publishing Company, Inc.: 15.

CBS News(2005). <http;//www.cbsnews.com/stories/2005/12/08/health/main1110165.shtml>.

Chargaff, E. (1998). *Heraclitean Fire: Sketches From a Life Before Nature.* Quoted in *Natural Law,* Accessed 14 October: <www.natural law.ca/genetic/ScientistssonDangers.html>.

Darwin, C. R. (1824). *The Autobiography of Charles Darwin 1809-1882 with Original Omission Restored* (1958). London: Collins.

Descartes. *Discourse on Method*: 120.

Farrington, B. (1949). *Francis Bacon: Philosophy of Industrial Science.* New York: Henry Schuman: 5.

Financial Times (2001). "The Danger of Knowing Too Much." (Weekend May 12/May 13): 11.

Flowers, E. B. (1998). "The Ethics and Economics of Patenting Human Genome." *Journal of Business Ethics.* Vol. 17, No. 15: 1737-1745.

French Bioresearchers (1998). "New Plants Threaten Bees." *The Futurist.* May Edition: 13.

Freud, Z. (1989) "Re-Examining Freud." *Psychology Today.* (September): 48-52.

Freud, Z. (1933). *"Lecture XXIII,"* New Introductory Lectures on *Pshychoanalysis.* New York: Norton, 48: 52, and 153-186.

Freud, Z. (1856-1939). "Re-Examining Freud." *Psychology Today.* (September)1989: 48-52.

Fox, M. W. (2001). *Bringing Life to Ethics: Global Bioethics for a Humane Society.* New York: State University of New York Press: 121.

Haeckel, E. (1905). *Die Weltratsel and Die Lebenswunder.* Germany, Stuttgart: Alfred Kroener Verlag.

Haldane, J. B. S. (1938). *Heredity and Politics.* London: Allen and Unwin.

Hoyle, F. (1965). *Galaxies, Nuclei and Quasars.* New York: Harp.

Kass, L. R. (2002). *Life, Liberty and the Defense of Dignity: The Challenge for Bioethics.* San Francisco: Encounter Books: 17 and 29.

Kimbrell, A. (1994). "Biological Patents Affront Human Values." In Bender, D. and Leone, B. (Eds.). *Biomedical Ethics: Opposing Viewpoints.* San Diego, CA: Greenhaven Press, Inc.

Matare', H. F. (1999). *Bioethics: The Ethics of Evolution and Genetic Interference.* Westport, Connecticut: 3, 19, and 63.

Meilaender, G. C. (1995). *Body, Soul, and Bioethics.* Notre Dame: University of Notre Dame Press: 13.

Murray, T. H. (1983). "Warning: Screening Workers for Genetic Risk." *Hastings Center Rep.* No. 13, (February): 5-8.

Parhizgar, K. D. (2002). *Multicultural Behavior and Global Business Environments.* New York: Haworth Press: 36, 51, and 125.

Parhizgar, R. R. and Parhizgar, S. S. (2000). "Analysis of Three Types of Personhood: Genotype, Phenotype, and Phylontype in Biotech Enterprise." In Maniam, B. and Metha, S. A. (Eds.). *Proceedings of the 31st Annual Conference of the Decision Sciences Institute Southwest Region.* San Antonio, Texas: 185-

187.
Plato, *Republic* VII, 514A ff.
Psychology Today (1989). "Re-Examining Fraud." September: 48-52.
Siewing, R. (1987). *Evolution.* 3rd Edition. New York: Gustav Fischer Verlag.
Tulka, T. (1977). *Time, Space, and Knowledge: A New Vision of Reality.* California: Dharma Press: 73.
Wald, G. (1979). "The Case Against Genetic Engineering." In Jackson, D. D. and Stich, S. (Eds.). *The Recombinant DNA Debate.* Englewood Cliffs, N.J.: Prentice Hall: 127-128.
Wilfond, B. S. and Fost, N. (1990). "The Cystic Fibrosis Gene: Medical and Social Implications for Hetrozygote Detection." *JAMA.* Vol. 263: 2777-2783.
Zadeh, L. A. (1965). "Fuzzy Sets." *Information Control.* Vol. 8: 338-353.

Chapter 8

Adler, N. (1986). *International Dimensions of Organizational Behavior.* Boston, Massachusetts: The Kent International Publishing Company: 18.
Adiga, A. (2000). "Dads Hope to Have Nice DNA: US Fathers Flock to Patiently Test Labs. The Book of Life." *Financial Times.* (Monday, June 26): 16.
Annas, G. J. (1994). "Individuals Own All Rights to Their Body Cells." In David Bender and Bruno Leone (Eds.). *Biomedical Ethics: Opposing Viewpoints.* San Diego: Greehaven Press, Inc.: 34-39.
Bacon, F. (1620). *The Novum Organumm or New Methods of Acquiring Knowledge.*
Barrett, M. (1991). *The Politics of Truth: From Marx to Foucault.* Stanford, CA: Stanford University Press: Viii.194.
Bender, D. and Leone, B. (Eds.), (1994). *Biomedical Ethics: Opposing Viewpoints.* San Diego: Greehaven Press, Inc.: 13 & 34-39.
Berzinsky, Z. (1970). *Between Two Ages: America's Role in the Technocratic Era.* New York: Penguin Books: 72, 83, and 300-304.
Buchholz, R.A. and Rosenthal, S. B. (1998). *Business Ethics.* Upper Saddle River, NJ: Prentice Hall: 111, 401, and 396.
Buchman, , E. S. (1980). *The Use of Humor in Psychotherapy.* Boston, Mass.: Boston University: Dissertation Abstract International, Vol. 41, No. 5-B: 1715.
Butler, J. (1849). "Advertisement" Prefixed to *The Analogy of Religion, Natural and Revealed, to the Constitution and Course of Nature.* New York: Robert Carter.
Butler, J. K. and Cantrell, R. S. (1984). "A Behavioral Decision Theory Approach to Modeling Dyadic Trust in Supervisors and Subordinates." *Psychological Reports.* August: 19-28.
Caplan, A. L. (1993). "Beasty Conduct: Ethical Issues in Animal Experimentation." In Bulger, R. E., Heitman, and Reiser (Eds.). *The Ethical*

Dimensions of the Biological Sciences.   Cambridge: Cambridge University Press: 175-185.

Chaudhry, P. E. and Walsh, M. G. (1995). "Intellectual Property Rights." *Columbia Journal of World Business.* Vol. 30, No. 2: 80.

CNN.com (2002).<wysiwyg://http://www.cnn.com/2002/WORLD/europe/07/19/shipman.victims/index.html>.

CNN.com (2004). <http://www.cnn.com/2004/TECH/science/10/20/how.many.genes.ap/index.html>.

CNN.com (2002).<wysiwyg://http://www.cnn.com/2002/WORLD/Europe/07/19/shipman.victims/index.html>.

CNN.com (2005). <http://money.cnn.com/2005/12/08/news/fortune500/nejournal.reut/index.htm?cnn'yes>.

Coser, L. R. (1960). "Laughter Among Colleagues." *Psychiatry.* Vol. 23, No. 1: 81-95.

Dooley, L. (1941). "The Relation of Humor to Masochism." *Psychoanalytic Review.* Vol. 28: 37.

Eichenwald, K. (1993). "Commissions Are Many, Profits Few." *New York. Times.* May 24: C1.

Epstein, M. A. (1989). *Modern Intellectual Property.* New York: Law & Business, Inc./Harcourt Brace Jovanovich: 3, n.3.

Financial Times. (2000). "Freedom to Grow." (Friday June 30): 12.

Financial Times. (2000). "The Book of Life." (Monday June, 26): 16.

Financial Times. (2000). "World News." (Friday, April 28): 1.

Freud, S. (1960). *Jokes and their Relation to the Unconscious.* New York: W. W. Norton. (Originally Published in 1905).

Freud, S. (1928). "Humour." *International Journal of Psychoanalysis.* Vol. 9: 2.

Grotjahn, M. (1956). *Beyond Laugher.* New York: McGraw-Hill.

Guerrera, F. and Jennen, B. (2001). "European Groups Face Record Fines for Roles in Price-Fixing." *Financial Times.* (Wednesday, November 21).

Hegel, G. W. F. (1965). *Hegel's Philosophy of Rights.* Translated by T. M. Knox, London: Oxford University Press: Section 54.

Heidigger, M. (1962). *Being and Time.* (Trans.) Macquarrie, J., and Robinson, E., (1962). New York: Harper & Row Publishers, Inc.

Holbrook, M. B. (1994). "The Nature of Customer Value." In R. T. Rust and R. L. Oliver (Eds.). *Service Quality: New Directions in Theory and Practice.* Thousand Oaks, CA: Sage Publications: 21 and 71.

Jackson, J. H., Miller, R. L., and Shawn, G. M. (1997). *Business and Society Today: Managing Social Issues.* Cincinnati, Ohio: West Publishing Company: 195.

Jonas, H. (1974). *Philosophical Essays: From Ancient Creed to Technological Man.* Chicago: University of Chicago Press: xvi, 117-119.

Kalupahana, D. J. (1975). *Causality: The Central Philosophy of Buddhism.* Honolulu, Hawaii: The University of Hawaii, Honolulu.

Kant, I. (1898). *Fundamental Principles of the Metaphysic of Morals.* (Trans.) Abbott, T. K. *From Kant's Critique of Practical Reason and Other Works on the Theory of Ethics.* London: Longmans, Green.

Kempton, W., Boster, J. S., and Hartley, J. A. (1995). *Environmental Values in American Culture.* Cambridge, Massachusetts: The MIT Press: 1and 27.

Kimbrell, A. (1994). "Biological Patents Affront Human Values." In David Bender and Bruno Leone (Eds.). *Biomedical Ethics: Opposing Viewpoints.* San Diego: Greehaven Press, Inc.: 26 and 31.

Knight, F. (1921). *Risk, Uncertainty and Profit.* Houghton Mifflin Company.

Lane, R. E. (1962). *Political Ideology: Why the American Common Man Beliefs What He Does.* New York: Free Press: 3, 15.

Laredo Morning Times (2000). "CC Trustees Tabs Trial a Witch Hunt." (Friday, May 19): 10A.

Locke, J. (1924). *An Essay Concerning Human Understanding.* (Abr. and Edeted By Pringle-Pattison, A. S.) Oxford: Clarendon Press.

Marger, M. N. (1985). *Race and Ethnic Relations: American and Global Perspectives.* Belmont, California: Wadsworth Publishing Company: 16.

Marx, K. (1938). *Critique of the Gotha Program.* New York: International Publisher: 3.

McKenny, G. P. (1997). *To Relieve the Human Condition: Bioethics, Technology, and the Body.* New York: State University of New York Press: 39.

Mullins, E. (1985). *The World Order.* Staunton, VA: Ezra Pound Institute of Civilization: 33-34 and 196.

Mullins, W.A. (1972). "On the Concept of Ideologies in Political Science." *American Political Science Review.* Vol. 66: 498-511.

Nietzsche, F. (1917). *The Will to Freedom.* New York: Charles Scribner's.

Nietzsche, F. (1917). Common, T. (Trans.), New York: Modern Library, Prologue, No. 3, as Found in Titus and Keeton. *Ethics for Today:* 178.

Norton, M. B., Katzman, D. M., Escott, P. D., Chudacoff, H. P., Peterson, H. P., and Tuttle, Jr., W. M. (1990). *A People and a Nation: A History of the United States.* Boston: Houghton Mifflin Company: 215.

Oesterle, J. A. (1957). *Ethics: The Introduction to Moral Science.* Englewood Cliffs, NJ: Prentice Hall: 17 and 156.

Olasky, M. N. (1985). "Ministers or Panderers: Issues Raised by the Public Relations Society Code of Standards." *Journal of Mass Media Ethics.* Vol. 1, No. 1.

Paikoff, L. (1999)."The Evil of Respecting Nature." In Ralston, R. (Ed.). *Why Businessmen Need Philosophy?* United States of America: The Ayn Rand Institute Publication: 9 and 66 - 67.

Parhizgar, K. D. and Parhizgar, F. F. (2002). "Analysis of Ecological Business Ethics Commitments." In Mostapha Abdelsamad (Ed.). *Proceedings Society for Advancement of Management BSA:* 826-833.

Punnett, B. J. and Ricks, D. A. (1992). *International Business.* Boston:

PWS-Kent Publishing Company: 237.

Rosenbloom, B. (1999). *Marketing Channels: A Management View*. New York: The Dryden Press: 336.

Rosner, F. (1979). "The Jewish Attitude Toward Euthanasia." In Fred Rosner and J. D. Bleich (Eds.). Jewish *Bioethics*. New York: Sanherin: 260-264.

Ross, W. D. (1930). *The Rights and the Good*. London: Oxford University Press: 42.

Royce, J. (1916). *The Philosophy of Loyalty*. The MacMillan Co.: 16-17 and 25.

Salameh, W. A. (1983). "Past Outlooks, Present Status, and Future Frontiers." In McGhee, P. and Goldstein, J. (Eds.). *Handbook of Humour*. New York: Springer, Verlag.

Schindler, P. L. and Thomas, C. C. (1993). "The Structure of Interpersonal Trust in the Workplace." *Psychological Reports*. October: 563-573.

Schwartz, R. (1996). "Genetic Knowledge: Some Legal and Ethical Questions." In Thomasma, D. C. and Kushner, T. (Eds.). *Birth and Death: Science and Bioethics*. Cambridge: Cambridge University Press: 22.

Sethi, S. P. (1982). *Up Against the Corporate Wall, Modern Corporations and Social Issues of the Eighties*. 4th Edition. Englewood Cliffs, NJ: Prentice Hall: 288.

Shaw, W. H. (1996). *Business Ethics*. Belmont, CA: Wadsworth Publishing Company: 61.

Sonnenberg, F. K. (1993). "Trust Me...Trust Me Not." *Industry Week*. (August 16): 22.

Spanner, R. A. (1986). *Who Owns Innovation?* Homewood, IL: Dow Jones-Irwin: 10.

Sproul, L. S. (1981) "Beliefs in Organizations" in P. C. Nystrom and W. H. Starbuck (Eds). *Handbook of Organizational Design*. New York: Oxford University Press: 204.

Stewart, D. (1996). *Business Ethics*. New York: The McGraw-Hill Companies, Inc.: 281-282.

Swain, M. S. and Marusyk, R. W. (1994). "Scientists Should Be Able to Own Cells They Have Altered." In David Bender and Bruno Leone (Eds.). *Biomedical Ethics: Opposing Viewpoints*. San Diego: Greehaven Press, Inc.: 40 - 46.

The Economist (1992). "Fake Drugs." (May, 2): 85.

Waldmeir, P. (2001). Copyright Extended to Digital Data." *Financial Times*. (Tuesday June 26): 4.

Chapter 9

Abrahams, P. (1999). "Debt Collector Told Client to Sell a Kidney." *Financial Times*. November 1: 1.

AMA (1968). "A Definition of Irreversible Coma, Report of the Ad Hoc Committee of the Harvard Medical School to Examine the Definition of Brain Death." Vol. 205: 337-340.

Apple, J. Z., M.D. (1968). "Ethical and Legal Questions Posed by Advances in Medicine." *JAMA*. Vol. 205, No. 7, (August 12): 102.

British Transplantation Society Working Party. "Guidelines on Living Organ Donation," (1986). *BMJ*. Vol. 293: 257-258.

Buchholz, R. A. and Rosenthal, S. B. (1998). *Business Ethics: The Pragmatic Path Beyond Principles to Process.* New York: McGraw-Hill Book Company: 30 and 297.

Cairncross, F. (1991). *Costing the Earth.* Boston: Harvard Business.School Press: 56.

CNN.com (2003). "Teen Mother Wakes Up, After Year in Coma." <http://www.cnn.com/2003/US/West/04/07/california.coma.ap/index.html>.

Engelhardt, Jr., H. (996). *The Foundation of Bioethics. Second Edition, New York: Oxford University Press:* 122-124.

Firm, D. (2001). "Pioneer of Heart Transplant Surgery." *Financial Times.* (Monday September 3): 4.

Fletcher, J. (1960). "The Patient's Right to Die." *Harper.* Vol. 140: 141-143.

Fried, M. H. (1967). *The Evolution of Political Society: An Essay in Political Anthropology.* New York: Random House.

Haring, B. (1973). *Medical Ethics.* Notre Dame, Ind.: Fides Publishers Inc.
Hill, T. P. (1996). "Care of the Dying: From an Ethics Perspective." In David C. Thomasma and Thomasine Kushner (Eds.). *Birth to Death: Science and Bioethics.* Cambridge, UK: Cambridge University Press: 198-206.

JAMA. "An Appraisal of the Criteria of Cerebral Death – a Summary Statement – a Collaborative Study." *JAMA,* Vol. 237, No. 10, (March 7): 982-986.

Hegel, G. W. In Loewenberg, J. (Ed.), (1929). *Hegel Selections.* New York: Harper, 468.

Jonas, H. (1980). "Philosophical Reflections on Experimenting with Human Subjects." In Thomas A. Shannon. *Bioethics.* N. J.: Papulist Press: 235-261.

Kant, I. (1898). *Fundamental Principles of the Metaphysic of Morals.* Translated by T. K. Abbott, from *Kant's Critique of Practical Reason and Other Works on the Theory of Ethics.* London: Longmans, Green: 1st Sec.: 10, and 12-14.

Leuba, J. H. (1950). *The Reformation of the Churches.* Boston, Mass.: The Bacon Press: 213.

Levine, C. (1999). *Taking Sides: Clashing Views on Controversial Bioethical Issuers.* New York: Dushkin/McGraw-Hill: 2.

Locke, J. (1924). *An Essay Concerning Human Understanding.* A. S. Pringle-Pattison (Abr. and Ed.). Oxford: Clardon Press.

Malinowski, B. (1925). In Needham, J. (Ed.). *Science, Religion, and Reality.* New York: The Macmillan Company: 49-50.

McFadden, C. J. (1976). *The Dignity of Life: Moral Values in a Changing Society*. Hungtinton, Ind: Our Sunday Visitor Inc.: 202.

Meiklejohn, A. (1942). *Education Between Two Worlds*. New York: Harper: 57 & 83.

Minnesota Statutes. Patients and Residents of Health Care Facilities: Bill of Rights. 144.651: Subd.: 6.

Nelson, J. R. (1994). "Genetic Research Broadens the Understanding of Humanness." In Bender, D. and Leone, B. (Series Editors) and O'Neill, T. (Book Editor). *Biomedical Ethics: Opposing Viewpoints*. San Diego, CA: Greenhaven Press, Inc.: 265.

Newsweek (1968). "Redefining Death." May 20: 68.

New York Times (1968). "Physicians Adopt a Code on Death." (August 10): 25.

Olson, S. (1989). *Shaping The Future: Biology and Human Values*. Washington D.C.: National Academy Press: 47.

Pope Puis XII (1957). "Allocation Delivered to the International Congress of Anesthesiologists." *Acta Apostolicae Sedis*. Vol. 24, (November 24): 1027-1033.

Ramsey, P. (1970). *The Patient as Person: Exploration in Medical Ethics*. New Haven, Conn.: Yale University Press: 101-112.

Rothman, D. J. (1998). "The International Organ Traffic." *The New York Review of Books*. (March 26): 14-17.

Rutstein, D. D. (1969). "The Ethical Design of Human Experiments." *Daedalus,* Vol. 98, (Spring): 526.

Smith, S. J., Evans, R. M., Sullivan-Fowler, M. and Hendee, W. R. (1988). "Use of Animals in Biomedical Research: Historical Role of the American Medical Association and the American Physician." *Arch Intern Med.* Vol. 148: 1849-1853.

Stanford Daily (1993). "Pioneering Heart Transplant Surgeon Retires." (January 25): 1.

Steiner, G. A. and Steiner, J. F. (1994). *Business, Government, and Society: A Managerial Perspective*. New York: Seventh Edition. McGraw-Hill, Inc.: 47.

Stevens, M. L. (2000). *Bioethics in America: Origins and Cultural Politics*. Baltimore and London: The John Hopkins University Press: 75.

The Council of the Transplantation Society, (1985). "Organ Sales." *Lancet.*, Vol. 2: 715-716.

Time (1966). "What Is Life? When Is Death?" May 27: 78.

Tina Stevens, M. L. (Ed.), (1991). *Transcript. Oral History of Daniel Callahan*. Briarcliff Manor, N.Y.: Hastings Center, (July 1) : 10-12.

Veith, F. J. (1981). "Brain Death." In Thomas A. Shannon (Ed.). *Bioethics*. Ramsey, NJ: Paulist Press: 171 and 175.

Veith, F. J, Jonas, H., Maguire, D., and Shannon, T. A. (1981). "Death and Dying." In Thomas A. Shannon (Ed.). *Bioethics: Basic Writings on the Key Ethical Questions That Surround the Major, Modern Biological Possibilities and Problems*. Ramsey, NJ: Paulist Press: 178.

Velasquez, M. G. (1992). *Business Ethics: Concepts and Cases.* 3rd Edition. Englewood Cliffs, NJ: Prentice Hall: 59.

Weber, C. O. (1960). *Basic Philosophies of Education.* New York: Rinehart and Winston: 29.

Weber, M. (1946). *The Theory of Social and Economic Organization.* Translated by T. Parsons. New York: Oxford University Press.

Weir, R.. F. and Peters, C. (1999). "Affirming the Decisions Adolescents Make About Life and Death." In Carol Levine (Ed.). *Taking Sides: Clashing Views on Controversial Issues.* Eight Edition. Dushkin/McGraw-Hill: 162-168.

Williamson, W. P., MD (1966). "Life or Death – Whose Decision?" *JAMA*, Vol. 197, No. 10, September 5: 139-141.

World Health Organization – WHO, (1992). "A Report on Developments Under the Auspices of WHO (1987-1991)." *WHO.* Geneva: 12-28.

Younger, S. J. (1988). "Who Defines Futility?" *JAMA.* Vol. 260, No. 14: 2094-2095.

Chapter 10

Arieti, S. (1993). "Science." In Ruth Ellen Bulger, Elizabeth Heitman, and Stanley Joel Reiser (Eds.). *The Ethical Dimensions of the Biological Sciences.* Cambridge, Cambridge University Press: 23.

Bernard, C. (1927). *An Introduction to the Study of Experimental Medicine.* Trans. By H. C. Greene. New York: Macmillan Co.

Blake, J. and Ernest, D. (1995). "Is Your Strategic Alliances Really a Sale?" *Harvard Business Review.* Vol. 73, January/February Edition: 97-105.

CNN.com (2004). *<http://www.cnn.com/2004/World/asiapcf/02/26/japan. sentence/index.html>.*

CNN.com (2005). <http://www.cnn.com/2005/HEALTH/12/15/skorea. stemcell.reut/index.html>.

Cookson, C. (1999). "US Biotech Group Buys Dolly Cloning Technology." *Financial Times.* May 5: 10.

Drucker, P. (1995). "The Network Society." *Wall Street Journal.* March 29: 12.

Fawler, C. and Mooney, P. (1990). *Shattering: Food, Politics, and the Loss of Genetic Diversity.* Tucson, Arizona: The University of Arizona Press: 123-24.

FOX NEWS.COM (2006). <http://www.foxnews.com/story/0,2933, 183593,00.html>.

Gert, B., Culver, C. M. and Clouser, K. D. (1977). *Bioethics: A Return To Fundamentals.* New York/Oxford: Oxford University Press, 98.

Glass, B. (1993). "The Ethical Basis of Science." In Ruth Ellen Bulger, Elizabeth Heitman, and Stanley Joel Reiser (Eds.). *The Ethical Dimensions of the Biological Sciences.* Cambridge: Cambridge University Press: 43.

Heidegger, M. (1962). *Being and Time.* (Trans.) Macquarrie, J., and Robinson, E., New York: Harper & Row Publishers, Inc.

Hobbes, T. (1839). *Leviathan and Philosophical Rudiments, From the English Works of Thomas Hobbes.* Vol. II and II. Sir William Molesworth (Ed.). London: John Bohn.

Kennedy, D. (1986). "The Social Sponsorship of Innovation." In Perpich, J. (Ed.). *Biotechnology in Society.* New York: Pergamon Press: 26-27.

National Education Association (NEA) Handbook, 1977-78, Washington, DC: National Education Association Press.

Nietzsche, F. (1917). *The Will to Freedom.* New York: Charles Scribner's.

Nietzsche, F. (1917). Common, T. (Trans.), New York: Modern Library, Prologue, No. 3, as Found in Titus and Keeton, *Ethics for Today:* 178.

Nietzsche, F. (1924). *The Complete Works of Friedrich Nietzsche.* Vol. XII. XIII, XVI, Levy, O. (Ed.). New York: Macmillan.

Petersdorf, R. G. (1993: 95). "The Pathogenesis of Fraud in Medical Science." In Ruth Ellen Bulger, Elizabeth Heitman, and Stanley Joel Reiser (Eds.), (1993). *The Ethical Dimensions of the Biological Sciences.* Cambridge: Cambridge University Press: 95.

Rifkin, J. (1998). *The Biotech Century: Harnessing the Gene and Remarking the World.* New York: Penguin Putman, Inc.: 37.

Rothman, B. K. (1999). "The Potential Cost of the Best Genes Money Can Buy." *The Chronicle of Higher Education.* (June 11): A52.

Strike, K. A. and Soltis, J. F. (1992). *The Ethics of Teaching.* Second Edition. New York: Teachers College Press, Columbia University: 57.

Wise, L. E. (1946). *Paper Industry & Paper World.* Vol. 28: 1299.

SUBJECT INDEX

ABOUT THE AUTHORS

Suzan S. Parhizgar has received her Ph. D. in Medical Pharmacology and Neurosciences, Texas Tech University, Lubbock, Texas in 2007. She obtained her undergraduate and graduate course works in the field of medical physiology from Texas A&M University, Kingsville, and Texas and A&M in College Station. She completed all Ph.D. course works in the field of Physiology, in the Graduate School of Sciences at the University of Texas Health Sciences Centers at San Antonio, Texas. Also, she has earned her Bachelor of Science, College of Biology, University of California, Irvine, California. She has published articles in the refereed *Journal of Cardiology, Journal of Advances in Competitiveness Research,* presented and published research papers in proceedings of the professional conferences of the *Decision Sciences Institutes, American Society for competitiveness, the World Business Congress, the International Management Development,* and *The International Trade and Finance Association.*

Kamal Dean Parhizgar, PhD, is Professor of Management at the Texas A&M International University, Texas. Previously in the United States, he has taught at California State University campuses, in Hayward, Dominguez Hills, and Los Angeles; The University of the District of Columbia; George Mason University; Georgetown University; YMCA College in Chicago; as well as at Iranian colleges and universities. Before the Iranian Islamic Revolution in 1979, he served as the Director of the Iranian Scientific Research Center for the Ministry of Sciences and Higher Education. Professor Parhizgar obtained his undergraduate and graduate degrees from the Universities of Shiraz and Teheran, and his PhD in 1972 from Northwestern University, Evanston, Illinois. His postdoctoral fellowship was at Northwestern University in 1983, and he spent his Hospital Administrative Residency and Intenrship Assignments in St. Paul Ramsey Hospital, University of Minnesota; National Iranian Oil Company (NIOC) Hospitals; and Firoozgar Medical Center.

Professor Parhizgar's extensive multicultural interests are illustrated by his research and teaching activities in the field of strategic cultural management. He has published numerous text books including 2002 Edition of *Multicultural Behavior and Global Business Environments,* 2006 Edition of *Multicultural Business Ethics and Global Managerial Moral Reasoning,* articles in refereed journals, conference proceedings research papers, and has presented papers at the regional, national, and international conferences in the United States and overseas. He has been Co-Program Chair, Division Chair, Track Chair, Session Chair, Discussant, and Reviewer for the ABI, IAoM, IMDA, SAM, ITFA, and GCA. He has served in the editorial review boards of the *Journal of Transnational Management Development, The Journal of Teaching in International Business*, and *Advances in Competitiveness Research Journal*. Finally, he has served McGraw Hill-Irvin Publishing Co., Prentice-Hall Publishing Co., Pregamon Publishing Co., South-West Publishing Co. and Haworth Press, Inc. as a book reviewer.